# THE
# HARRIET LANE
# HANDBOOK

A Manual for Pediatric House Officers

**ELEVENTH EDITION**

# THE HARRIET LANE HANDBOOK

A Manual for Pediatric House Officers

**ELEVENTH EDITION**

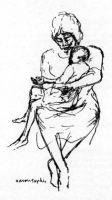

The Harriet Lane Service
Children's Medical and Surgical Center
of the
Johns Hopkins Hospital

Editor
Peter C. Rowe, M.D.

YEAR BOOK MEDICAL PUBLISHERS, INC.
Chicago • London • Boca Raton

3 4 5 6 7 8 9 0 MC 91 90 89 88


**Library of Congress Cataloging-in-Publication Data**

The Johns Hopkins Hospital/The Harriet Lane handbook.

  Rev. ed. of: The Harriet Lane handbook. 10th ed. c1984.
  Includes index.
  1. Pediatrics—Handbooks, manuals, etc.
I. Rowe, Peter C.  II. Johns Hopkins Hospital.
III. Harriet Lane handbook. [DNLM: 1. Pediatrics—
handbooks.  WS 29 J653]
RJ48.H35  1987      618.92        87-10603
ISBN 0-8151-7379-2

## NOTICE

**Every effort has been made to ensure that the drug dosage sched-
ules herein are accurate and in accord with the standards accepted
at the time of publication. However, as new research and experience
broaden our knowledge, changes in treatment and drug therapy occur. Therefore, the reader is advised to check the product information sheet included in the package of each drug he plans to administer to be certain that changes have not been made in the
recommended dose or in the contraindications. This is of particular
importance in regard to new or infrequently used drugs.**

Sponsoring Editor: Stephany S. Scott
Manager, Copyediting Services: Frances M. Perveiler
Production Manager, Text and Reference/Periodicals: Etta Worthington
Proofroom Supervisor: Shirley E. Taylor

# PREFACE
## TO THE 11th EDITION

The Harriet Lane Handbook originated in 1950 as a convenient repository of information useful to pediatric residents and practitioners. Since then, at intervals of approximately 3 years, the residents of the Harriet Lane Service have revised the content but not the purpose of the book. In preparing the 11th edition we have attempted to incorporate recent changes in pediatric practice while keeping the size of the book manageable.

To assist with the increasing complexity of inpatient care, we have added information on parenteral nutrition and pediatric sedation, and have expanded the table of cancer chemotherapy. The catalogue of new sections ranges from the use of magnetic resonance imaging to the technique for intraosseous infusion, from pulse oximetry to new blood pressure norms for children.

The formulary has been thoroughly revised and expanded to accommodate, among other things, the proliferation of new antimicrobials and new agents for the treatment of dysrhythmias. We have substantially revised the chapters on Genetics (removing obsolete tests and adding a section on dysmorphology), Perinatology (adding the biophysical profile as well as blood pressure norms for premature infants), Cardiology (new ECG norms, new charts on the differentiation of tachyarrhythmias and the interpretation of the oxygen challenge test), and Infectious Diseases (new vaccine schedules and recommendations on *H. Flu* prophylaxis). Virtually every other chapter has been revised, reorganized, and updated.

The seventeen Senior Assistant Residents listed below acted as contributing editors for this edition. Their dedication, creativity, and good cheer have made my task a rewarding one. My thanks go to the following for their work:

Bettina H. Ault (Nephrology)
Steve D. Barnes (Respiratory Care and Pulmonary Function)
Paul C. Brewer (Poisoning)
Barry Byrne (Formulary)
Ann M. Cadwalader (Formulary)
Christine T. Chiaviello (Procedures)
Debra R. Counts (Infectious Diseases)
Hal C. Dietz (Fluid and Electrolyte Therapy, Sedation)
Barbara T. Felt (Developmental Evaluation, Neurology)
J. Elica Kang (Cerebrospinal Fluid, Synovial Fluid, Microbiological
    Examinations, Gastroenterology, Growth and Development)
Ann Kavanaugh-McHugh (Perinatology)
John J. McCloskey (Radiology, Index)
Gregory E. Plautz (Hematology)
Ann M. Rasmusson (Endocrinology)

W. Reid Thompson (Cardiology)
Cynthia Tifft (Gastroenterology, Genetics, Burns)
Jennifer C. Wiebke (Nutrition, Normal Values)

I am grateful to the members of the Department of Pediatrics who offered suggestions and reviewed rough drafts, and I would like to thank the Chairman of the Department, Dr. Frank A. Oski, for his support and good counsel throughout the year.

This edition builds on the cumulative efforts of housestaff and chief residents who have worked on the Harriet Lane Handbook since 1950. I am indebted to the previous editors, Drs. Henry Seidel, Harrison Spencer, Herbert Swick, William Friedman, Robert Haslam, Jerry Winkelstein, Dennis Headings, Kenneth Schuberth, Basil Zitelli, Jeffrey Biller, Andrew Yeager, and Cynthia Cole. I particularly appreciate the efforts of my immediate predecessor as editor, Dr. Cole, who had the foresight to use a word processor for the 10th edition, thereby improving the accuracy and simplifying the production of subsequent editions.

A special note of appreciation goes to Ms. Cecilia Young, who has typed the bulk of the manuscript. Without her enthusiasm and her admirable devotion to detail, the handbook would not have been completed. I also want to thank Mrs. Terry Langbaum for administrative and artistic help. Ms. Stephany Scott from Year Book Medical Publishers, Inc., has been most helpful throughout.

Finally, I want to thank my wife, Carla, for her willingness to tolerate the long hours that made the book possible, and for her invaluable support.

Peter C. Rowe, M.D.
Chief Resident
Editor

Baltimore, 1987

## TABLE OF CONTENTS

PART IV - REFERENCE DATA

PART I

DIAGNOSTIC TESTS

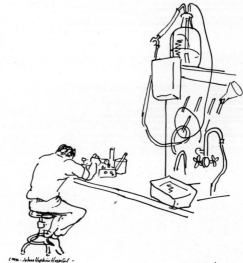

P R O C E D U R E S

The following are guidelines for common pediatric procedures. For a more detailed description see: Hughes WT, Buescher ES. Pediatric Procedures 2nd Edition. Philadelphia: WB Saunders, 1980; Fletcher, MA, et al. Atlas of Procedures in Neonatology. Philadelphia: J B Lippincott, 1983.

I.   Obtaining Blood

    A.   Capillary Blood
        The extremity should first be warmed in order to provide optimal blood flow and more accurate samples. To prevent burns, do not use a warming towel which is >40° C.

        1)   The lateral or medial side of the heel may be used; avoid heel pad. For digital artery sampling use the lateral surface of the distal phalanx of second, third, or fourth finger.
        2)   Use a 2.5 mm lancet or an Autolet for optimal skin penetration.
        3)   Wipe away first drop of blood with dry gauze. Alcohol used in cleansing skin may produce hemolysis.
        4)   Massage (but avoid squeezing) finger or heel.
        5)   Samples may be inaccurate with poor perfusion or polycythemia.

        Ref: Blumenfeld TA, et al. Lancet 1979; 1:230; Morgan EJ. Am Rev Resp Dis 1979; 120:795.

    B.   External Jugular Puncture
        1)   Wrap infant in mummified manner.
        2)   Turn head to one side and extend.
        3)   Prepare area carefully with iodine and alcohol.
        4)   Provoke child to cry in order to distend external jugular vein, which runs from angle of mandible to posterior border of lower third of sternocleidomastoid muscle.

    C.   Femoral Puncture

        NOTE: Careful skin antisepsis is needed to prevent septic arthritis. Femoral puncture is particularly hazardous in neonates and is not recommended in this age group. Avoid femoral punctures in children with thrombocytopenia, coagulation disorders, and those scheduled for cardiac catheterization.

        Ref: Asnes RS, et al. Pediatrics 1966; 38:837.

1) An assistant should hold the child securely.
2) The assistant stands behind the infant, leans over the head and trunk, and holds the legs in "semi-frogleg" position. The assistant also holds the infant's arms down by use of the upper arms and elbows.
3) Prepare area carefully as for blood culture.
4) After locating the femoral pulse just below the inguinal ligament, insert needle, aiming slightly medial to the pulse beat.
5) Insert needle slowly to a depth of approximately 0.5 to 0.75 cm.
6) While exerting suction, slowly withdraw needle until a small amount of blood enters syringe.
7) If flow ceases, push needle deeper and withdraw as before.
8) Hold both syringe and legs stationary to insure drawing the amount of blood needed.

D. Internal Jugular Puncture
1) Wrap infant securely in sheet.
2) Place child on table and adjust position so that head falls over the side. With the neck extended, turn head slightly to one side. This makes the posterior margin of the sternocleidomastoid muscle on the opposite side stand out.
3) Sterilize area.
4) Insert needle just deep to and behind posterior margin of sternocleidomastoid muscle, approximately halfway between its origin and insertion. Then advance needle under the muscle, parallel to skin surface and in direction of suprasternal notch, for a distance equal to width of sternocleidomastoid.
5) Slowly withdraw needle while keeping a negative pressure on syringe, until the point is reached at which blood enters syringe.
6) After obtaining blood, hold child upright and apply pressure.

2. Bone Marrow Aspiration

A. General Comments and Warnings
1) Always use sterile surgical technique for bone marrow aspirations.
2) In children from birth to 3 months of age, the tibia is the preferred site for aspiration.
3) In children over 3 months of age, the posterior iliac crest is a technically superior site.
4) Anesthetize skin, soft tissue, and periosteum with local anesthetic.
5) Insert needle with a boring motion and steady but not excessive pressure.

      6)    The classic description of a "give" when the marrow cavity is entered not only is unreliable, but also indicates loss of control.

      7)    Aspiration of more than 0.2 ml of marrow will result in dilution with sinusoidal blood.

B.    Femoral Marrow Technique

May be performed at either of two sites:

      1)    Midline and anteriorly, 2-3 cm above the external condyle in the distal third of the femur.

      2)    Lateral aspect of the midportion of the femur.

C.    Iliac Marrow Technique

      1)    The patient is placed on a firm table in the lateral recumbent position (with neck, knees and hips flexed), or prone with a pillow under the pelvis to elevate it slightly.

      2)    Enter the ileum at the posterior superior iliac spine which is a visible and palpable bony prominence superior and lateral to the intergluteal cleft. It is inferior and medial to the crest.

D.    Tibial Marrow Technique

Best obtained from medial aspect of the head of the tibia, below medial condyle and tibial tuberosity. Insert needle perpendicular to outer table.

E.    Smear Technique

      1)    Eject marrow from syringe onto clean slide.

      2)    With another syringe and needle, aspirate excessive blood and plasma from marrow to concentrate it.

      3)    Use remaining marrow to make multiple smears in usual way.

3.    Chest Tube Placement in the Neonate for Pneumothorax

A.    Position the infant with the affected side up. The desired location for chest tube insertion is in the third or fourth intercostal space in the midaxillary line. Avoid breast tissue.

B.    Temporary decompression may be obtained by using a "butterfly" or angiocath in the same location or in the ipsilateral anterior 2nd intercostal space.

C.    After anesthetizing the area locally with 0.5% lidocaine, make an 0.5 cm incision directly over the rib below the desired interspace. Then use the trochar or a small curved clamp to bluntly dissect a track over the superior margin of the higher rib through the intercostal muscles and into the pleural cavity.

D. Place clamp 0.5-1.0 cm from tip of chest tube and pass through previously punctured space into pleural cavity. Angle tube anteriorly and superiorly and insert tube desired distance.

E. Secure tube to chest wall with suture through skin incision and then around tube. (Cover incision with petroleum gauze and a sterile dressing.)

F. Connect tube to 15-20 cm water suction for decompression via one-way valve.

G. Confirm position and function with chest x-ray.

COMPLICATIONS: lung perforation, hemorrhage, scarring, and malpositioning of tube.

Ref: Henderson R. Pediatrics 1976; 58:861.

4. Endotracheal Intubation

A. Endoctracheal Tube Sizes

| | Internal diameter (mm) |
|---|---|
| Premature infant | 2.5 - 3.0 (see note 2) |
| Term infant | 3.0 - 3.5 |
| 3 months - 1 year | 3.5 - 4.0 |
| 2 years | 4.0 - 4.5 |
| 2 - 15 years | [16 + age (years)] ÷ 4 |
| Adult women | 7.0 - 8.0 (average) |
| Adult men | 8.0 - 9.0 (average) |

Notes

1) Most premature neonates can accept a 3.0 ETT. 2.5 ETT's have increased airway resistance and are difficult to suction adequately.
2) The head should not be extended for placement of the ETT in newborns due to anatomic differences compared to adults.
3) Cuffed ETT's are used only in older patients (>10 years) because of the increased risk of subglottic stenosis. The subglottic region is the narrowest portion of the airway in young children, whereas the larynx is the narrowest portion in older children and adults.
4) If no leak is present, change to the next smaller tube.

Ref: Gregory GA. Pediatric Anesthesia. New York: Churchill Livingston, 1983:371; Fleisher GR et al. (eds.): Pediatric Emergency Medicine. Baltimore: Williams & Wilkins, 1983:1251; Yaster M, Personal Communication, 1986.

B.  Laryngoscope Blades

    Premature infant            Straight 0
    Term - 1 year (2-5 kg)      Straight 1
    1-1½ years (5-12 kg)        Straight 1½
    1.5-12 years              Straight 2
    13 years + (>50 kg)         Straight 3 or curved 3

    Note:  The following are straight laryngoscope blades:
            Miller, Wis-Hipple, Seward and Flagg.
            The curved blade is MacIntosh.

    Ref:  Fleisher GR, et al. (eds.):  Pediatric Emergency
    Medicine.  Baltimore:  Williams & Wilkins, 1983:1251;
    Scarpelli EM, et al. (eds.):  Pulmonary Disease of the
    Fetus, Newborn and Child. Philadelphia: Lea & Febiger,
    1978:106; Yaster M, Personal Communication, 1986.

C.  Suctioning

    The following suctioning equipment should be available:
        <6 months - 14 french catheter
        >6 months - Yankauer catheter

D.  Drugs for Intubation (see chart, next page)

E.  Endotracheal Intubation Technique

    1.    The patient should be well oxygenated and lying on
         his back on a firm surface with the head midline.

    2.    Hold the laryngoscope blade in the left hand.  With
         the patient's head extended, insert the blade on the
         right side of the mouth and sweep the tongue to
         the left out of the line of vision.

    3.    Advance the blade to the vallecula and gently raise
         the epiglottis by lifting the laryngoscope straight
         up.  The cords can now be visualized.

    4.    Advance the endotracheal tube from the right
         corner of the mouth and pass it through the cords
         while maintaining direct visualization.  In infants,
         the tip of the tube may be palpated in the
         suprasternal notch after it passes through the
         cords.

7

D. Drugs for Intubation:
NOTE: The dosage and frequency of administration of these agents is variable and should be individualized according to patient response. These agents should be used only by an experienced physician knowledgeable of their indications and effects.

| | Dosage | Contraindications/Side Effects |
|---|---|---|
| Atropine | 0.01-0.02 mg/kg Min 0.1 mg; Max 0.5 mg (can be injected intralingually if no IV access) | |
| Pavulon (defasciculating dose) | 0.01 mg/kg | Not usually necessary in children <4 years May cause complete paralysis. |
| Thiopental Sodium (Pentothal) | 4-6 mg/kg | Contraindicated in hemodynamically unstable patients secondary to hypotensive effects. The more ill the patient, the lower the dose which should be used (usually ¼-½ the dose). |
| OR | | |
| Ketamine | 1-2 mg/kg | Alternative to pentothal in hemodynamically unstable patients. Forbidden in head trauma because of its effect in increasing cerebral blood flow. Antidote to hallucinogenic effects = valium. Caution in use with propranolol and α-blockers. |
| Succinylcholine | 1 mg/kg (onset 30-45 sec) (lasts 3-10 min) | Dosage = 2 mg/kg in <1 year old. Hyperkalemia possible. Contraindicated in burns, massive trauma, neuromuscular disease. Can cause bradycardia and cardiac dysrhythmia (always give atropine first). Increases intraocular pressure - contraindicated in eye injuries. |
| OR | | |
| Pavulon (paralyzing dose) | 0.04-0.1 mg/kg (onset 1-2 min) (lasts 1 hour) | Reversal drugs: Atropine 0.02 mg/kg Neostigmine 0.07 mg/kg *Reversal not possible for 40 min following administration. |

f: Steward DJ. Some Aspects of Paediatric Anaesthesia. Amsterdam: Excerpta Medica, 1982:64-74; Gregory GA. Pediatric Anesthesia. New York: Churchill Livingston, 1983:467-70; Yaster M, Personal Communication, 1986.

5.  Exchange Transfusion in Newborns

    NOTE: CBC, reticulocyte count, peripheral smear, bilirubin, Ca, glucose, total protein, infant blood type, and Coombs test should be performed on pre-exchange sample of blood since they are no longer of diagnostic value on post-exchange blood. If indicated, also save pre-exchange blood for serologic or chromosome studies.

    A.  Routine Exchange: for removal of sensitized cells or bilirubin.
        1)  Cross match donor blood against maternal serum for first exchange and against post-exchange blood for subsequent exchanges.
        2)  Blood:
            a)  Type: O negative (low titer) anytime; infant's type if no chance of maternal-infant incompatibility.
            b)  Anticoagulant: ACD or CPD unless infant is acidotic or hypocalcemic.
            c)  Temperature: room temperature.
            d)  Age: fresh up to 48 hours old.
        3)  Infant feeding: N.P.O. during exchange. Empty stomach if infant was fed within 4 hours of exchange. Maintain infant N.P.O. for 4 hours after exchange.
        4)  Procedure:
            a)  Provide for: cardiorespiratory monitoring and frequent temperatures. Have resuscitation equipment ready.
            b)  Prep and drape patient for sterile procedure.
            c)  Insert umbilical artery catheter as per page 14.
            d)  Insert umbilical vein catheter as per page 15.

    Note: During the exchange, blood should be removed via the umbilical artery catheter and infused via the venous catheter. If unable to pass an arterial catheter, a single venous catheter will suffice.

            e)  Prewarm blood in quality-controlled blood warmer if available; do not improvise with a water bath!
            f)  Use 15 ml increments in vigorous full-term infants, smaller volumes for smaller, less stable infants. Do not allow cells in donor unit to sediment.
            g)  Rate: 2-3 ml/kg/min avoiding mechanical trauma to patient and donor cells.
            h)  Calcium gluconate 10% solution: 1-2 ml slowly IV for EKG evidence of hypocalcemia. (i.e. prolonged Q-Tc intervals see page 65).

Flush tubing with NaCl before and after calcium infusion. Observe for bradycardia during infusion.

    i)    Total volume exchanged should be 160 ml/kg for a full-term infant and 160-200 ml/kg for a preterm (double volume exchange).

    j)    Use last withdrawal for: Hct, smear, glucose, bilirubin, potassium, $Ca^{++}$, and future cross-matching.

Ref: Kitterman JA, et al. Pediatr Clin North Am 1970; 17:895

B.  **Exchange Transfusion for Anemic Heart Failure in Newborns**
Have O-negative concentrated RBCs in the delivery room. Perform a partial exchange with packed RBCs to correct anemia and failure (30-50 ml/kg). Allow infant to stabilize if possible before attempting a full two volume exchange.

C.  **Complications of Exchange Transfusion**
1)  Cardiovascular: thrombo- or air emboli, thromboses, dysrhythmias, volume overload, and cardiorespiratory arrest.
2)  Chemical: hyperkalemia, hypernatremia, hypocalcemia, hypoglycemia, and acidosis.
3)  Hematologic: thrombocytopenia, DIC, over-heparinization (may use 3 micrograms protamine for each unit of heparin in donor unit), and transfusion reaction.
4)  Infectious: hepatitis and bacteremia.
5)  Physical: injury to donor cells (especially from overheating), vascular or cardiac perforation, and blood loss.

6.  **Intraosseous Infusion**

A.  Indication:
A method for intravascular access that may be especially useful when peripheral IV access is unobtainable or unacceptably delayed.

B.  Technique:
1)  The tibia is the preferred site, approximately 1-2 cm below the tubercle on the anteromedial surface. The femur is an alternate site, in the midline 2-3 cm superior to the lateral condyle.
2)  Prep and drape the patient for a sterile procedure.
3)  Anesthetize the puncture site down to the periosteum.
4)  The needle should be a large bore bone marrow needle or an 18-gauge spinal needle.

5) Insert the needle perpendicular to the skin and advance to the periosteum. Now with a boring motion penetrate into the marrow.

6) Remove the stylet, and aspirate some marrow into a saline-filled syringe. Next, infuse some saline to insure location and remove any clotted material from the needle.

7) Standard IV tubing is attached and saline or drugs may be infused.

<u>Ref</u>: Rosetti VA, et al. Ann Emerg Med 1985; 14:885-88.

7.   <u>Lumbar Puncture</u>

<u>Indications</u>
Examination of spinal fluid for suspected infection or malignancy, or installation of intrathecal chemotherapy.

<u>Contraindications</u>
Bleeding diathesis, infection of skin overlying site, cerebral mass lesion, or increased intracranial pressure.

A.   Position the child in either the sitting position or lateral recumbent position with hips, knees, and neck flexed. Have the patient's head on the nondominant side of the person performing the technique. Care should be taken to ensure that small infants' cardiorespiratory status is not compromised by positioning.

B.   Locate the desired interspace (either L3-L4 or L4-L5) by drawing a line between the top of the iliac crests.

C.   Prepare the skin by cleaning with iodophor and draping conservatively so as to be able to monitor the infant. Use a spinal needle with stylet (epidermoid tumors from introduced epithelial tissue have been reported).

D.   Anesthetize overlying skin with 0.5% lidocaine (not necessary in infants).

E.   Puncture skin in midline just below palpated spinous process, angling slightly cephalad. Use two fingers to guide needle and thumbs to slowly advance. Advance several mm at a time and withdraw stylet frequently to check for CSF flow. In small infants, one may <u>not</u> feel a change in resistance or "pop" as the dura is penetrated.

F.   If resistance is met, withdraw needle to skin surface and redirect angle slightly.

G.   Send CSF for appropriate cultures, glucose, protein, cell count and differential, antigen detection tests, and cytospin (if suspected malignancy).

8. Paracentesis
   Valuable as a diagnostic or therapeutic test for abnormal collection of fluid within the peritoneal cavity.

   A. Precautions
      1) In performing a paracentesis for therapeutic measures, do not remove a large amount of fluid too rapidly because hypovolemia and hypotension may result from rapid fluid shifts.
      2) Avoid scars from previous surgery; localized bowel adhesions increase the chances of entering a viscus in these areas.
      3) The bladder should be empty to avoid perforation.

   B. Technique
      Prepare and drape the abdomen as for a surgical procedure. Anesthetize puncture site.
      1) With patient in supine position, perform needle aspiration just lateral to the rectus muscle in either the right or left lower quadrants, a few centimeters above the inguinal ligament.
      2) With patient in semi-Fowler or cardiac position, employ a midline subumbilical aspiration technique, approximately midway between the umbilicus and pubis.
      3) The use of an intravenous catheter is preferable in this procedure. Apply negative pressure as catheter is inserted into the peritoneal cavity. Use a "Z" tract technique in most instances.
      4) Once fluid appears in the syringe, remove introducer needle and leave catheter in place. Continue aspiration slowly with negative pressure until an adequate amount of fluid has been obtained for diagnostic studies.
      5) If upon entering the peritoneal cavity air is aspirated, withdraw the needle immediately. Aspirated air indicates entrance into a hollow viscus. (In general, penetration of a hollow viscus during paracentesis does not lead to complications.) Then repeat paracentesis with sterile equipment.
      6) Send fluid for lab studies, including: electrolytes, glucose, protein, cell count, differential, Gram stain, culture (AFB, if suspected), and cytospin (if malignancy suspected).

9. Pericardiocentesis

   A. Indications: To remove effusion fluid, purulent material or blood for diagnostic and or therapeutic purposes.

B.  Technique:
1)  Unless contraindicated, the patient should be sedated.
2)  The patient is seated at a 60° angle. The extremities should be held by an assistant.
3)  The site should be prepped and draped in sterile fashion. A drape across the upper chest is unnecessary and may obscure important landmarks.
4)  Anesthetize the puncture site.
5)  An 18 or 19 gauge needle (6.3-8.8cm in length) is inserted either subxiphoid or at the xyphocostal angle. Direct the needle toward the left shoulder keeping it close to the chest wall.
6)  Advance needle until the tip reaches the inner aspect of the rib cage, then depress the needle so the tip points to the left shoulder. Advance needle another 5-10 mm and depress the needle so that it is a few millimeters from the inner aspect of the ribs. Continue to advance the needle until the fluid source is reached.
7)  Upon entering the pericardial space clamp the needle at the skin edge to prevent further penetration. Attach a 30 ml syringe with a stopcock.
8)  Gently and slowly remove the fluid. Too rapid a withdrawal of the pericardial fluid can result in shock or myocardial insufficiency.

10. Radial Artery Catheterization

A.  Use the right radial artery because it is more representative of preductal blood flow. Perform a modified Allen test to assess adequate ulnar blood flow to the entire hand: passively clench the hand and simultaneously compress the ulnar and radial arteries. Release the ulnar artery and note the degree of flushing of the blanched hand. Catheterization may be performed if the entire hand flushes while the radial artery is still compressed. Avoid inadvertent compression of the ulnar artery while compressing the radial vessel.

B.  Secure the hand to an armboard with the wrist extended. Leave the fingers exposed to observe any color changes. Under sterile conditions, palpate the radial artery at the wrist and note the point of maximum impulse. Use a 20 gauge needle to make a small skin puncture at the point of maximal impulse.

C.  Place a 22 gauge intravenous catheter through the puncture site at a 30° angle to horizontal and pass the needle through the artery to transfix it. Withdraw the inner needle. Very slowly withdraw the catheter until free flow of blood is noted, then advance the catheter.

Apply an antibiotic ointment and pressure dressing over the puncture site and secure the catheter with adhesive tape.

D. Firmly attach the catheter to a T-connector to permit a continuous infusion of heparinized isotonic saline (1 unit heparin/ml saline) at a rate of 1 ml/hour via a constant infusion pump. A pressure transducer may be connected in order to monitor blood pressure.

E. To obtain samples, occlude the distal end of the T-connector with the attached clamp. Clean the rubber end of the T-connector with an antiseptic solution and insert a 22 or 25 gauge needle. Allow 3 to 4 drops of blood and fluid (0.3 - 0.5 ml) to drip out to clear line. Attach a 1 ml syringe and withdraw 0.3 - 0.5 ml of blood.

NOTE: Do not infuse any fluids (other than the flushing fluid), medications, or blood products through the arterial line.

Ref: Todres ID, et al. J Pediatr 1975; 87:273.

11. Sweat Electrolyte Test Using Pilocarpine Iontophoresis

Refer to The Harriet Lane Handbook, Tenth Edition, 1984.

12. Thoracentesis

Valuable as a diagnostic or therapeutic test for an abnormal collection of fluid within the pleural space.

Ideally, perform procedure with the patient sitting on the side of the bed, and with an assistant standing in front to support the patient. Select the interspace to be tapped on the basis of dullness to percussion and the level of effusion on the erect chest x-ray. In the event of a small effusion the patient may be tilted laterally toward the affected side to maximize yield.

A. Technique
1) Carry out surgical preparation and draping of the chest.
2) Use a local anesthetic infiltrating the skin down to the periosteum.
3) A large bore needle or intravenous catheter attached to a 3-way stopcock and syringe are the necessary equipment. With needle bevel down, insert into skin at lower edge of the selected rib and "walk" needle over superior edge into the pleural space.

4) Upon entering the pleural space, apply negative pressure on the syringe and slowly withdraw the desired amount of fluid.

5) At the end of the procedure, withdraw the needle or catheter and place dressing over the thoracentesis site.

6) Obtain follow-up chest x-ray after thoracentesis to rule out pneumothorax.

NOTE: Send the fluid obtained for routine lab studies (see above, Paracentesis).

13. Tympanocentesis
A. Restrain patient in standard fashion.

B. Sedation is not usually necessary in infants and toddlers. Sedation may be used with the larger child, more for the allaying of fear than for analgesia.

C. If necessary, gently remove cerumen with a wire curette.

D. Attach 1 ml plastic syringe (containing approximately 0.2 ml nonbacteriostatic saline) to an 18 gauge, $3\frac{1}{2}$ inch spinal needle that has a double bend to permit visualization of needle point.

E. Visualize the posterior inferior quadrant of tympanic membrane using an otoscope with operating head.

F. Perforate the tympanic membrane and apply negative pressure for 1-2 seconds. Then remove needle quickly.

G. The first drop is sent for culture. The next drop is used for the Gram stain. One drop each on blood and chocolate agar plates and the rest into thioglycolate broth.

14. Umbilical Artery Catheterization
A. Restrain infant appropriately. Prepare and drape umbilical cord and adjacent skin in sterile fashion. Place sterile drapes sparingly so as to avoid unnecessary cooling of small infants. Make exterior measurements needed to determine length of catheter insertion for either high (T6-T9) or low ($L_3$ to $L_4$) position. Place marker (sterile bandage or tape) on catheter at desired length (see page 291). Flush catheter with sterile saline solution prior to insertion.

NOTE: Catheter length is approximately 1/3 of crown-heel length.

B.  Place sterile umbilical tape around base of cord.  Cut through cord horizontally approximately 1.5-2.0 cm from skin; tighten umbilical tape so as to prevent bleeding.

C.  Identify large, thin-walled umbilical vein and smaller, thick-walled arteries.  Use one tip of open curved iris forceps to gently probe and dilate one artery.  Then gently probe with both points of closed forceps and dilate artery by allowing forceps to open gently.  Grasp catheter 1 cm from tip with toothless forceps and insert catheter into lumen of artery.  Gently feed catheter in to desired distance.  DO NOT FORCE.  (If resistance is encountered, try loosening umbilical tape, steady gentle pressure, or manipulating angle of umbilical cord to skin.)

D.  The catheter should be secured by means of a suture through the cord and marker tape, and a tape bridge.  The position of the catheter tip should be confirmed radiologically.

COMPLICATIONS:  blanching or cyanosis of lower extremities, perforation, thrombosis, embolism, and infection.

Ref:  Mokrohisky ST, et al.  New Engl J Med 1978; 299:561.

15.  Umbilical Vein Catheterization

(Refer to section on Umbilical Artery Catheterization, above.)

1)  Refer to chart on page 292 to determine proper catheter length for insertion.
2)  Upon isolating the thin-walled vein, clear thrombi with forceps and insert catheter.
3)  Obtain an abdominal radiograph to confirm that the catheter tip is in the inferior vena cava.

16.  Urinary Bladder Catheterization

A.  Prepare the urethral opening using sterile technique.

B.  In the male, gentle traction is applied to the penis in a caudal direction to straighten the urethra.

C.  A lubricated catheter is gently inserted into the urethra.  Slowly advance the catheter until resistance is met at the external sphincter.  Continued force will overcome this resistance and the catheter will enter the bladder.  In the female only a few centimeters of advancement is required to reach the bladder.

D.  Carefully remove the catheter once the specimen is obtained.

17. Suprapubic Aspiration of Urine
    Used for obtaining urine for culture in suspected urinary
    tract infection or sepsis.  Avoid in children with genito-
    urinary tract anomalies.

    A.  The infant's diaper should be dry and the infant should
        not have voided in the 30-60 minutes before the
        procedure.  Anterior rectal pressure in females, or
        gentle penile pressure in males may be used to prevent
        urination during the procedure.

    B.  Restrain the infant in the supine, frog-leg position.
        Clean the lower abdomen suprapubic area with iodine and
        alcohol.

    C.  The site for puncture is just above the symphysis pubis
        (0.5-1 cm) in the midline.  Use a syringe with a 22
        gauge 1½ inch needle and puncture at 10-20° to the
        perpendicular aiming slightly caudad.  Exert suction
        gently as the needle is advanced until urine enters
        syringe.  Aspirate the urine with gentle suction.

18. Venous Cutdown

    Readily accessible veins are the external jugular as it crosses
    the sternocleidomastoid muscle below the angle of the man-
    dible, and the long saphenous just anterior and superior to
    the medial malleolus.  A venous cutdown should be performed
    under careful aseptic conditions and thereafter treated as a
    potential source of local and/or systemic infections.

    NOTE:  In small premature infants bilateral jugular vein cut-
    downs have been associated with superior vena cava syndrome
    and chylothoraces, and should be avoided if possible.

    Prepare the skin for surgical procedure and make a trans-
    verse incision directly over the vein selected.  Isolate the
    vein by blunt dissection and place two 4-0 silk sutures
    around the vein.  Tie the distal ligature and use for traction.
    Make an oblique incision in the vein and insert the appropri-
    ate beveled Silastic catheter (previously filled with saline) to
    the desired length and tie the proximal ligature snugly about
    the vein and catheter.  Close the skin incision with fine silk
    and an additional silk ligature about the catheter in the skin
    to secure the catheter externally.  Place an antibiotic oint-
    ment over the wound and apply a dressing.

19. Punch Skin Biopsy

    A.  Prep site in sterile fashion.  Use alcohol and avoid
        surgical gloves when the skin biopsy is being obtained
        for fibroblast culture.  Iodine and the glove talc can
        interfere with growth of cells.

B.  Anesthetize biospy site.

C.  Use one-punch biopsy device and insert into skin with a rotational motion. The biopsy should penetrate the subcutaneous tissues.

D.  Withdraw punch carefully removing a core of skin.

E.  Carefully remove the biopsy specimen with fine tissue forceps and send the specimen to pathology.

F.  If a biopsy punch larger than 3 mm is used, or there is excessive bleeding, close the wound with a single stitch of 5-0 nylon.

18

H E M A T O L O G Y

1.   Routine <u>Hematology</u> (methods adapted from Williams WJ, et al., eds. Hematology. New York: McGraw-Hill, 1983). For normal values see pages 359-60.

A.   <u>Microhematocrit Determinations</u>
Fill standard microhematocrit tube with blood and seal one end with clay. Centrifuge (12,000 g) for 5 minutes. Falsely high hematocrits caused by increased plasma trapping occur when centrifugation time is short and in disorders with decreased red cell deformability (e.g., sickle cell anemia, thalassemia, spherocytosis).

B.   <u>Wright's Staining Technique</u>
1)   Place air-dried blood smears, film side up, on a staining rack.
2)   Cover smear with undiluted Wright's stain and leave for 2 to 3 minutes.
3)   Add equal volume of distilled water and blow gently on the surface until a greenish metallic sheen appears. Leave diluted stain on smear for 2 to 6 minutes. Without disturbing the slide, flood with water and wash until stained smear is pinkish-red.

C.   <u>Hematologic Indices</u> (for normal values, see p. 359-60)
1)   Mean Corpuscular Volume (MCV): average RBC volume. Usually measured directly by electronic counters. Expressed in femtoliters (fl, $10^{-12}$L).

$$MCV = \frac{Hct\ (\%)\ x\ 10}{RBC\ count\ (millions/mm^3)}$$

2)   Mean Corpuscular Hemoglobin (MCH): average amount of Hb per red cell expressed in picograms (pg, $10^{-12}$g) per cell.

$$MCH = \frac{Hb\ (gm\ \%)\ x\ 10}{RBC\ count\ (millions/mm^3)}$$

3)   Mean Corpuscular Hemoglobin Concentration (MCHC): grams of Hb per 100 ml packed cells.

$$MCHC = \frac{Hb\ (gm\%)\ x\ 100}{Hematocrit\ (percent)}$$

High in congenital spherocytic hemolytic anemias; may be low in iron deficiency and HbSC.

4) Coefficient of Variation (CV) or Red Cell Distribution (RDW):  $\underline{\text{Standard deviation of MCV} \times 100}$
$$\text{MCV}$$
Statistical description of heterogeneity of red cell size. Increases with anisocytosis. In adults, normal 11.5-14.5%. Increased in reticulocytosis, iron deficiency, newborns. Normal in thal minor.

NOTE: Many automated cell counters can display a histogram showing frequency distribution relative to MCV, delineating subpopulations. This can be very helpful in evaluating evolving conditions (e.g. recovery from iron deficiency).

D. Reticulocyte Count
Technique: Mix equal amounts new methylene blue or brilliant cresyl blue with whole blood. Let stand 10-20 minutes then prepare thin smears. Count the number of reticulocytes (cells containing reticulum or blue granules) per 1000 red cells and report as % of RBCs.

E. Platelet Estimation
Approximation of platelet count may be made by examination of Wright's stained blood smear. Presence of platelets on a smear usually excludes severe thrombocytopenia. Always examine periphery of smear or coverslip as platelet clumps may be deposited there.

NOTE: For rough approximation, 1 platelet/oil immersion field corresponds to 10,000-15,000 platelets/$\text{mm}^3$. Platelet clumps usually indicate >100,000 plts./$\text{mm}^3$.

2. Approach to the Anemic Patient

A. Evaluation of Anemia
Is the patient anemic? Anemia is defined by age specific norms (see page 359). These data are derived from white children. Black children's Hb levels average 0.5 gm/dl lower.

1) Is the Hb alone depressed or are other cell lines (plts, wbc) also affected? (Pancytopenia suggests bone marrow failure or general immune-mediated destruction.)
2) Are the red cells large or small, or normal in size?
   a) Microcytosis suggests iron deficiency, thalassemia, and lead poisoning. Can also be seen with ↓copper, ↓pyridoxine, and chronic disease.

  b) Normocytic anemias include congenital hemolytic anemias (hemoglobinopathies, enzyme deficiencies), acquired hemolytic anemias, acute blood loss, bone marrow dysfunction, and the anemia of chronic disease.

  c) Macrocytic anemias occur with reticulocytosis, bone marrow dysfunction, hypothyroidism, folate and $B_{12}$ deficiency, and Down's syndrome.

3) Is red cell production increased or decreased?

$$\text{Reticulocyte Index} = \text{Retic \% X} \frac{\text{Patient's Hct}}{\text{Expected Hct}}$$

If polychromasia is present, correct for early released cells, divide by 2.

Retic index >2 indicates hemorrhage or hemolysis

Retic index <2 indicates hypoproliferative or maturation disorder.

4) Are there characteristic red cell morphologic changes? e.g., spherocytes in immune hemolysis and hereditary spherocytosis; sickled cells in the sickle hemoglobinopathies; fragmented cells in DIC; or target cells in HbC, thalassemias.

B. Specific Tests of Value in the Evaluation of the Anemic Patient

1) Therapeutic trial of iron

Adequate iron therapy should result in reticulocytosis peaking between seventh and tenth day of therapy. Significant increase in Hb concentration should be evident after 3-4 weeks of therapy.

2) Ferritin

Measurement is accurate reflection of total body iron stores after 6 months of age; it is more reliable than serum iron and total iron binding capacity. Normal values, 6mo-15yr: 10-150 ng/ml.

NOTE: Ferritin may be falsely elevated with infection or inflammation.

Ref: Siimes MA, et al. Blood 1974;43:581.

3) Serum iron/total iron binding capacity. Generally replaced by ferritin because of diurnal variability, poor reproducibility, and poor predictive value. Normal serum iron age 6mo-17yr:>20 mcg/dl (adults >50). Normal transferrin saturation, >7% (adults >16%).

Ref: Koerper MA, et al. J Pediatr 1977; 91:870.

4) Free erythrocyte protoporphyrin (FEP).

Accumulates when the conversion of protoporphyrin to heme is blocked by elevated lead levels or iron deficiency. Normal values: <3 mcg/gm Hb, <50 mcg/dl whole blood, <130 mcg/dl PRBC's. Elevated in iron deficiency, plumbism, and erythropoietic protoporphyria (rare). Levels >300 mcg/dl PRBC generally found only with lead intoxication. See p. 252 (lead poisoning).

5) Screening tests for sickle hemoglobin.

   a) Principle: any substance which reduces $O_2$ tension will cause HbS containing red cells to sickle. A positive "sickle prep" is found in the sickle hemoglobinopathies (SS, SC, Sβthal, and others) as well as in sickle trait. All positive tests should be confirmed with cellulose acetate electrophoresis.

   b) Sulfite solution: Mix one or two drops of 2% sodium metabisulfite or sodium hyposulfite on a slide with one drop of blood; apply coverslip. Read preparation at 30 minutes and again at 3 hours. Positive test: presence of sickled cells.

   c) "Sickledex": a solubility test using dithionate reduction of HbS. Used in many commercial and hospital diagnostic laboratories.

   NOTE: Venous blood will sickle more readily than capillary blood. False negatives may be obtained with either test in neonates.

   d) Cellulose acetate electrophoresis: separation of hemoglobin variants based on molecular charge. The initials of the hemoglobins found are listed in order of relative abundance in the sample; e.g., sickle cell trait is ASA2, sickle cell disease SFA2.

6) Indicators of hemolysis

   a) Haptoglobin: binds free hemoglobin. Normal levels: 100-300 mg/dl (after 3 months of age) Interpretation: decreased with intravascular and extravascular hemolysis, and hepatocellular disease. Falsely normal or increased levels may occur in association with inflammation, infection or malignancy.

   b) Hemopexin: binds free heme groups.
      Normal levels: premature 2- 26 mg/dl
                     newborn   8- 42 mg/dl
                     1-12 yrs  40- 70 mg/dl
                     >12 yrs   50-100 mg/dl
      Interpretation: decreased with intravascular hemolysis. Low levels also seen with renal disease and hepatocellular disease. Hemopexin is usually not increased in states of inflammation, infection, or malignancy.

3.  Coagulation (See coagulation cascade page 23.)

A.  Normal clotting depends on adequate platelet number and function as well as intact coagulation cascade.

B.  Adequacy of platelet function and number can be measured by bleeding time.
    1)  Bleeding time IVY technique
        Blood pressure cuff is placed on upper arm and inflated to 40 mm Hg. The forearm is cleaned with alcohol and allowed to dry. A standardized incision is made, taking care to avoid a superficial vein, with a nonheparinized long point disposable lancet (3 mm deep) or with a commercially available template. Gently absorb the blood onto filter paper every 30 seconds, without disturbing the wound. The time required for bleeding to cease is the bleeding time. Normal <9 minutes.

    NOTE: Aspirin ingestion within past week may prolong bleeding time in normal subjects. A prolonged bleeding time in a non-hemophiliac patient with normal platelet count indicates von Willebrand's disease or platelet dysfunction.

C.  Activated Partial Thromboplastin Time, APTT
    Measures intrinsic system; requires factors XII, XI, IX, VIII, V, II, I. Prolongation may occur with polycythemia, inadequate sample volume, blood drawn from heparin containing catheter.

D.  Prothrombin time, PT
    Measures extrinsic and common pathway; requires factors VII, X, V, II, I. Yields information about current synthetic capacity of liver, adequacy of vitamin K absorption, and inhibition of clotting factor synthesis by warfarin. False positives may occur from inadequate sample volume and drawing from heparin containing catheter. Systemic heparin has little effect at usual therapeutic doses.
    Normal values (seconds):

|     | Pre-term | Term Newborn | Child |
|-----|----------|--------------|-------|
| PT  | 12-21    | 13-30        | 12-14 |
| PTT | 70-145   | 45-70        | 30-45 |

NOTE: APTT and PT are useful for evaluation of both abnormal bleeding and anticoagulant therapy. APTT useful for monitoring heparin therapy. PT useful for monitoring warfarin therapy.

Ref: Suchman AL, et al. Ann Intern Med. 1986; 104:810. Bleyes WA, et al. J Pediatr 1971;79:838.

23

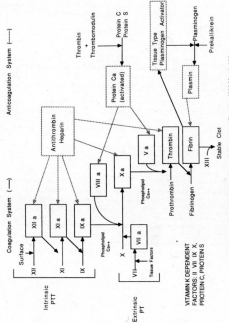

Coagulation System (——→)    Anticoagulation System (------→)

Surface

XII → XII a
XI → XI a
IX → IX a

Intrinsic PTT

Antithrombin Heparin

VIII a

X a

Phospholipid Ca++

X → VII a

Extrinsic PT

VII ← Tissue Factors

V a

Thrombin

Fibrin → Stable Clot
XIII

Prothrombin

Fibrinogen

Phospholipid Ca++

Thrombin + Thrombomodulin → Protein C Protein S

Protein Ca (activated)

Tissue Type Plasminogen Activator

Plasmin

Plasminogen

Prekallikrein

VITAMIN K DEPENDENT FACTORS: II VII IX X, PROTEIN C, PROTEINS

Modified from Rosenberg RD, Bauer KA. Hospital Practice 1986;March:133

E. Disseminated Intravascular Coagulation

If DIC is suspected clinically the following laboratory results will usually be seen: 1) Fragmented RBCs and low or decreasing platelet count. 2) Pink plasma indicating hemoglobinemia. 3) PT and APTT are prolonged, and fibrinogen is low or decreasing.

   1) Confirmatory tests
      a) Fibrin split products (FSP): present
      b) Factor V assay: decreased
      c) Factor VIII assay: decreased

4. Miscellaneous Hematologic Studies

A. Erythrocyte Sedimentation Rate (ESR)

   1) Collect venous blood in EDTA containing or oxalated tube. Determine ESR within one hour of blood drawing.

   2) Place 1 ml in a Wintrobe tube, using long Pasteur pipette. Fill carefully; do not shake tube or allow air bubbles to form in column of blood.

   3) Place tube in its special upright rack, which is exactly vertically aligned.

   4) Read depth of fall of RBC column at the end of 60 minutes.

   5) Normal values (mm/hr):

| | |
|---|---|
| New born (0-48 hrs.) | 0-4 |
| Children | 4-20 |
| Men | 0-10 mean = 4 |
| Women | 0-20 mean = 10 |

   6) Factors which will artificially increase rate of fall: anemia, tilting, warming, and shaking.

Factors associated with decreased rate of fall: hypo- or afibrinogenemia, old or cold blood, excessive anticoagulant, sickle cell anemia (oxygenate sickle cell blood sample before performing ESR), congestive heart failure, polycythemia, trichinosis, pertussis. Elevated in newborn period with infection and ABO hemolysis.

Ref: Cartwright GE. Diagnostic Laboratory Hematology 4th Ed. New York: Grune and Stratton, 1968.

B. Cold Agglutinins - Rapid Screening Test

   1) Method:
      a) Collect 4-5 drops of blood in 60X7mm Wasserman tube containing $\sim$ 0.2 ml of 3.8 NaEDTA.
      b) Cap tube and place in ice water bath for 30-60 seconds.
      c) Tilt tube and observe blood as it runs down wall of tube.

d)  Definite floccular agglutination (seen with the unaided eye) with disappearance thereof upon warming to 37°C is considered a positive (3-4+) test. A control sample is useful for interpretation of test.

2)  Interpretation: positive test frequently correlates with cold agglutinin titer of >1:64. 75-85% of patients with atypical pneumonia and a positive rapid screening test will develop serologic evidence of mycoplasma pneumonia infection.

Ref: Griffin JP. Ann Intern Med 1969; 70:701; Coradero L, et al. J Pediatr 1967; 71:1.

C.  Mononucleosis "Spot Test"
1)  Basis of test: Heterophile (mono) antibody, unlike Forssman antibody, is not adsorbed by guinea pig kidney extract. Both antibodies will agglutinate sheep or horse erythrocytes.
2)  Test for heterophile antibodies:
a)  Obtain test card (Monosticon, Organon Laboratories) and place one drop of water onto blue spot (horse erythrocyte antigen). Stir to suspend the antigen.
b)  Add one drop of serum to buff spot (guinea pig kidney antigen). Mix thoroughly and let stand (one minute) to fully adsorb Forssman antibody.
c)  Mix buff and blue spots together and rock slide gently for 2 minutes. Read results under strong, glare-free light; look for agglutination.
d)  Interpretation of test: Positive "card" test correlates with horse cell titer of >1:244 or a sheep cell titer (Davidsohn) of 1:28 to 1:56.

5.  Blood Component Replacement Guidelines

A.  Estimation of Blood Volume
| | |
|---|---|
| Premature infants | 85-100 ml/kg |
| Term newborns | 85 ml/kg |
| >1 month | 75 ml/kg |

Ref: Oski FA; In: Nathan DG, Oski FA: Hematology of Infancy and Childhood. Philadelphia: WB Saunders, 1981; 29,1507.

B.  Quantity of Packed Cells Needed to Raise Hematocrit

$$\text{Vol of cells (ml)} = \frac{\text{Est Bld Vol (ml)} \times \Delta\text{Hct desired}}{\text{Hct of packed cells (60-70\%)}}$$

Infused no faster than 2-3 ml/kg/hr or in 10 ml/kg aliquots infused over several hours.

C.  <u>Partial Exchange Transfusion for Symptomatic Poly-cythemia</u> (e.g., symptomatic newborns, cyanotic congenital heart disease)

Vol of Exchange (ml) =
$$\frac{\text{Est Blood Vol (ml) x } \Delta\text{Hct desired}}{\text{obs Hct}}$$

Exchange patient's blood for fresh frozen plasma or 5% albumin solution.

D.  <u>Partial Exchange Transfusion Formula for Rapid Correction of Severe Anemia</u> (e.g., preoperatively, severe congestive heart failure)

Exchange Vol (ml) =
$$\frac{\text{Bld Vol (ml) x desired rise in Hb}}{22 \text{ gm/dl} - \text{HbR}}$$

Where HbR =
$$\frac{\text{Hb (initial) + Hb (desired)}}{2}$$

Perform exchange with PRBC (est. Hb 22 gm/dl)

<u>Ref</u>:  Nieburg PI, et al.  Am J Dis Child 1977;131:60.

E.  <u>Partial Exchange Transfusion to Reduce Load of Sickle Cells</u> (e.g., in stroke, lung infarction, priapism)

Exchange volume = Est Bld Vol x Pt. Hct (%) x 2

Usually reduces sickle cells to <40%

<u>Ref</u>:  Zinkham WH, Personal Communication, 1986.

F.  <u>Platelet Transfusions</u>
Usually give 4 units/$M^2$.  Hemorrhagic complications due to thrombocytopenia are rare with platelet counts >20,000/$mm^3$.  Platelet counts >50,000/$mm^3$ are advisable before performing lumbar punctures.  One unit of platelets per $M^2$ will raise the platelet count 10,000/$mm^3$ in the absence of platelet destruction or antiplatelet antibodies.

Platelet increment (expected)/$mm^3$ =
$$\frac{30,000 \text{ x (number of units)}}{\text{Est blood volume (Liters)}}$$

G. Coagulation Factor Replacement Guidelines

1 unit Factor activity equals amount of activity in 1 ml normal plasma.

For Factor VIII deficiency 1 unit/kg raises VIII levels 2%

For Factor IX deficiency 1 unit/kg raises IX levels 1%

FFP - contains all of the clotting Factors in a concentration of 1 unit/ml Cryoprecipitate-protein precipitate contains 5-10 units/ml of Factor VIII. Factor VIII and Factor IX concentrates contain a variable number of units/ml.

| Type of Hemorrhage | Approximate Level Desired (%) |
|---|---|
| Hemarthrosis, simple hematoma | 20-40% |
| Simple dental extraction* | 50% |
| Major soft tissue bleeding Serious oral bleeding* | 80-100% |
| Head injuries Major surgery (dental, orthopedic, other) | 100+% |

*Aminocaproic Acid, 100 mg/kg IV or PO q6h (up to 24 gm/d) is useful in oral bleeding and prophylactically for dental extractions.

H. Irradiation of Blood Products

Principle: Many blood products (PRBC, platelet preparations, leukocytes, FFP, and others) contain viable lymphocytes capable of sustained survival in recipient. Irradiation of all blood products with $\geq$1500 rad prior to transfusion is advisable to prevent graft vs. host disease in children with severe immunosuppression. Indications include:

1) Intensive chemotherapy
2) Leukemia and lymphoma
3) Bone marrow transplantation
4) Known or suspected T-cell deficiencies e.g. SCIDS, DiGeorge Syndrome, Wiscott-Aldrich Syndrome.
5) Intrauterine transfusions for erythroblastosis fetalis.
6) Possibly, exchange transfusions in neonates

Ref: Von Fliedner V, et al. Am J Med 1982;72:951.

I. Use of CMV negative blood desirable in neonates who are CMV antibody negative.

Ref: Yeager A, et al. J Pediatr 1981;98:281.

# NEPHROLOGY

1. <u>Routine Urinalysis</u> - should be done on freshly voided specimen (within 1 hour), ideally the first morning void.

   A. <u>Color</u>
      <u>RED</u>: RBC's, hemoglobin, porphyrins, urates, Adria-
      mycin, food coloring, beets, blackberries, Povan,
      phenazopyridine (acid urine), phenolphthalein (above
      pH8), desferoxamine (with elevated serum iron),
      Aldomet, phenothiazines, Dilantin, red diaper syndrome
      (nonpathogenic <u>Serratia marcescens</u> producing red
      pigment).
      <u>YELLOW TO BROWN</u>: bilirubin, carotene, B-complex
      vitamins, metronidazole, antimalarials (pamaquine,
      primaquine, quinacrine), sulfonamides, azulfidine (in
      alkaline urine), nitrofurantoin, cascara.
      <u>BROWN-BLACK</u>: old blood, hemosiderin, myoglobin,
      homogentisic acid (alkaptonuria), melanin (especially in
      alkaline urine), quinine.
      <u>PURPLE-BROWN</u>: porphyrins (after specimen stands a
      few days).
      <u>DEEP YELLOW</u>: riboflavin.
      <u>ORANGE</u>: rifampin, urates, warfarin, phenazopyridine.
      <u>BLUE-GREEN</u>: methylene blue; biliverdin (seen in
      chronic obstructive jaundice); riboflavin, amitriptyline,
      Adriamycin, <u>Pseudomonas</u> UTI (rare), blue diaper
      syndrome (familial metabolic disease associated with
      hypercalcemia and nephrocalcinosis), indomethacin (due
      to biliverdin).

   B. <u>Clarity</u>

   C. <u>Specific Gravity</u>
      1) Hydrometer (urinometer). Must be free-floating in
         sample.
      2) Refractometer (American Optical Company T.S.
         Meter). Requires only 1 drop of urine. Principle:
         Refractive index of a solution is related to content
         of dissolved solids. The presence of glucose or
         large amounts of protein in the urine elevates the
         specific gravity. Iodine - containing contrast
         material can give readings >1.035.

   D. <u>pH</u> - Nitrazine paper, dipstick (Combistix, Bili-Labstix,
      Ames Co.)

   E. <u>Albumin</u>
      1) Sulfosalicylic Acid (SSA) Test:
         a) Add 0.5-0.8 ml (5-8 drops) 20% SSA to 5 ml
            of urine (pH should be 4.5-6.5) and examine
            after one minute for turbidity. Barely
            evident turbidity is ±, increasing amounts of

turbidity are graded 1-4+.

b) False positives: tolbutamide, sulfonamides, penicillins and cephalosporins, i.v. contrast material, PAS, phosphates, gross hematuria, concentrated urine.

2) Heat Coagulation Test: Add 3% acetic acid to 7-10 ml of clear urine until pH is 4.0-4.6 (check with bromcresol green pH paper). Heat until boiling begins. Any turbidity, cloudiness or precipitate indicates the presence of protein. Most sensitive of the three tests.

| Appearance | Reading | Approx. Protein Concentration (mg/100 ml) |
|---|---|---|
| No turbidity | negative | 0.4 |
| Slight turbidity | ± | 4-10 |
| Definite turbidity - light print readable | 1+ | 15-30 |
| Light cloud - heavy print readable | 2+ | 40-100 |
| Moderate cloud with slight precipitate | 3+ | 200-500 |
| Heavy cloud with precipitation | 4+ | over 800 - 1000 |

3) Albustix (Ames Co.) May give false positives in presence of concentrated or highly alkaline urine or in patients treated with phenazopyridine; confirm with SSA.

Ref: Tietz NW. Fundamentals of Clinical Chemistry. Philadelphia: W B Saunders, 1976: 358-359.

F. Sugars
1) Clinistix (Ames Co.) or Tes-Tape (Eli Lilly Co.): specific for glucose; cannot use for quantitation.
2) Clinitest tablets (Ames Co.): not specific for glucose. 5 drops urine, 10 drops water, 1 tablet. Compare with scale supplied. Reducing substances such as glucose, fructose, galactose, pentoses (e.g. xylulose), lactose, ascorbic acid, chloramphenicol, chloral hydrate, penicillin, PAS, uric acid, creatinine, cysteine, ketone bodies, oxalate, hippurate, homogentisic acid, glucuronates, isoniazid, salicylates, nitrofurantoin, streptomycin, sulfonamides, tetracycline, and amino acids, all give positive tests with Clinitest. Sucrose is not a reducing sugar and does not react with Clinitest.

|                |                        |
|----------------|------------------------|
| Blue           | Negative               |
| Greenish blue  | Trace                  |
| Green          | 0.5% reducing substance |
| Greenish brown | 1% reducing substance  |
| Yellow         | 1.5% reducing substance |
| Brick red      | 2% reducing substance  |

G. Acetone
   1) Acetest tablets (Ames Co.): directions from manufacturer - measures acetone but not B-hydroxybutyrate.
   2) Ketostix (Ames Co.): directions from manufacturer.

H. Urine Hemoglobin and Myoglobin
   1) The reagent found in dipstick methods (Hemastix, Bili-Labstix, Ames Co.) reacts positively with intact red blood cells, hemoglobin and myoglobin; can detect as little as 3-4 RBC/hpf.
   2) Perform a microscopic examination to differentiate hemoglobinuria or myoglobinuria from hematuria (intact RBC's).
   3) Distinguish myoglobinuria from hemoglobinuria.
      a) By history
         Hemoglobinuria - seen with intravascular hemolysis, hematuric urine that has been sitting a long time.
         Myoglobinuria - crush injuries, after vigorous exercise or major motor seizures, fever and malignant hyperthermia, electrocution, snakebite, ischemia, metabolic causes (DKA, hypokalemia, carbon monoxide poisoning, barbiturate poisoning), inflammatory or hereditary muscle disorders.
      b) Laboratory methods
         Qualitative differentiation can be done in clinical lab by a variety of methods.

Ref: Tietz NW. Fundamentals of Clinical Chemistry. Philadelphia: W B Saunders, 1976: 448-51.

   4) If one suspects pigment nephropathy secondary to myoglobinuria, obtain both a CPK and serum urea nitrogen/serum creatinine ratio. This ratio should be very low in myoglobin nephropathy due to release of creatinine from damaged muscle.

Ref: Hamilton R, et al. Ann Int Med 1972; 77:77.

   5) False Positive Hemastix
      a) Microbial peroxidase associated with urinary tract infections.
      b) Ascorbic acid concentrations >5 mg% (used

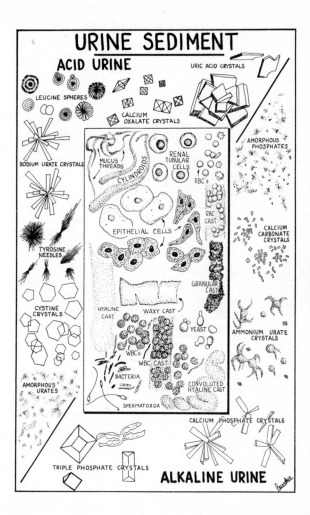

as a preservative for certain antibiotics).
c)   Betadine (Povidone - iodine), particularly
     on the fingers of medical and nursing staff.

Ref:  Ames Co.; Rasoulpour M, et al.  J Pediatr
1978; 92:852.

I.   Urine Bilirubin - Bili Labstix (Ames Co.)

J.   Urine Gram Stain
     1)   Purpose:  to screen for suspected urinary tract
          infections.
     2)   Interpretation:  Almost all uncentrifuged urine
          specimens with bacterial colony counts of $10^5$/ml
          or greater will have positive Gram stains.  A
          urine culture should be taken to confirm these
          results.

     Ref:  Greenhill A, et al.  Pediatr Clin North Am
     1976; 23:661.

K.   Sediment
     Examine all fields for red cells, white cells, casts,
     and crystals.  Area at edge of coverslip should also
     be examined as formed elements collect there.  See
     illustration on page 31.

2.   Renal Function Tests

     A.   Endogenous Creatinine Clearance (Ccr)
          1)   Purpose:  This is a standard measure of
               glomerular filtration rate (GFR) and closely
               approximates the inulin clearance in the normal
               ranges of GFR.  With the low GFR of advanced
               renal disease, Ccr is greater than the inulin
               clearance.  (See section 2A4).  Results are not
               accurate in children with obstructive uropathy.
          2)   Method:  Timed collection of urine is made for
               any time period, recording the nearest minute.
               (Have patient empty bladder and discard this
               specimen before beginning collection.  Collect all
               urine during the timed period and have the
               patient void at the end of the collection period,
               keeping this specimen.)  Draw a single blood
               specimen during the collection period unless the
               patient's renal function is rapidly changing.  In
               the latter condition, draw specimens at the
               beginning and end of the period.

3)  Calculation:

$$Ccr = \frac{UV}{P} \times \frac{1.73}{S.A.}$$

U = urinary concentration of creatinine in mg/dl
V = total volume of urine divided by number of minutes in the collection period = ml/min (<u>NOTE</u>: 24 hrs = 1440 mins)
P = serum creatinine level (or average of 2 levels) in mg/dl
S.A. = surface area in square meters (see nomogram on p. 330)

4)  With decreased renal function (Ccr <25), creatinine clearance is elevated over true GFR because of tubular secretion of creatinine. The method of choice for measuring low GFR is a renal scan with a GFR study using $^{99M}$Technetium-labelled DTPA.

<u>Ref</u>: Chervu LR, et al. Semin Nucl Med 1982; $\overline{12}$:224; Rubovsky EV, et al. Semin Nucl Med 1982; 12:308 with permission.

5)  Normal values:
a)  Newborns, 27-43 weeks gestation, first 24 hours of life: mean GFR (measured by inulin clearance) expressed as a function of body weight is fairly constant regardless of gestational age: 1.07 ± 0.12 ml/min/kg.
b)  Prematures >24 hours of age - GFR correlates with gestational age; no good reference values available.
c)  5 - 7 days  :  50.6 ± 5.8 ml/min/1.73 M²
d)  1 - 2 months:  64.6 ± 5.8 ml/min/1.73 M²
e)  5 - 8 months:  87.7 ± 11.9ml/min/1.73 M²
f)  9 -12 months:  86.9 ± 8.4 ml/min/1.73 M²
g)  1½ years to Adult:
1)  Males:   124 ± 25.8 ml/min/1.73 M²
2)  Females: 108.8 ± 13.5 ml/min/1.73 M²
h)  Adults
1)  Males:   105 ± 13.9 ml/min/1.73 M²
2)  Females:  95.4 ± 18 ml/min/1.73 M²

<u>Ref</u>: Robillard JE et al. Pediatrics Update - Reviews for Physicians. New York: Elsevier North Holland, 1980; 168-9; Schwartz GJ et al.: J Pediatr 1984; 104:849; Fobias GJ et al. New Engl J Med 1962; 266:317; Winberg J. Acta Pediatr Scand 1959; 48:443.

B.  Estimating Creatinine Clearance with Length
    and Plasma Creatinine (a useful alternative when a
    timed urine specimen can not be collected; correlates
    well with standard creatinine clearance for children >1
    year of age).
        An estimate of the creatinine clearance can be
        obtained using the formula: 0.55 L/Pcr, where L
        = length in centimeters; Pcr = plasma creatinine
        in mg/dl. A constant of 0.7 is more appropriate
        in postpubertal boys (who have larger muscle
        mass).
        This formula is not accurate for infants < 6
        months of age and must be used with caution in
        patients with severe reduction of muscle mass.

    Ref:  Schwartz GJ, et al.  Pediatrics 1976; 58:259;
    Schwartz GJ, et al.  J Pediatr 1985; 106:522.

C.  BUN:Cr ratio
    1)    normally 10 - 15
    2)    >20:  suggests prerenal azotemia (see p. 236) or
                GI bleeding
          <5:   suggests liver disease, starvation, inborn
                error of urea metabolism.

    Ref:  Greenhill A, et al., Ped Clin North Am 1976;
    23:661.

D.  Concentration Test
    1)    Concentration:  A random urine S.G. of 1.023 or
          more indicates intact concentrating ability within
          the limits of clinical testing and no further tests
          are indicated.  A first-voided specimen following
          an overnight fast is adequate to test concentrat-
          ing ability.

    Ref:  Edelmann CM, et al.  Am J Dis Child 1967;
    114:639

    2)    Technique:  See Water Deprivation Test, page
          96.

E.  Proteinuria
    1)    24-hour urine protein - normally <100 mg/$M^2$.
          Nephrotic range proteinuria - $\geq$ 40mg/$M^2$/hr.
    2)    Proteinuria by dipstick
          a)   Transient - most common cause in children,
               associated with exercise, changes in
               posture, exposure to cold, fever, emotional
               stress; not associated with renal disease.
          b)   Orthostatic - another common cause, also
               not associated with renal disease.
               (1)  Method for diagnosis:

    (a)   No food or fluids after 9 p.m.
    (b)   Empty bladder immediately before retiring; label this sample #1.
    (c)   Void without rising at 12 midnight and at 5 a.m. (samples #2 and #3).
    (d)   Void at 7 a.m. (may arise to void). Label this sample #4.
    (e)   Walk about actively from 7 to 9 a.m. (no food or fluids until test is completed). Void at 9 a.m.; label this #5.

For each specimen record the specific gravity and the protein content (by the sulfosalicylic acid or other simple test).

Orthostatic proteinuria is confirmed if samples 1 and 5 contain protein, and samples 3 and 4 do not. Sample 2 may contain some protein.

   c)   Persistent proteinuria - requires evaluation for associated renal disease.

Ref: Rudolf AM. Pediatrics. Norwalk: Appleton-Century-Crofts, 1982: 1165-6; Dodge WF, et al. J Pediatr 1976; 88:327.

F.   Estimation of proteinuria using albumin/Cr ratio
   1)   Collect random sample during normal ambulation
   2)   95th percentile for normals (mcg albumin/mg Cr)
          <2 years: 492.1
          2 years to adult: 178.1
   3)   If >95th percentile, confirm with standard 24 hour collection.

Ref: Ginsberg JM et al. New Engl J Med 1983; 309:1543; Houser M. J Pediatr 1985; 104:845.

G.   Urine Calcium

   1)   Hypercalciuria: 24 hour urinary calcium excretion >4 mg/kg/24 hrs. Seen in RTA, vitamin D intoxication, immobilization (associated with hypercalcemia and hypertension), excessive calcium intake, loop diuretics; can be idiopathic (associated with hematuria and renal stones).
   2)   Can screen spot urine for Ca/Cr ratio (mg $Ca^{2+}$/mg Cr). Normal <0.21; mean 0.08 (boys), 0.06 (girls). No standards for prematures.

Ref: Moore ES et al. J Pediatr 1978; 92:906; Stapleton FB et al. New Engl J Med 1984; 310:1345.

H.  Urine Acidification Test

1)  Purpose:  To evaluate the renal tubular acidification mechanisms when random urine pH values are >6 in the presence of systemic metabolic acidosis.  Acidification defect should be confirmed by simultaneous venous or arterial pH, plasma bicarbonate concentration, and pH meter (not dipstick) determination of pH of <u>fresh</u> urine.  Ammonium chloride loading test should be done only in a well hydrated child, preferably under the guidance of a nephrologist.

2)  Method:
   a)  Give ammonium chloride 75 mEq/M$^2$.
   b)  Over the next 5 hours measure urine pH with pH meter every hour if possible.
   c)  Measure plasma bicarbonate concentration 3 hours after ingestion of ammonium chloride.

3)  Results:  The urine pH should fall below 5.5 and plasma bicarbonate should fall 4-5 mEq/L.  If urine pH is not lower than 5.5 and the plasma bicarbonate is not below 20 mEq/L (18 for an infant), larger doses (100 mEq/M$^2$) of ammonium chloride may be necessary to produce a plasma bicarbonate concentration below an abnormal renal bicarbonate reabsorption threshold. Extreme care should be taken when using larger doses of ammonium chloride.

   <u>Ref</u>:  Edelmann CM et al. Pediat Res 1967; 1:452.

4)  Interpretation:
   <u>Normal Response</u>
   a)  Fall in plasma bicarbonate concentration.
   b)  Fall in urine pH to below 5.5.

   <u>Type 1 Renal Tubular Acidosis</u> - <u>Distal</u> - defect in distal tubular excretion of hydrogen ion.

   a)  Fall in plasma bicarbonate concentration.
   b)  Urine pH remains above 6.0.

   <u>Type 2 Renal Tubular Acidosis</u> - <u>Proximal</u> - defect in proximal tubular reabsorption of bicarbonate.

   a)  Fall in plasma bicarbonate concentration (see above).
   b)  Fall in urine pH below 5.5.

   <u>Type 3 Renal Tubular Acidosis</u> - probably a variant of Type 1 RTA; a defect in distal tubular hydrogen ion excretion <u>plus</u> bicarbonaturia (bicarbonate leak subsides after adolescence).

Type 4 Renal Tubular Acidosis – hyperchloremic acidosis, hyperkalemia, and acid urinary pH. Has five subtypes. Associated with adrenal insufficiency, obstructive uropathy, diabetic nephropathy, pyelonephritis and other disorders.

For more detailed information on renal tubular acidosis, the best references are: McSherry E. Kidney Int 1981; 20:799; Chan JCM. J Pediatr 1983; 102:327.

3. Acute Peritoneal Dialysis

A. Indications: acute renal failure with life-threatening electrolyte imbalance, severe lactic acidosis, hyperammonemia, dialyzable toxins or poisons.

B. Procedure (Whenever possible, catheter insertion should be performed by a surgeon or nephrologist.)

   1) Place patient in supine position, prep and shave from xiphoid to groin after the bladder has been emptied by catheterization.

   2) Inject local anesthesia (1% xylocaine) in the midline, down 1/3 of the distance from the umbilicus to the symphysis pubis.

   3) Make a small puncture with a #11 scalpel point in the anesthetized area down to the linea alba but not through the peritoneum.

   4) Insert an 18 gauge needle into the peritoneal cavity.

   5) Introduce a quantity of 1.5% dialysis fluid (warmed to 37°) into the peritoneal cavity sufficient to distend the abdomen slightly and allow the intestines to float (approximately 20 ml/kg).

   6) Remove the needle and push the trocar (with the dialysis catheter fitted over it) through the existing perforation. This may require considerable force; rotation of the trocar may help. Lifting the peritoneal membrane with pickups and making a small incision with a scalpel can make insertion more controlled in difficult cases. One hand should be used to control the depth of the initial entry. Remove the trocar and angle the catheter to the right or left lower quadrant. After making sure all the perforations on the dialysis catheter are within the peritoneal cavity, cut the catheter to an appropriate length. Connect catheter to the warmed dialysis solution, support the entire apparatus by gauze squares and cover with a dressing. The quantity of fluid for each pass varies according to the weight of the child; 40-50 ml/kg is commonly

used, but neonates and infants may need less (30-40 ml/kg). Final volume should be limited by abdominal distention.

7) It should take no longer than 10 minutes to run in each pass. The fluid should remain in the peritoneal cavity 30-45 minutes, and run out in 10-15 minutes.

8) 24-36 passes have been used as a standard number. The catheter should not be left in beyond 72 hours because of the danger of peritonitis. Need for prolonged peritoneal dialysis is an indication for the surgical insertion of a soft subcutaneous catheter (Tenckhoff catheter).

9) All fluid should be warmed and maintained at 37°C. Cold dialysate can cause arrythmias.

10) Venous access should be established during acute peritoneal dialysis. Equipment for emergency airway management and rapidly acting anticonvulsants should be on hand. Careful records of vital signs, time and amounts of fluid in and out, with cummulative deficits in either direction, must be kept. Twice daily weights should be obtained. Electrolytes, Ca, $PO_4$, BUN and Cr should be monitored frequently. Culture and cell count of outflow should be sent twice daily.

11) Major risks - perforation of viscera and/or major vessels, infection.

C. Available Fluids and Additives

1) Solutions with 1.5% dextrose: contents (mEq/L):

|  | Na | Ca | Mg | Cl | acetate | lactate |
|---|---|---|---|---|---|---|
| McGaw: | 141 | 4.0 | 2.0 | 103 | 45 | --- |
| Dianeal (Travenol): | 141 | 3.5 | 1.5 | 101 | --- | 45 |

2) Solution with 4.25% dextrose and the same electrolyte composition as the 1.5% solution. Much higher osmolality (550 mOsm/L) for taking off large quantities of fluid rapidly. Must be used carefully and sparingly due to large fluid shifts and subsequent hypotension.

3) Heparin is added (100 - 500 units/liter) to initial dialysate to prevent clots from forming; this can be discontinued when outflow is clear.

4) If the serum potassium is < 3.5 mEq/L, then $K^+$ may be given IV or added to the dialysis fluid (4 mEq/L).

5) Most fluids commercially available are prepared with lactate or acetate as a bicarbonate precursor. In situations where there is hepatic failure, metabolic acidosis, or lactic acidosis, a

solution prepared with acetate is better. In some of these patients conversion of acetate to bicarbonate is also impaired and an acetate-free dialysate may be preferable (prepared as follows).

| | |
|---|---|
| 916 ml | 0.45 N NaCl |
| 12 ml | NaCl (2 mEq/ml) |
| 40 ml | NaHCO$_3$ (1 mEq/ml) |
| 30 ml | D$_{50}$W |
| 1.8 ml | 10% Mg SO$_4$ |

1000 ml   (D$_{1.5}$; 140 mEq Na; 100 mEq Cl; 50 mEq HCO$_3$; 1.5 mEq Mg$^2$ )

Note: Contains no calcium; must monitor Ca$^{2+}$ carefully.

Ref: Nash MA et al. J Pediatr 1977; 91:101.

Ref: Rubin M ed. Pediatric Nephrology. Baltimore: Williams and Wilkins, 1975; 833; Edelmann CM. Pediatric Kidney Disease. Boston: Little, Brown 1978; 499-500.

CEREBROSPINAL FLUID

Caution: Lumbar puncture may be dangerous in the presence of the following:

Increased intracranial pressure
Prior to lumbar puncture, perform a fundoscopic exam. The presence of papilledema/hemorrhage calls for extreme caution and may be a contraindication to the procedure. A sudden drop in intraspinal pressure by rapid release of CSF may cause fatal herniation.

Bleeding tendency
A platelet count of >50,000/mm³ is desirable prior to L.P. Correct any clotting factor deficiencies.

Overlying skin infections
May result in inoculation of CSF with organisms.

A. Cerebrospinal Fluid Pressure
Accurate measurement of CSF pressure can only be made with the patient lying quietly on his side. Once free flow of spinal fluid is obtained, attach the manometer and measure CSF. (Normal values, see page 358.)

B. Collection of Cerebrospinal Fluid
Collect 3 tubes of spinal fluid under sterile conditions (save a fourth tube if possible for additional studies). The first tube is for culture, the second for chemistry determinations, and the third for cell count. About 1-2 ml in each tube will suffice for routine examinations, but cell count and Gram stain can be done on less than 1 ml. Collect larger amounts of fluid if special studies are contemplated (i.e., IgG, myelin basic protein, antigen studies, cytology).

C. Appearance
Record:
1) Color
2) Clarity
3) Coagula, pellicles, or sediments. Time required for their formation will vary with different diseases; coagula may form in a short time in suppurative meningitis, whereas T.B. meningitis may take 12-24 hours to produce pellicle.

D. Culture
Most microbiology laboratories are open 24 hours a day, seven days a week, and CSF is treated as a major medical emergency.

However, whenever immediate culture is not available through the hospital laboratory, see pages 44-46 for culture techniques.

E.  Cell Count, Differential WBC and Cell Morphology
    The appropriate CSF tubes should be sent immediately to
    the hospital laboratories for these studies. (Normal
    values, see page 358.)

F.  Examination for Bacteria
    1)  If pellicle forms, remove and crush it between 2
        clean slides. Pull the slides apart, giving 2
        smears. Stain one with Gram stain and the other
        for acid-fast bacilli (see page 44).
    2)  Spin uncontaminated CSF, smear the sediment on a
        slide and Gram stain it.

G.  Examination for Fungus
    Place one drop of CSF and one of India ink on a slide
    and mix well. Cover with coverslip and press out
    excess fluid. Ring with vaseline. Examine for round
    organisms with large halos. If the index of suspicion
    for fungi is high, incubate the preparation at 37°C and
    reexamine at 24 and 48 hours.

H.  Chemical Determination
    The appropriate CSF tubes should be sent immediately to
    the hospital laboratories for sugar and protein deter-
    minations.

I.  Serologic Studies
    May be performed in serology laboratory.

# SYNOVIAL FLUID

## Examination of Synovial Fluid

A.  **Appearance**
    Note quantity, turbidity, pH, clot formation, viscosity, and icterus.

B.  **Microscopic**
    Examine undiluted for total RBC and WBC count and crystals. Dilute with saline to obtain WBC if necessary. The use of acidic WBC diluting fluids may produce clotting. Any cell count >50,000/mm³ must be assumed to represent septic arthritis until proven otherwise. Crystal induced synovitis is rare in children. The exception is acute gout in Lesch-Nyhan syndrome or glycogen storage diseases. Please see page 43 for normal values.

C.  **Chemical**
    Obtain sugar and protein determinations. Sugar should be within 10 mg/dl of blood sugar. Be sure to obtain blood sugar before procedure. Normal joint fluid contains little protein.

D.  **Mucin**
    A qualitative test for hyaluronic acid. To 1 ml of synovial fluid, from which the cells have been centrifuged, add 4 ml water, then 2-3 drops glacial acetic acid, and stir. A tight rope of mucin is normal. In infection and rheumatoid arthritis no precipitate, or a loose fibrillar precipitate, is formed.

E.  **Bacteriologic**
    Gram stain sediment; culture aerobically, anaerobically, and for AFB.

F.  **Icterus**
    May indicate trauma. Send sample to chemistry lab for bilirubin.

    NOTE: A portion of the fluid may be placed in a heparinized tube to prevent clotting.

SYNOVIAL FLUID ASSESSMENT

| Etiology | Appearance | Leukocytes /mm³ | % Neutrophils | Mucin | Blood glucose / Synovial glucose |
|----------|------------|-----------------|---------------|-------|------------------|
| Normal | clear, straw | <2,000 | <40% | good | <2 |
| Inflammatory | clear – turbid | 2,000 – 100,000 | ≥50% | loose friable | ≥2 |
| Infectious | turbid | >50,000 | >75% | loose friable | >2 |

Adapted from: Hoekelman RA, et al. (eds.): Principles of Pediatrics. New York: McGraw Hill, 1978, p. 1099.

# MICROBIOLOGICAL EXAMINATIONS

1.  <u>Examination of Fresh Preparations and Stained Smears</u>
    One of the most important steps in the laboratory
    identification of microorganisms is the staining of slide
    preparations. Staining makes the organisms clearly visible
    under the microscope and also differentiates them on the
    basis of their staining characteristics. The three most
    important screening methods available are:

    A.  The Gram stain
    B.  The acid-fast stain
    C.  India ink stain

    The following guidelines are helpful when performing the
    above stains:
    > When making smears for staining, it should be remem-
    > bered that <u>thin smears give the best results</u>.
    > Always allow the smears to air dry before they are
    > fixed. (Heating wet smears will usually distort orga-
    > nisms and cells.)
    > The smears are fixed in gentle heat by quickly passing
    > slide through a bunsen burner flame (no more than
    > four times). Test heat by tapping slide on the back
    > of your hand. It should feel just warm.
    > Allow slide to cool before staining.

    A.  <u>Gram Stain</u>
        1)  Flood slide with gentian (Crystal) violet - 1 min.
        2)  Wash with gently running water
        3)  Flood with Iodine solution - 1 min.
        4)  Wash with gently running water
        5)  Decolorize with acetone/alcohol - 3-4 sec.
        6)  Wash with water immediately
        7)  Counterstain with safranin - 30 sec.

        <u>Gram Stain - Rapid Method</u>
        Fix as above except for
        1)  gentian violet - 10 sec.
        3)  Iodine solution - 10 sec.
        7)  Safranin counterstain - 10 sec.

    B.  <u>Acid Fast Stain</u>
        1)  Flood slide with Kenyoun's stain - 5 minutes.
            Wash with water.
        2)  Decolorize with acid alcohol - 2 minutes. Wash
            with water.
        3)  Counterstain with 1/2% methylene blue - 2
            minutes.

    C.  <u>India Ink</u>
        A negative stain used mainly for identification of
        <u>Cryptococcus</u>. Mix one drop of test fluid and one
        drop of India ink and examine for presence of

organism identified as a refractile image against a black background. (See technique under CSF examination for fungus, page 41).

2. Culture Methods
When immediate culturing is not available through the hospital laboratory, culture as follows:

A. Culture the Following Materials Immediately
   1) Blood: The sample volume should equal 10% of the volume of the culture medium. When patient is treated with penicillin request that the laboratory add penicillinase, if desired. (The use of penicillinase is of questionable validity).
   2) CSF:
      a) Chocolate blood agar (place in $CO_2$ jar)
      b) 5% sheep blood agar
      c) MacConkey
      d) Thioglycolate broth
      e) Original fluid
   3) Cavity Fluid:
      a) Culture the same as CSF.
      b) Peritoneal and abscess cultures should be placed in special anaerobic containers.

B. To Expedite Cultures the Following Media May Be Used Directly (in order of plating when multiple plates are used)
   1) Nasopharynx, eye and ear:
      a) Chocolate blood agar
      b) 5% sheep blood agar
      c) MacConkey (or Thayer-Martin in infants)
      * Separate swab in transport media
   2) Throat:
      a) 5% sheep blood agar
      b) MacConkey
      * Separate swab in transport media
   3) Vagina and urethra:
      a) Chocolate blood agar
      b) Thayer-Martin agar
      c) Broth - institution specific
   NOTE: Always culture immediately, and always do Gram stain as well.
   4) Skin:
      a) 5% sheep blood agar
      b) MacConkey
      c) Inoculate thioglycolate broth
      d) Swab in transport media

C. Fungus Preparation
Scrape the edges of a lesion in which fungus is suspected with a scalpel onto a glass slide. Cover the scrapings with 10% to 20% KOH or NaOH and apply a

coverslip. Warm over light bulb for a few minutes (15 min. ideal). Examine for fragments of mycelia and spores.

D.  Culture for Chlamydia Trachomatis
    All specimens should be sent in the Chlamydia transport media if that is available from the hospital microbiology or virology laboratory. If swabs are used to collect the specimen, they should be immediately extracted into the transport medium and discarded. Extraction is done by pressing and rotating the swab against the wall of the specimen container. Dacron swabs must be used. Cotton-wood swabs and calcium alginate swabs are unacceptable.
    1)  Specimen
        a)  Genital: urethral swab, urethral scrapings, prostatic secretions from males, cervical swabs from females.
        b)  Conjunctival: conjunctival scrapings or swab.
        c)  Respiratory: throat, NP swabs, lung biopsy.
        d)  Other: inner ear secretions, synovial fluid, pus from LGV-suspected lesions and lymph nodes.
    2)  Specimen storage
        For best results, specimens should be inoculated without delay onto cell cultures. However, the following is done if this is not possible.
        a)  If inoculation will take place within 24 hours of collection, the specimen should be refrigerated at 4°C.
        b)  If inoculation will take place after 24 hours of collection, the specimen should be frozen at -70°C in the mechanical freezer.

E.  Tzanck Test
    This test can be used to identify the multinucleated giant cells that are seen in lesions of herpes simplex, herpes zoster, and varicella infections. The lesions tested must be vesicular or bullous. The vesicle or bulla should be unroofed, the fluid blotted off, and the base curetted gently with the blunt end of a scalpel. The scraping should be spread on a glass slide, fixed in methyl alcohol, then stained with a Giemsa or Wright stain.

F.  Antigen/Antibody Test
    Ag/Ab detections are available by Immunofluorescent, ELISA, Latex and other techniques for bacteria, viruses and fungi. Consult with the processing laboratory for availability of the tests and specimen preparation.

# GASTROENTEROLOGY

I. Stool Examination

    A. Parasitology Preparations
       See page 48 for illustrations.

       1. Direct Smear
          Add small amount of feces to drop of saline, mix and remove feces with applicator stick. Cover. Examine under low power to locate the parasite and high dry for identification. Species identification of protozoan cysts can be made by adding iodine stain (KI 1.0% saturated with crystalline iodine) to smear, or by making an additional prep in a drop of stain.

       2. Preservatives
          Specimens should be delivered to the laboratory immediately. If delays are expected, place in either polyvinylalcohol fixatives or formalin.

       3. Giardia Lamblia
          The use of string test collection system (Entero/Test) can be helpful. The Entero/Test is available in sizes for both children and adults.

    B. Examination for Pinworms

       1. Parents inspect perianal area at night about an hour after the child retires, looking for thread-like white worms (1/4 to 1/2 inch).

       2. Pinworm Smear (Cellophane Tape Method)
          a) Obtain smear in morning before bath.
          b) Cover one end of a tongue depressor with clear cellophane tape, sticky side out.
          c) Apply to perianal area with mild pressure.
          d) Put 1 drop xylol on glass slide, then apply tape to slide.
          e) Look for ova under microscope.

    C. Test for Occult Blood in Stool (Guaiac Method)

       1. Reagents
          a) Glacial acetic acid
          b) Guaiac
          c) Hydrogen peroxide (fresh)

       2. Method
          Make thin stool smear on filter paper. Serially apply 2 drops of each in this order: acetic acid, guaiac, hydrogen peroxide. A royal blue color is

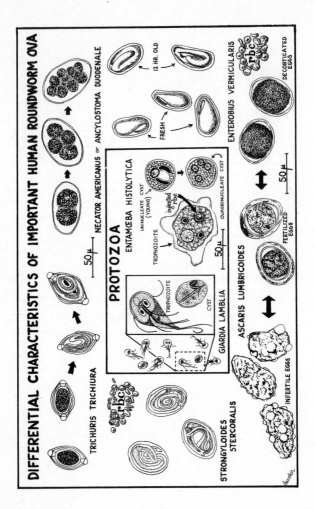

# DIFFERENTIAL CHARACTERISTICS OF IMPORTANT HUMAN ROUNDWORM OVA

NECATOR AMERICANUS or ANCYLOSTOMA DUODENALE

12 HR. OLD

FRESH

TRICHURIS TRICHIURA

STRONGYLOIDES STERCORALIS

## PROTOZOA

### ENTAMOEBA HISTOLYTICA

UNINUCLEATE CYST (YOUNG)

QUADRINUCLEATE CYST

ingested rbc

TROPHOZOITE

### GIARDIA LAMBLIA

TROPHOZOITE

CYST

50 μ

ASCARIS LUMBRICOIDES

FERTILIZED EGGS

INFERTILE EGGS

ENTEROBIUS VERMICULARIS

rbc

DECORTICATED EGGS

50 μ

49

4+; a green color is negative.  Other gradations of blue are 1-3+.

NOTE:  Medicinal iron does <u>not</u> give a positive guaiac reaction.

D.  <u>Apt Test for Fetal Hemoglobin</u>

1.  <u>Purpose</u>
To differentiate fetal blood from swallowed maternal blood.

2.  <u>Method</u>
Mix specimen (stool, vomitus, etc.) with an equal quantity of tap water.  Centrifuge or filter. Supernatant must have pink color to proceed.  To 5 parts of supernatant, add 1 part of 0.25 N (1%) NaOH.

3.  <u>Interpretation</u>
A pink color persisting over 2 minutes indicates fetal hemoglobin.  Adult hemoglobin gives a pink color that becomes yellow in 2 minutes or less indicating denaturation of hemoglobin.

<u>Ref</u>:  Apt L, Downey WS.  J Pediatr 1955; 47:6.

E.  <u>Test for Sugar in Stool (Reducing Substances)</u>

1.  <u>Purpose</u>
Detection of carbohydrate malabsorption by measuring reducing substances in stool.  Since sucrose is not a reducing substance modify test as noted.

2.  <u>Method</u>
a)  Place a small amount of fresh liquid stool in a test tube.
b)  Dilute with twice its volume of water. To look for sucrose malabsorption use 1 N HCl instead of water and boil briefly.
c)  Place 15 drops of this suspension in second test tube containing a Clinitest tablet.
d)  Compare the resulting color with the chart provided for urine testing.

3.  <u>Interpretation</u>
Normally <0.25% reducing substances in the stool. Values of 0.25% to 0.5% are questionable.  The finding of >0.5% reducing substances in the stool is abnormal and suggests carbohydrate malabsorption. Stool pH may be <6.0 if carbohydrate malabsorption is occurring.

F.   Fecal Leukocyte Exam

1.   Purpose
     To aid in the early diagnosis of diarrhea by noting
     the presence or absence of leukocytes.

2.   Method
     a)  Place a small fleck of stool or mucus (ideally
         from a rectal swab) on a clean glass slide.
     b)  Mix thoroughly with 2 drops of 0.5% methylene
         blue stain.
     c)  Wait 2-3 minutes for good nuclear staining,
         cover with coverslip and examine under low
         power.

3.   Interpretation
     PMNs are seen with any inflammatory enterocolitis,
     most commonly shigellosis, salmonellosis, Yersinia,
     Campylobacter, invasive E. coli infections, and
     ulcerative or granulomatous colitis. A predominance
     of mononuclear cells is seen in typhoid fever.

Ref:  Harris JC, et al. Ann Intern Med 1973; 76:697.

II.  Tests of Malabsorption
     A.   D-Xylose Test
          1.  Purpose:  To estimate the surface area of the
              duodenojejunal intestinal mucosa by measuring the
              absorption of an oral dose of D-xylose. Either the
              elevation in serum concentration or the % urinary
              excretion of xylose may be used to quantitate
              D-xylose absorption. Absorption is independent of
              bile salts, pancreatic exocrine secretions, and
              intestinal mucosal disaccharidases. The test is
              unreliable in patients with edema, renal disease,
              delayed gastric emptying and severe diarrhea.

          2.  Method:
              a.  Preparation:  Older children fast for 8 hours
                  prior to the test; younger infants need fast
                  for only 4-6 hours.
              b.  Test dose:  Give D-xylose in a dose of 14.5
                  $gm/M^2$ BSA (max: 25 gm) as a 10% water
                  solution orally or via a gastric tube.
              c.  Measurement of urinary excretion:  Patient
                  voids and all urine for 5 hours is collected.
                  Insure adequate urine flow by supplementary
                  oral or IV fluid. The quantity of xylose is
                  determined colorimetrically.

Normal values:  5 hour urinary excretion of
25% or greater of the administered dose is
normal for children over 6 months.  Values
between 15 and 23% are questionable.  Urinary
excretion of less than 15% is abnormal.  In
infants less than 6 months values below 10%
are considered abnormal.

d.  Measurement of serum concentration (infants):
Obtain serum samples for determination of
xylose concentration in fasting state and at 30,
60, 90, and 120 minutes following the xylose
dose.
Normal values:  A  normal  response  is
associated with a serum level exceeding 25
mg/dl in any of the post absorptive specimens.
Ref:  Santiago-Borrero P, et al.  Pediatrics 1971;
48:55.  Anderson CM, Burke A.  Pediatric Gastroenterology.  St Louis:  CV Mosby 1975:  623-70.
Silverman  A,  Roy  CC.  Pediatric  Clinical
Gastroenterology. CV Mosby, 1983:894.

C.  Mono- and Disaccharide Absorption Tests
1.  Purpose:  To diagnose malabsorption of a specific
carbohydrate by measuring the change in blood
glucose following an oral dose of the carbohydrate
in question.
2.  Method:
a)  The patient fasts 4-6 hours prior to test.
b)  The  test  carbohydrate  (lactose,  sucrose,
maltose, glucose, galactose) is given orally or
by gastric tube in a dose of 2.0 gm/kg as a
10% solution (maximum dose of 100 gms.)  For
maltose, the dose is 1.0 gm/kg.
c)  Measure serum glucose prior to the carbohydrate dose and at 30, 60, 90, and 120 minutes
following the dose.
d)  Note the number and character of the stools.
Perform a Clinitest determination for reducing
substances on all stools passed during the test
and for 8 hours after the test is completed.
3.  Interpretation:
a)  A rise in the blood glucose level of  25 mg/dl
over the fasting level within the test period is
considered normal.  An increase of < 20 to 25
mg/dl is questionable.  Increases of < 20 mg/dl
are abnormal and suggest malabsorption of the
test carbohydrate.

b)  Malabsorption is also suggested if during the test or subsequent 8 hour period one notes:
    (1) The onset of diarrhea.
    (2) Stool pH of 6.0 or less.
    (3) > 0.50% reducing substances (Clinitest) in the stool. Sucrose is not a reducing substance.
    (4) Crampy abdominal pain or abdominal distention.

Ref: Silverman A, Roy CC. Pediatric Clinical Gastroenterology. CV Mosby, 1983:895.

D.  Breath Hydrogen Test
    Principle: $H_2$ gas is produced by bacterial fermentation of carbohydrate, then absorbed, and excreted in the breath. Elevation in breath content of $H_2$ correlates with malabsorption of delivered carbohydrate.
    Procedure:
    1.  Fast infants for 4-6 hrs and older children for 8 hrs
    2.  Give 2 gm/kg (max. 50 gm) of carbohydrate.
    3.  End-expired air is collected by aspirating 3.5 ml of air after each breath to a total of 30 ml via nasal prongs attached to a gas-tight syringe or via gas balloon attached to a face mask.
    4.  $H_2$ is measured by gas chromatography on baseline sample (before carbohydrate load) and on Ω30min samples for 3 hrs.
    5.  Elevation in $H_2$ content > 20 ppm above baseline is considered significant.
    6.  An elevated basal value after a fast is sometimes observed in patients with bacterial overgrowth.

    NOTE: Prior antibiotic use can obliterate normal enteric flora needed for fermentation and cause a false negative result.

Ref: Perman JA, et al. J Pediatr 1978; 93:17. Solomon NW. Current Concepts in Gastroenterology 1977; 2:38. Barr RG, et al. Pediatrics 1981; 68:526.

E.  Quantitative Fecal Fat
    1.  Purpose: Quantitative determination of fecal fat excretion to aid in diagnosis or management of fat malabsorption syndromes.

    2.  Method:
        a)  Patient should be on a normal diet with adequate fat content (35% of diet) and caloric intake for 2 days before beginning the test.

No meals should be omitted and no medications given during the test period. Exclude medium chain triglyceride oil from diet.

NOTE:    Adjust amount of fat administered to the child according to age. Attempt to deliver:
> 25 gm/day in infants
> 50 gm/day in toddlers
100 gm/day in school-aged children

b) All stools passed within a 72 hour period should be collected and kept in a freezer.
c) Determine total fecal fatty acid content. (For children with steatorrhea and constipation, caramine red markers (0.6 to 0.9 gms) can be given at the beginning of the test and again 72 hours later. All stools appearing between the markers regardless of time interval are collected).

3. Normals:
a) Total fecal fatty acid (FA) excretion for children >2 yrs. is <5.0 gm fat/24 hrs.
b) Fat absorption can be more accurately expressed as the coefficient of absorption (CA) and is independent of the amount of dietary fat intake. Its determination requires a strict record of dietary fat intake and is therefore best reserved for patients whose fecal fat excretion is borderline abnormal.

$$CA = \frac{\text{gms fat ingested} - \text{gms fat excreted}}{\text{gms fat ingested}} \times 100$$

| | |
|---|---|
| premature infants | 60-75% |
| newborn infants | 80-85% |
| 10 mo. - 3 yrs. | 85-95% |
| > 3 yrs. | 95% |

Ref: Silverman A, Roy CC. Pediatric Clinical Gastroenterology. CV Mosby, 1983:901. Shmerling DH, et al. Pediatrics 1970; 46:690.

## G E N E T I C S

I.  Karyotypes
    A.  Indications:
        1.  Two or more major malformations (consider small for gestational age and mental retardation as major malformations if no other etiology is obvious).
        2.  Features of specific chromosomal syndromes.
        3.  At risk for a familial chromosomal aberration.
        4.  Disorders of sexual malformation
        5.  Malignancies
        6.  Recurrent spontaneous abortions (>2) or history of infertility (karyotype both husband and wife).
    B.  Method (JHH lab):  Draw 1-2cc of blood into a green top tube which contains sodium heparin (a heparinized syringe is less desirable but adequate).  Keep the tube at room temperature.

II. Normal Morphology
    A.  Palpebral fissure size in newborns (mean ± 2SD).

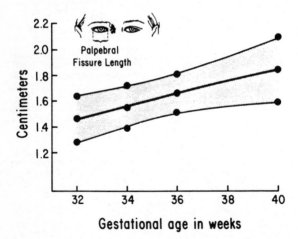

Palpebral
Fissure Length

Ref:  Jones KL, et al. J Pediatr 1978; 92:787.  (With permission)

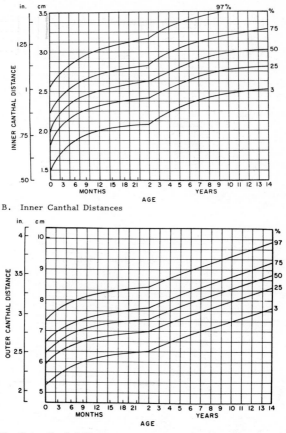

B. Inner Canthal Distances

C. Outer Canthal Distances

Ref: Feingold M, Bossert WH. Birth Defects: Original Article
Series 1974; 10(13):8-9. (With permission).

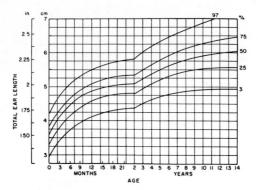

D.  Total Ear Length

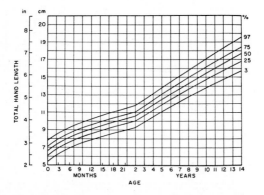

E.  Total Hand Length

Ref: Feingold M, Bossert WH.  Birth Defects:  Original Article
Series 1974; 10(13):11,13.  (With permission).

F.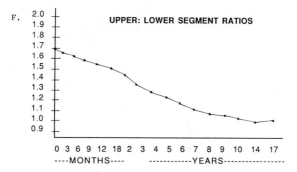

**UPPER: LOWER SEGMENT RATIOS**

0 3 6 9 12 18 2 3 4 5 6 7 8 9 10 14 17
----MONTHS---- -----------YEARS-----------------

Ref: Pediatrics Endocrinology division, Johns Hopkins Hospital.

III. Detection of Inborn Errors of Metabolism (IEM)
   A. Initial lab tests:
      Blood: CBC (neutropenia, thrombocytopenia seen in organic acidemias), serum electrolytes, anion gap, arterial blood gas, glucose, plasma ammonium.
      Urine: odor, pH, ketones, reducing substances.

   B. If above tests are abnormal:
      Blood: plasma amino acids, plasma carnitine.
      Urine: metabolic screen, organic acids, amino acids.

      The JHH urine metabolic screen includes: pH, spec. gravity, prot, glu, ketones, reducing substances (clinitest), ferric chloride, DNPH (for ketoacids), nitrosonapthal (for tyrosine metabolites), nitroprusside (for sulfhydryl groups), and a mucopolysaccharide spot test.

NOTE: 1. Plasma amino acids and plasma carnitine each require 3cc of blood in a green top (sodium heparin) tube. Samples should be drawn after an overnight fast (or at least a 4 hour fast in an infant). Deliver on ice or separate and freeze plasma for later analysis.
2. Urine amino and organic acid assays each require 5-10 ml of urine. If fresh urine cannot be delivered immediately to the lab, freeze samples.
3. Plasma ammonium values increase rapidly on standing. Collect on ice and deliver immediately to lab.
4. Skin biopsy for fibroblasts studies (see p 16 for method): Specimen should be stored in tissue culture medium at 4°C. When this is unavailable, store the specimen in the patient's serum. Refrigerate, but do not freeze specimen. Keep the tissue immersed in the culture media.

B.  Metabolic Diseases Associated with an Unusual Odor:

| Acute Disease | Odor |
|---|---|
| Maple Syrup urine disease | Maple syrup, burned sugar |
| Isovaleric Acidemia | Cheesy, or sweaty feet |
| Multiple carboxylase def. | Cat's urine |
| 3-OH, 3 methyl glutaryl CoA lyase deficiency | Cat's urine |

| Non-Acute Disease | |
|---|---|
| Phenylketonuria | Musty |
| Hypermethioninemia | Rancid butter, or rotten cabbage |

C.  Ferric Chloride Reaction
    Ferric iron forms colored derivatives when combined with
    many organic compounds. Results depend on
    methodology.
    a.  Use fresh urine.
    b.  Standard reagent: 10% ferric chloride
    c.  Mix 2 drops of $FeCl_3$ to 1 ml of urine, mix and
        observe color immediately and upon standing.

NOTE: The test is relatively insensitive and usually requires
high concentrations of the reacting metabolite. Salicylate is
an exception. Phosphate ions yield cloudy precipitates which
may mask positive results. A negative test does not rule out
the disease.

Urine Color with FeCl: Interpretation
Green:  PKU, tyrosinemia, direct hyperbilirubinemia, L-dopa
Blue-Green:  Histidinemia, pheochromocytoma
Gray-Green:  MSUD, forminimotransferase deficiency
Purple:  Salicylates, methionine malabsorption
Blue-Purple:  phenothiazines

Ref:  Buist NRM. Brit Med J 1968; 2:745; Thomas GH,
Howell RR. Selected screening tests for genetic metabolic
diseases. Chicago: Year Book, 1973.

D.  Urine reducing substances
    For method see p 29. Metabolic disorders associated
    with a positive test include:
    galactose - galactosemia, galactokinase deficiency, severe
                liver disease
    fructose - hereditary fructose intolerance, essential
               fructosuria
    glucose - diabetes mellitus, renal glycosuria, Fanconi's
              type RTA
    xylulose - pentosuria
    p-hydroxyphenyl pyruvic acid - tryrosinemia

Ref:  Burton BK, Nadler HL. Pediatrics 1978; 61:398; Aleck
KA, Shapiro LJ. Pediatr Clin North Am 1978; 25:431.

E.  Diagnosis of hyperammonemia in the neonate.

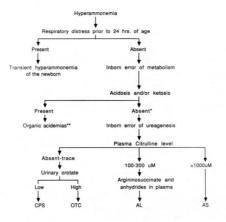

*  Respiratory alkalosis is present early.
**  Detected by gas chromatography – mass spectroscopy.
Includes propionic, methylmalonic, and isovaleric acidemia,
type II glutaric acidemia, and others.  Hyperglycinemia is
characteristic of propionic and methylmalonic acidemia.

CPS – carbamyl phosphate synthetase deficieny;  OTC –
ornithine transcarbamylase deficiency;  AL – argininosuccinase
deficiency;  AS – argininosuccinic acid synthetase deficiency.

Ref: Brusilow SW, Valle DL. In:  Nelson N, ed. Current
Therapy in Neonatal-Perinatal Medicine 1985-1986.  B.C.
Decker, 1985:211.  (With permission)

# C A R D I O L O G Y

1.  Cardiac Cycle
    See illustration on p 61.

2.  X-Ray Contours, Normal Pressures and Saturations
    See illustration on p 62.

3.  Electrocardiography

    A.  Placement of Leads (see illustration on page 63.)
        1)  Bipolar leads
            a)  Lead I:   right arm-left arm
            b)  Lead II:  right arm-left leg
            c)  Lead III: left arm-left leg
        2)  Unipolar leads
            a)  aVR:  right arm
            b)  aVL:  left arm
            c)  aVF:  left foot
        3)  Precordial leads
            a)  V 1:  4th RICS at right sternal border
            b)  V 2:  4th LICS at left sternal border
            c)  V 3:  midway between V 2 and V 4
            d)  V 4:  5th LICS at mid-clavicular line
            e)  V 5:  5th LICS at anterior axillary line
            f)  V 6:  5th LICS at mid-axillary line
            g)  V3R:  V3 on right chest
            h)  V4R:  V4 on right chest
            i)  V 7:  posterior axillary line (use if no Q
                      wave in V6)

    B.  Terminology
        See illustration on page 61.

        The P wave represents atrial depolarization.
        The QRS Complex represents ventricular depolar-
        ization.
        Waves in the QRS Complex are as follows:
        1)  Q Wave  -  the first negative deflection before a
                       positive deflection
        2)  R Wave  -  the first positive deflection
        3)  S Wave  -  the negative deflection following the R
                       wave
        4)  QS Wave -  a monophasic negative complex
        5)  R' Wave -  the second positive deflection
        6)  S' Wave -  the second negative deflection
        7)  T Wave  -  represents ventricular repolarization
        8)  U Wave  -  may follow the T wave

    C.  Rate
        ECG paper speed should be set at 25 mm/second.
        Obtain rate by multiplying by 20 the number of com-
        plexes between two vertical lines (3 seconds) at the

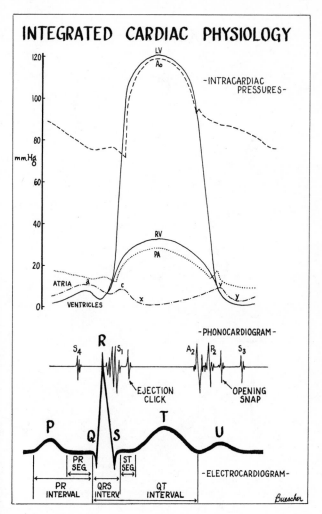

INTEGRATED CARDIAC PHYSIOLOGY

- INTRACARDIAC PRESSURES -

LV
Ao
RV
PA
ATRIA
VENTRICLES
a
c
x
v
y

mm.Hg

- PHONOCARDIOGRAM -

$S_4$   R   $S_1$        $A_2$ $P_2$   $S_3$

EJECTION CLICK        OPENING SNAP

- ELECTROCARDIOGRAM -

P   Q   S   T   U

PR SEG.   ST SEG.

PR INTERVAL   QRS INTERV   QT INTERVAL

Buescher

62

# X-RAY CONTOUR OF THE HEART

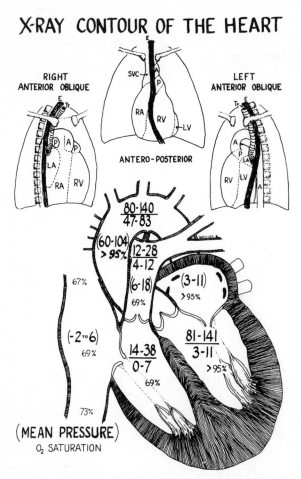

RIGHT ANTERIOR OBLIQUE

ANTERO-POSTERIOR

LEFT ANTERIOR OBLIQUE

(MEAN PRESSURE)
O₂ SATURATION

BASED ON NORMAL PATIENTS 2 MONTHS TO 20 YEARS OF AGE

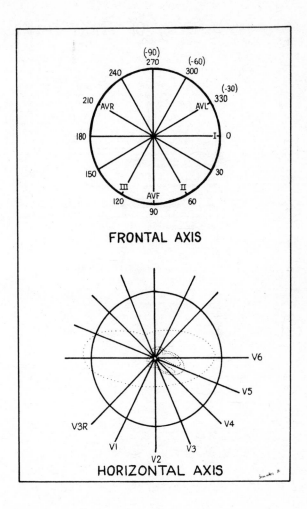

FRONTAL AXIS

HORIZONTAL AXIS

top of the strip. If rate is slow or irregular, a more accurate reflection of rate is obtained by multiplying by 10 the number of complexes between three vertical lines (6 seconds). Record atrial and ventricular rates when AV block is present. An exact heart rate also can be obtained by dividing 60,000 by the number of milliseconds between complexes (40 msec between small boxes, 200 msec between large boxes). Alternatively the rate may be estimated from the R-R interval in increments of 0.2 sec:

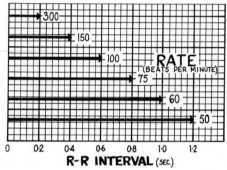

## AGE-SPECIFIC HEART RATES

| | Heart Rate (beats/min) | | |
| Age | 2% | Mean | 98% |
| --- | --- | --- | --- |
| Less than 1 day | 93 | 123 | 154 |
| 1-2 days | 91 | 123 | 159 |
| 3-6 days | 91 | 129 | 166 |
| 1-3 weeks | 107 | 148 | 182 |
| 1-2 months | 121 | 149 | 179 |
| 3-5 months | 106 | 141 | 186 |
| 6-11 months | 109 | 134 | 169 |
| 1-2 years | 89 | 119 | 151 |
| 3-4 years | 73 | 108 | 137 |
| 5-7 years | 65 | 100 | 133 |
| 8-11 years | 62 | 91 | 130 |
| 12-15 years | 60 | 85 | 119 |

D.  Intervals
    1)  P-R Interval

| Age | P-R Interval (sec) in Lead II | | |
|---|---|---|---|
| | 2% | Mean | 98% |
| Less than 1 day | .08 | .11 | .16 |
| 1 - 2 days | .08 | .11 | .14 |
| 3 - 6 days | .07 | .10 | .14 |
| 1 - 3 weeks | .07 | .10 | .14 |
| 1 - 2 months | .07 | .10 | .13 |
| 3 - 5 months | .07 | .11 | .15 |
| 6 - 11 months | .07 | .11 | .16 |
| 1 - 2 years | .08 | .11 | .15 |
| 3 - 4 years | .09 | .12 | .16 |
| 5 - 7 years | .09 | .12 | .16 |
| 8 - 11 years | .09 | .13 | .17 |
| 12 - 15 years | .09 | .14 | .18 |

2)  $QT_c$ (corrected QT interval)
    $$QT_c = \frac{\text{measured QT (in seconds)}}{\sqrt{\text{R-R interval}}}$$
    $QT_c$ should not exceed:
    0.45 in infants < 6 months old,
    0.44 in children,
    0.425 in adolescents and adults

E.  Axis
    1)  P Wave Axis. Frontal axis calculated using diagram page 63 is 0-90° and defines sinus rhythm.
    2)  QRS Axis: Frontal axis is age specific.

| Age | Frontal Plane QRS Mean Vector (degrees) | | |
|---|---|---|---|
| | 2% | Mean | 98% |
| Less than 1 day | 59 | 137 | -167 |
| 1-2 days | 64 | 134 | -161 |
| 3-6 days | 77 | 132 | -167 |
| 1-3 weeks | 65 | 110 | 161 |
| 1-2 months | 31 | 74 | 113 |
| 3-5 months | 1 | 60 | 104 |
| 6-11 months | 1 | 56 | 99 |
| 1-2 years | 1 | 55 | 101 |
| 3-4 years | 1 | 55 | 104 |
| 5-7 years | 1 | 65 | 143 |
| 8-11 years | 1 | 61 | 119 |
| 12-15 years | 1 | 59 | 130 |

### 3) T Wave Orientation

#### NORMAL ORIENTATION OF T WAVE

| Age | V1, V2 | aVF | I, V5, V6 |
|---|---|---|---|
| Birth - 1 day | ± | + | ± |
| 1 - 4 days | ± | + | + |
| 4 days - adolescence | - | + | + |
| Adolescence - adulthood | + | + | + |

+ = T wave positive
- = T wave negative
± = T wave may normally be positive OR negative

F.  Atrial Enlargement
    1) Right atrial enlargement (RAE) - suggested by:
       Peaked P wave, >2.5 mm in any lead (best seen
       in L-2, L-3, V3R, and V1)
    2) Left atrial enlargement (LAE) - suggested by
       either:
       a) P wave duration >0.08 seconds; may have
          "plateau" or "notched" contour
       b) Terminal and deep inversion of the P wave
          in V3R or V1

G.  Ventricular Hypertrophy
    1) Normal range for R and S waves:

| | Amplitude in $V_1$ (mm at normal standardization) | | | | | |
|---|---|---|---|---|---|---|
| | R Wave | | | S Wave | | |
| Age | 2% | Mean | 98% | 2% | Mean | 98% |
| Less than 1 day | 5.2 | 13.8 | 26.1 | 0.0 | 8.5 | 22.7 |
| 1-2 days | 5.3 | 14.4 | 26.9 | 0.0 | 9.1 | 20.7 |
| 3-6 days | 2.8 | 12.9 | 24.2 | 0.0 | 6.6 | 16.8 |
| 1-3 weeks | 3.2 | 10.6 | 20.8 | 0.0 | 4.2 | 10.8 |
| 1-2 months | 3.3 | 9.5 | 18.4 | 0.0 | 5.0 | 12.4 |
| 3-5 months | 2.7 | 9.8 | 19.8 | 0.0 | 5.7 | 17.1 |
| 6-11 months | 1.4 | 9.4 | 20.3 | 0.4 | 6.4 | 18.1 |
| 1-2 years | 2.6 | 8.9 | 17.7 | 0.7 | 8.4 | 21.0 |
| 3-4 years | 1.0 | 8.1 | 18.2 | 1.8 | 10.2 | 21.4 |
| 5-7 years | 0.5 | 6.7 | 13.9 | 2.9 | 12.0 | 23.8 |
| 8-11 years | 0.0 | 5.4 | 12.1 | 2.7 | 11.9 | 25.4 |
| 12-15 years | 0.0 | 4.1 | 9.9 | 2.8 | 10.8 | 21.2 |

| Age | Amplitude in $V_6$ (mm at normal standardization) | | | | | |
|---|---|---|---|---|---|---|
| | R Wave | | | S Wave | | |
| | 2% | Mean | 98% | 2% | Mean | 98% |
| Less than 1 day | 0.0 | 4.2 | 11.1 | 0.0 | 3.2 | 9.6 |
| 1-2 days | 0.0 | 4.5 | 12.2 | 0.0 | 3.0 | 9.4 |
| 3-6 days | 0.3 | 5.2 | 12.1 | 0.0 | 3.5 | 9.8 |
| 1-3 weeks | 2.6 | 7.6 | 16.4 | 0.0 | 3.4 | 9.8 |
| 1-2 months | 5.2 | 11.6 | 21.4 | 0.0 | 2.7 | 6.4 |
| 3-5 months | 6.4 | 13.1 | 22.4 | 0.0 | 2.9 | 9.9 |
| 6-11 months | 5.8 | 12.6 | 22.7 | 0.0 | 2.1 | 7.2 |
| 1-2 years | 5.9 | 13.3 | 22.6 | 0.0 | 1.9 | 6.6 |
| 3-4 years | 8.1 | 14.8 | 24.4 | 0.0 | 1.5 | 5.2 |
| 5-7 years | 8.4 | 16.3 | 26.5 | 0.0 | 1.2 | 4.0 |
| 8-11 years | 9.2 | 16.3 | 25.4 | 0.0 | 1.0 | 3.9 |
| 12-15 years | 6.5 | 14.3 | 23.0 | 0.0 | 0.8 | 3.7 |

2) Right ventricular hypertrophy (any of below, singly or in combination):
   a) R in V1 above 98th percentile for age
   b) S in V6 above 98th percentile for age
   c) Upright T in V1 after 4 days
   d) qR in V3R or V1
   e) Normal duration RSR' in V3R or V1 with R' > 15mm if < 1 yr, > 10 mm thereafter. (This is suggestive of diastolic volume overload – eg. ASD)
   f) Tall R with asymmetrically inverted T in V1 suggests right ventricular strain.

3) Left ventricular hypertrophy (any of below, singly or in combination):
   a) R in V6 above 98th percentile for age (suggests volume overload)
   b) Q wave >4 mm in V5 or V6 (suggests volume overload)
   c) R in V1 below 5th percentile for age (suggests pressure overload)
   d) S in V1 above 98th percentile for age (suggests pressure overload)
   e) Asymmetric T wave inversion in V5 or V6 suggests LV strain.

4) NOTE: In the event of abnormal conduction, abnormal cardiac position, or complex congenital heart disease, these criteria may not be applicable. There is a gradual progression from LV to RV predominance as an infant approaches term. Therefore these conventional electro-

cardiographic criteria for interpretation of
ventricular hypertrophy are not reliable in the
premature neonate.

H. Disorders of Conduction and Rhythm

1) Sinus Arrhythmia
Normal respiratory variation of the RR interval
without morphological changes of the P wave or
QRS complex.

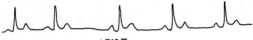

LEAD II

2) Low Atrial Pacemaker ("coronary sinus rhythm").
Shortened to normal PR interval with negative P
in L-2, L-3, aVF, and upright in V6. P wave
axis is 180-360°.

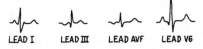

LEAD I        LEAD III        LEAD AVF        LEAD V6

3) Left Atrial Rhythm
Varying P configurations in limb leads depending
on site of origin (high, low, mid); however,
frequently negative in L-2, L-3, aVF, and always
negative in V6. Dome and dart configuration
diagnostic of left atrial rhythm with the dome
representing the left atrium and the dart the
right atrium. Best seen in L-2 and V1. P wave
axis is 90-270°.

LEAD I

LEAD II        LEAD V1        LEAD V6

4)  Premature Atrial Contraction (PAC)
    a)  Premature beat with abnormal P wave, normal
        QRS complexes, and usually not followed by
        a fully compensatory pause.

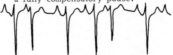

    b)  PAC (with aberrancy) - similar to 4a, but
        with wide QRS usually resembling a RBB
        pattern. The initial vector is in the same
        direction as the normal sinus QRS.

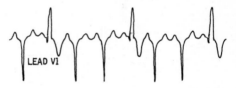

5)  Supraventricular Tachycardia (PAT or SVT)
    Normal QRS complexes at a rapid rate with or
    without discernible P waves. After the first
    10-20 beats, the QRS in SVT almost always has
    the same morphology as the QRS in sinus rhythm.
    If after the first 10-20 beats the QRS has a BBB
    pattern, think V tach. (see chart p 73)

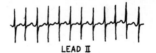

6)  Atrial Flutter
    Normal QRS complexes, absence of P waves,
    "flutter waves" between QRS complexes.
    (see p 73)

LEAD V1

7) Atrial Fibrillation
   Normal QRS complexes, absence of P waves,
   irregularly irregular RR interval.

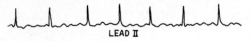

LEAD II

8) First Degree AV Block
   Prolongation of the PR interval beyond normal for
   age and rate (see page 65).

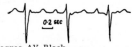

0·2 sec

9) Second Degree AV Block
   Atrial rate greater than the ventricular rate with
   conduction of the atrial impulse at regular
   intervals, i.e., every other (2:1 block), every
   third (3:1 block), three atrial for every 2
   ventricular (3:2 block).
   a) Type I (Wenckebach): Progressive
      lengthening of the PR interval until an atrial
      impulse is not conducted and the beat is
      dropped.

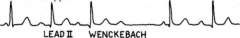

LEAD II    WENCKEBACH

   b) Type II: Dropped beats without lengthening
      of the PR interval.

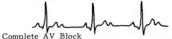

10) Complete AV Block
    No conducted atrial impulses (complete AV
    dissociation), with a slow unrelated junctional or
    ventricular rhythm.

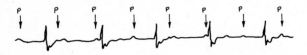

11) <u>A-V Dissociation with Junctional Tachycardia</u>
Failure of conduction of the atrial impulse through
the A-V node with a faster, independent nodal or
ventricular rhythm.

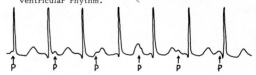

12) <u>Wolff-Parkinson-White</u> (WPW)
Prolonged QRS duration and shortened PR
interval secondary to initial slurring of the
upstroke of the QRS (delta wave). Type A has
predominantly positive QRS complexes in lead V1.
Type B has predominantly negative QRS
complexes in V1.

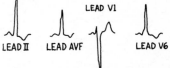

**LEAD V1**

**LEAD II**   **LEAD AVF**            **LEAD V6**

13.) <u>Complete Bundle Branch Block</u>
Longest QRS abnormally prolonged for age:
> 0.08 sec if < 2 yr
> 0.09 sec if 2-8 yr
> 0.10 sec if > 8 yr
a) LBBB: Monophasic R wave in L-1; absence
of Q wave in V6. (LBBB is rare in children.
W-P-W frequently mimics LBBB)

**LEAD V1**

**LEAD I**   **LEAD II**            **LEAD V6**

b) RBBB: Wide S wave in L1, V6; M-shaped
QRS in V-1, RAD.

**LEAD I**   **LEAD II**   **LEAD V1**   **LEAD V6**

14) Left Anterior Hemiblock
   Normal QRS duration, left axis deviation; qR in
   L1, rS in L3.

15) Premature Ventricular Contraction (PVC)
   QRS complexes are usually prolonged but always
   differ morphologically from sinus, ST segments
   slope away from QRS, and T waves are inverted.
   PVC's occur before the expected atrial beat and
   are usually followed by a compensatory pause.
   Bigeminy is alternating normal and abnormal
   ventricular complexes.

16) Fusion Beat
   Characteristics of both a sinus beat and a PVC.
   It has the same early activation of a sinus beat
   and late activation of a PVC (see illustration 17).

17) Ventricular Tachycardia (VT)
   Three or more serial PVC's at a rapid rate. P
   waves, if present, may be dissociated. Usually
   no Q wave in V5-6. Presence of fusion beats
   prior to onset or at termination of V. tach. is
   usually diagnostic. The QRS in VT may not be
   wide in children. If (after 10-20 beats) the
   morphology of the QRS differs from the sinus
   QRS, the diagnosis is probably VT (see p. 73).

## I. Distinguishing Tachyarrhythmias in Children

|  | Sinus Tach | SVT | Atrial flutter | V. Tach |
|---|---|---|---|---|
| History | Sepsis,fever, hypovolemia, etc. | Usually otherwise normal | 92% have abnormal heart | 70% have abnormal heart |
| Rate | Almost always <230/min. | 60% > 230/min. Infants usually 260-300 | Atrial 250-500. Vent 1:1 to 4:1 conduction | Usually rate <250/min. Infants 200-500 |
| Ventricular rate variation | Over several seconds may get faster and slower | After first 10-20 beats, extremely regular | May have variable block (1:1, 2:1, 3:1) giving diff. ventricular rates | Slight variation over several beats |
| P wave axis | Same as sinus almost always visible P waves | 60% visible P waves, usually P waves do not look like sinus P waves | Flutter waves (best seen in L2, L3, AVF, VI) | May have sinus P waves continuing unrelated to VT (AV diss.), retrograde P waves, or no visible P waves |
| QRS | Almost always same as slower sinus rhythm | After first 10-20 beats, almost always same as sinus | Usually same as sinus, may have occasional beats different from sinus | Different from sinus (not necessarily "wide") |

Tables and values for electrocardiography section adapted from:
- Adams FH, Emmanouilides GC eds. Moss' Heart Disease in Infants, Children and Adolescents, 3rd Edition. Baltimore: Williams and Wilkins, 1983: 18-57.
- Garson A Jr. The Electrocardiogram in Infants and Children: A Systematic Approach. Philadelphia: Lea Febiger, 1983: 99-118,172,396-403 and personal communication.
- Davignon A, et al. Normal ECG Standards for Infants and Children. Pediatr Cardiol 1979; 1:123-131.

J. Systemic Effects on the Electrocardiogram

| | Short QT | Long QT-U | Prolonged QRS | ST-T Changes | Sinus Tachy | Sinus Brady | AV Block | V. Tachy | Miscellaneous |
|---|---|---|---|---|---|---|---|---|---|
| **CHEMISTRY** | | | | | | | | | |
| Hyperkalemia | | | X | X | | | X | X | low voltages Ps peaked Ts. |
| Hypokalemia | | X | X | X | | | | | |
| Hypercalcemia | X | | | | | | X | | |
| Hypocalcemia | | X | | | X | | X | X | |
| Hypermagnesemia | | | | | | X | X | | |
| Hypomagnesemia | | X | | | | | | | |
| **DRUGS** | | | | | | | | | |
| Digitalis | X | | | X | | T | X | T | |
| Phenothiazines | | T | | | | | | T | |
| Phenytoin | X | | | | | | | | |
| Propranolol | | | | | | X | X | | |
| Quinidine | | X | X | | T | T | T | T | |
| Tricyclics | | T | T | T | | | T | | |
| Verapamil | | | | | | X | X | | |
| **CNS** | | | | | | | | | |
| Jervell-Lange-Neilson | | X | | | | X | | | |
| Romano-Ward | | X | | | | X | | | |

NOTE: X = present; T = present only with drug toxicity

Ref:  Garson A Jr. The Electrocardiogram in Infants and Children: A Systematic Approach. Philadelphia: Lea and Febiger, 1983.

4. Echocardiography

A. 2-D Echocardiogram
   The two-dimensional echocardiogram can define many
   structural abnormalities of the heart. These include
   abnormalities of the great vessels, semilunar valves,
   A-V valves, atria and atrial septum, ventricles and
   ventricular septum, the venae cavae, and the proximal
   coronary arteries.

B. M-Mode Echocardiogram
   M-Mode echocardiography is useful especially for accurate measurement of structures, and for calculation of
   standardized indices. These can be used serially
   following changes in an individual (e.g. size of the
   aortic root in a Marfan syndrome patient, or the right
   systolic time interval in a patient with cor pulmonale),
   or can be compared to the normal ranges for age.

C. Systolic Time Intervals
   The ratio of the ventricular pre-ejection period (ie.
   from beginning of QRS to opening of aortic or
   pulmonary valve) to the ejection time (ie. from opening
   of valve to valve closure). These ratios vary directly
   with changes in ventricular afterload and electro-
   mechanical delay and inversely with changes in preload
   and contractility.

|  | Normal Range | Average |
|---|---|---|
| $\frac{LVPEP}{LVET}$ | 0.3 - 0.39 | 0.35 |
| $\frac{RVPEP}{RVET}$ | 0.16 - 0.30 | 0.24 |

D. Doppler
   Utilizes Doppler principle to convert changes between
   transmitted and received ultrasound frequencies to
   velocity (V) of blood stream from which US beam is
   reflected. Using modified Bernoulli's equation,
   gradients (Δ P) across valves may be estimated:
   $$\Delta P = 4 V^2.$$

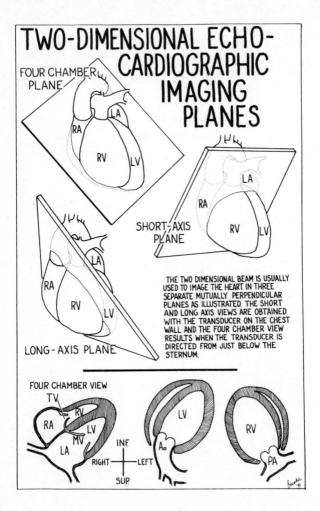

# TWO-DIMENSIONAL ECHO-CARDIOGRAPHIC IMAGING PLANES

FOUR CHAMBER PLANE

LA
RA
RV
LV

SHORT-AXIS PLANE

LA
RA
RV
LV

LONG-AXIS PLANE

LA
RA
RV
LV

THE TWO DIMENSIONAL BEAM IS USUALLY USED TO IMAGE THE HEART IN THREE SEPARATE MUTUALLY PERPENDICULAR PLANES AS ILLUSTRATED. THE SHORT AND LONG AXIS VIEWS ARE OBTAINED WITH THE TRANSDUCER ON THE CHEST WALL AND THE FOUR CHAMBER VIEW RESULTS WHEN THE TRANSDUCER IS DIRECTED FROM JUST BELOW THE STERNUM.

FOUR CHAMBER VIEW

TV
RV
RA
LV
MV
LA

INF.
RIGHT ─┼─ LEFT
SUP.

LV
Ao

RV
PA

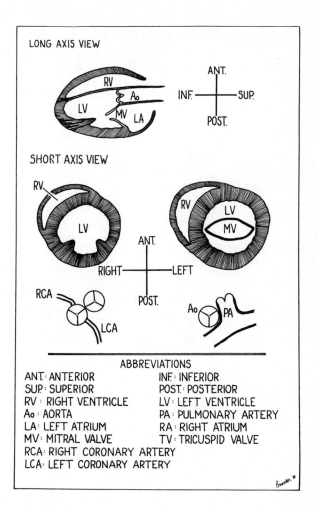

LONG AXIS VIEW

SHORT AXIS VIEW

ABBREVIATIONS

| | |
|---|---|
| ANT: ANTERIOR | INF: INFERIOR |
| SUP: SUPERIOR | POST: POSTERIOR |
| RV: RIGHT VENTRICLE | LV: LEFT VENTRICLE |
| Ao: AORTA | PA: PULMONARY ARTERY |
| LA: LEFT ATRIUM | RA: RIGHT ATRIUM |
| MV: MITRAL VALVE | TV: TRICUSPID VALVE |
| RCA: RIGHT CORONARY ARTERY | |
| LCA: LEFT CORONARY ARTERY | |

5. <u>Oxygen Challenge Test for Cyanotic Neonates</u>

| | $F_iO_2=.21$ $PaO_2$ | $F_iO_2=1.00$ $PaO_2$ | $PaCO_2$ |
|---|---|---|---|
| <u>Normal</u> | 70 | >200 | 35 |
| <u>Pulmonary Disease</u> | 50 | >150 | 50 |
| <u>Neurologic Disease</u> | 50 | >150 | 50 |
| <u>Methemoglobinemia</u> | 70 | >200 | 35 |
| Cardiac Disease | | | |
|   -Right to Left Shunt Lesions (eg. D-TGA with IVS, TA with PS or PA, PA with IVS, severe PS or TOF) | <40 | <50 | 35 |
|   -Admixture Lesions (eg. Truncus, TAPVR, Sing.vent., HLH, D-TGA with VSD, TA without PS or PA) | 50 | <150 | 35 |

Persistent Pulmonary Hypertension

| | Preductal | Postductal | | |
|---|---|---|---|---|
| - without PFO | 70 | <40 | variable | 35-50 |
| - with PFO | <40 | <40 | variable | 35-50 |

Ref: Lees MH, J. Pediatr 1970; 77:484-98. Kitterman JA, Pediatr Rev 1982; 4:13-23. Jones RWA, et al. Arch Dis Child 1976; 51:667-73.

6. <u>Glossary of Selected Cardiac Surgical Procedures and Shunts</u>

    A. Procedures
1) Blalock-Hanlon - closed heart atrial septectomy.
2) Brock - closed heart pulmonary valvulotomy or infundibulotomy.
3) Fontan - an anastomosis of the right atrial appendage to the pulmonary artery used to separate the circulations in admixture lesions without an adequate RV.
4) Mustard - intra-atrial baffle (usually pericardium) for repair of simple transposition of great arteries.
5) Park - knife-tipped cardiac catheter enlarges the intraatrial communication at the foramen ovale.

6) Rashkind - use of a balloon-tipped cardiac catheter which is rapidly pulled across the foramen ovale to create a defect in the atrial septum.

7) Rastelli -
   a) Placement of a valved conduit or graft between right ventricle and pulmonary arteries; used for pulmonary atresia and complex transposition.
   b) Repair of A-V canal by resuspension of mitral and tricuspid valves upon the newly-created ventricular septum.

8) Senning - intraatrial baffle constructed using flaps of native atrial septum and atrial wall as a repair for TGA.

9) Waldhausen - use of left subclavian artery as an on-lay patch for repair of coarctation of the aorta.

10) Norwood - (palliation for hypoplastic left heart)
    Stage 1: Anastomosis of proximal pulmonary artery to aorta; B-T shunt; atrial septectomy.
    Stage 2: Modified Fontan.

11) Damus-Kaye-Stansel - (for double outlet right ventricle with subpulmonic VSD): VSD patched to right of PA; anastomosis of pulmonary artery to aorta; conduit placed between RV and distal main PA.

12) Arterial Switch (of Jatene) - (for TGA) - Pulmonary artery and aorta transected above valves and switched. Coronary arteries moved from old aortic root to new aorta (former pulmonary root).

B. Shunts
   1) Blalock-Taussig - subclavian to pulmonary artery
   2) Glenn - superior vena cava to right pulmonary artery
   3) Potts - descending aorta to left pulmonary artery
   4) Waterston - ascending aorta to right pulmonary artery

Ref: Arciniegas E. Pediatric Cardiac Surgery, Chicago: Year Book Medical Publishers, 1985.

7. <u>Emergency</u> <u>Management</u> <u>of</u> <u>Paroxysmal</u> <u>Hyperpnea</u> <u>in</u> <u>Cyanotic</u> <u>Heart</u> <u>Disease</u> (e.g. "Tetralogy Spells")

| TREATMENT | RATIONALE |
|---|---|
| <u>Knee-chest</u> <u>position</u> | Decreases venous return and increases systemic resistance. |
| <u>Propranolol</u>:<br>Acute 0.15-0.25 mg/kg IV over 2-5 min; may repeat in 15 min x 1. Chronic - 1 mg/kg/dose PO divided Q6h. | Negative inotropic effect on (infundibular) myocardium. May block drop in systemic vascular resistance. |
| <u>Morphine</u>: 0.1-0.2 mg/kg IV or SC; may repeat in 1 hr | Decreases venous return, depresses respiratory center, relaxes infundibulum. |
| <u>Phenylephrine</u> HCl: 0.1 mg/kg/ dose SC or IM Q1-2h PRN; 0.01 mg/kg IV | Increases systemic vascular resistance. |
| <u>Methoxamine</u>: 0.1 mg/kg IV | Increases systemic vascular resistance. |
| <u>Sodium</u> <u>bicarbonate</u>: 1-2 mEq/ kg/dose IV | Reduces metabolic acidosis. |
| <u>Oxygen</u> | Reduces hypoxemia (LIMITED VALUE). |
| <u>NO</u> <u>digitalis</u> <u>preparations</u> | Avoid positive inotropic effect on myocardium. |
| <u>Correct</u> <u>anemia</u> | Increases delivery of oxygen to tissues. |
| <u>Correct</u> <u>pathological</u> <u>tachyarrhythmias</u> | May abort hypoxic spell. |
| <u>Glucose</u> <u>infusion</u> | Avoids hypoglycemia resulting from increased utilization and depletion of glycogen stores. |

8. Prophylaxis Against Bacterial Endocarditis in Patients With Structural Cardiac Disease

A. Cardiac Conditions
Endocarditis Prophylaxis Recommended:
Prosthetic cardiac valves (including biosynthetic valves)
Most congenital cardiac malformations
Surgically constructed systemic-pulmonary shunts
Rheumatic and other acquired valvular dysfunction
Idiopathic hypertrophic subaortic stenosis (IHSS)
Previous history of bacterial endocarditis
Mitral valve prolapse with insufficiency
Permanent endocardial pacemaker electrode
Endocarditis Prophylaxis Not Recommended:
Isolated secundum atrial septal defect
Secundum atrial septal defect repaired without a patch six or more months earlier
Patent ductus arteriosus ligated and divided six or more months earlier
Permanent epicardial pacemaker electrode

B. Procedures for which Endocarditis Prophylaxis is Indicated
All dental procedures likely to induce gingival bleeding (not simple adjustment of orthodontic appliances or shedding of deciduous teeth)
Tonsillectomy and/or adenoidectomy
Surgical procedures or biopsy involving respiratory mucosa
Bronchoscopy, especially with a rigid bronchoscope
Incision and drainage of infected tissue
Genitourinary and gastrointestinal procedures including cystoscopy, urethral catheterization, urinary tract surgery, gall bladder surgery, colonic surgery, esophageal dilatation, colonoscopy, upper GI endoscopy with biopsy or proctosigmoidoscopic biopsy. In high risk patients or if infection is suspected, also for percutaneous liver biopsy, upper GI endoscopy or proctosigmoidoscopy without biopsy, barium enema, uncomplicated vaginal delivery, in and out bladder catheterization, uterine dilatation and curettage, Caesarian section, therapeutic abortion, sterilization procedures, and IUD insertion or removal.
Endotracheal intubation alone does not require prophylaxis.

C. Recommended Antibiotic Regimens for Dental/Respiratory Tract Procedures
1. Standard Regimen
Penicillin V 1.0 g PO one hour before procedure, then 500 mg six hours after initial dose (double the Pen V doses if patient > 27 kg).

or, if unable to take oral medication,

Aqueous penicillin G 50,000 U/kg (max. 2 million U) IM or IV 30-60 minutes before the procedure and 25,000 U/kg (max. 1 million U) six hours after initial dose.

2. When Maximal Protection Desired (e.g. for patients with prosthetic valves)
Ampicillin 50 mg/kg (max. 2.0 g) IM or IV, plus
Gentamicin 2.0 mg/kg (adults 1.5 mg/kg) IM or IV one-half hour before procedure, then
Penicillin V 500 mg PO six hours after initial dose (double the Pen V dose if patient > 27 kg).
Alternatively, the parenteral regimen may be repeated once 8 hours after the initial dose.

3. For Penicillin Allergic Patients
Erythromycin 20 mg/kg (max 1.0 g) PO one hour before procedure then 10 mg/kg (max. 500 mg) 6 hours after initial dose,

or, if unable to take oral medication,

Vancomycin 20 mg/kg (max. 1.0 g) IV slowly over one hour starting one hour before procedure. No repeat dose needed.

D. Recommended Regimens for Gastrointestinal/Genitourinary Procedures

1. Standard Regimen
Ampicillin 50 mg/kg (max. 2.0 g) IM or IV, plus
Gentamicin 2.0 mg/kg (adults 1.5 mg/kg) IM or IV 30-60 minutes before procedure. May be repeated once 8 hours after initial dose.

2. For Minor or Repetitive Procedures in Low-Risk Patients
Amoxicillin 50 mg/kg (max. 3.0 g) PO one hour before preocedure and 25 mg/kg (max 1.5 g) PO 6 hours after initial dose.

3. For Penicillin Allergic Patients
Vancomycin 20 mg/kg IV slowly over one hour, plus
Gentamicin 2.0 mg/kg (adults 1.5 mg/kg) IM or IV one hour before procedure. May be repeated once 8-12 hours after initial dose.

Note: Modify antibiotic doses in patients with significant renal insufficiency (see pages 223-8).

Adapted from: Committee on Rheumatic Fever and Infective Endocarditis, American Heart Association; Circulation 1984; 70:1123A-27A.

ENDOCRINOLOGY

## NORMATIVE DATA

I. Laboratory Values

NOTE: Normal values may differ among laboratories because
of variation in technique and in the type of radioimmunoassay
used.

A. Gonadotropins

|  | FSH mIU/ml | LH mIU/ml |
|---|---|---|
| Adult males | 1.5-16.0 | 3.9-18.0 |
| Adult females | 2.0-17.2 | 2.0-22.6 |
| Adult females (mid cycle) | variable | variable |
| Prepubertal children | <5.0 | <5.0 |

Ref: Johns Hopkins Hospital Pediatric Endocrine Labs, 1986.

B. Steroid Hormones
   1) Plasma
      a) Total Testosterone ng/dl (mean ± SD)

|  |  |  |
|---|---|---|
| Adult male | = | 575 ± 150 |
| Adult female | = | 49 ± 13 |
| Pregnancy | = | 30 - 201 |
| At delivery | = | 135 ± 70 |
| Cord | = | 45 ± 25 |
| Prepubertal | = | 10 - 20 |
| Male Tanner 2 | = | 25 - 85 |
| 3 | = | 52 - 328 |
| 4 | = | 134 - 532 |

   b) Free Testosterone ng/dl RIA

|  |  |  |
|---|---|---|
| Adult male | = | 1.4 - 5.79 |
| Adult female | = | 0.2 - 0.73 |
| Prepubertal | = | 0.06- 0.38 |

   c) Estradiol pg/ml

|  |  |  |
|---|---|---|
| Adult male | = | 20 - 90 |
| Adult female |  |  |
| luteal phase | = | 60 - 170 |
| early follicular | = | 25 - 120 |
| late follicular | = | 80 - 300 |
| Prepubertal | = | <25 |

   d) Androstenedione ng/dl

|  |  |  |
|---|---|---|
| Adult male | = | 109 ± 20 |
| Adult female | = | 152 ± 39 |
| Pregnancy | = | 250 ± 80 |
| At delivery | = | 390 ± 175 |
| Cord | = | 125 ± 60 |
| Prepubertal | = | 20 ± 15 |

    e)  17OH-Progesterone ng/dl
          Adult male          = 95 ± 30
          Adult female (non-pregnant)
            follicular     = 58 ± 22
            luteal        = 268 ± 59
          Prepubertal
            male          = 33 ± 24
            female       = 42 ± 25
          CVAH in good control = 190 ± 120

    f)  Cortisol mcg/dl
          Any age/sex 8 AM   = 8 - 18
            pre-ACTH     = 8 - 18
            post-ACTH = twice pre-ACTH value

2)  Urine
    a)  17-ketosteroids mg/24h
          Adult male       = 6 - 18
          Adult female    = 4 - 13
          Prepubertal
            < 1 month     = <2.0
            1 mo - 5 yrs  = <0.5
            6-8 yrs      = 1.0-2.0
            >8 yrs       = gradually increases
                                    to adult levels

    b)  17 OH-corticosteroids
          Adult male       = 3 - 9 mg/24h
          Adult female    = 2 - 8 mg/24h
          Prepubertal     = 2.5 mg/24h
    c)  Pregnanetriol        = <2.5 mg/24h
    d)  Free cortisol mcg/24h = 25 - 125
                           (Any age/sex)

Ref: Migeon CJ. In Collu R, et al. (eds). Pediatric Endocrinology. New York, Raven Press 1981; 482, 484; Penny R. Pediatr Clin North Am 1979; 26:113. Johns Hopkins Hospital Pediatric Endocrinology Labs, 1986.

C. Tests for Pheochromocytoma

24 hour urine with results expressed as mg/g creatinine

| Age | VMA | HVA | Metanephrines |
|---|---|---|---|
| 1-12 mo | 1.40-15.0 | 1.20-35.0 | 0.001-4.6 |
| 1- 2 yr | 1.25- 8.0 | 4.0 -23.0 | 0.27 -5.38 |
| 2- 5 yr | 1.50- 7.5 | 0.7 -13.5 | 0.35 -2.99 |
| 5-10 yr | 0.50- 6.0 | 0.5 - 9.0 | 0.43 -2.7 |
| 10-15 yr | 0.25- 3.25 | 0.25-12.0 | 0.001-1.87 |
| 15-18 yr | 0.1 - 2.75 | 0.5 - 2.0 | 0.001-0.67 |
| Adult | 0.25- 3.5 | 0.25- 2.5 | 0.05 -1.20 |

Total free catecholamines: 20-270 mcg/g creatinine

Ref: Gitlow SE, et al. J Lab Clin Med 1968; 72:612.

#### D. Thyroid Function Tests

| Test | Normals | | Comment |
|------|---------|---|---------|
| $T_4$RIA mcg/dl | Cord | 7.4-13.0 | Direct measurement of total thyroxine by radioimmunoassay. See values for premature infants below. |
| | 1- 3 d | 11.8-22.6 | |
| | 1- 2 wk | 9.8-16.6 | |
| | 2- 4 wk | 7.0-15.0 | |
| | 1- 4 mo | 7.2-14.4 | |
| | 4-12 mo | 7.8-16.5 | |
| | 1- 5 yr | 7.3-15.0 | |
| | 5-10 yr | 6.4-13.3 | |
| | 10-15 yr | 5.6-11.7 | |
| | Adult | 4.3-12.5 | |
| $T_3$RU | 25-35% | | Measures thyroid hormone binding, not $T_3$ |
| T index | 1.63-4.73 | | $T_4$RIA X $T_3$ RU |
| Free $T_4$ | 0.7-1.7 ng/dl | | Metabolically active form |
| $T_3$RIA (ng/dl) | Cord | 15- 75 | Measures triiodothyronine by radioimmunoassay |
| | 1 - 3 d | 32-216 | |
| | 2 - 4 wk | 160-240 | |
| | 1 - 4 mo | 117-209 | |
| | 4 -12 mo | 110-280 | |
| | 1 - 5 yr | 105-269 | |
| | 5 -10 yr | 94-241 | |
| | 10 -15 yr | 83-215 | |
| | Adult | 70-204 | |
| TSH-RIA (MIU/ml) | | | Best sensitivity for primary hypothyroidism |
| | Cord | 0-17.4 | |
| | 1- 3d | 0-13.3 | |
| | Otherwise | 0-5.5 | |

Thyroid Antibodies   (High titers suggest Hashimoto's thyroiditis).

| | Antithyroglobulin | Antimicrosomal |
|------|-------------------|----------------|
| Insignificant | <1:40 | <1:400 |
| Borderline | 1:80 | 1:400 |
| Significant | 1:160-1:640 | 1:1600 - 1:6400 |
| Very Significant | >1:640 | >1:6400 |

Ref:  LaFranchi SH. Ped Clin North Am 1979; 26:46.
Johns Hopkins Hospital In Vitro Laboratory, 1986.

Thyroid Function Tests in Premature Infants
estimated gestational age (wks)

| Serum T$_4$ Mean ±1 SD | 30-31 | 32-33 | 34-35 | 36-37 | Term |
|---|---|---|---|---|---|
| Cord | 6.5±1.0 | 7.5±2.1 | 6.7±1.2 | 7.5±2.8 | 8.2±1.8 |
| 12-72 hr | 11.5±2.1 | 12.3±3.2 | 12.4±3.1 | 15.5±2.6 | 19.0±2.1 |
| 3-10 d | 7.7±1.8 | 8.5±1.9 | 10.0±2.4 | 12.7±2.5 | 15.9±3.0 |
| 11-20 d | 7.5±1.8 | 8.3±1.6 | 10.5±1.8 | 11.2±2.9 | 12.2±2.0 |
| 21-45 d | 7.8±1.5 | 8.0±1.7 | 9.3±1.3 | 11.4±4.2 | 12.1±1.5 |
| | | (30-37 wks) | | | |
| 46-90 d | | 9.6±1.7 | | | 10.2±1.9 |

Ref: Cuestas RA. J Pediatr 1978; 92:963-967.

    E.   Miscellaneous

        a)   Somatomedin C, RIA U/ml

| Age | | Males | Females |
|---|---|---|---|
| 0-3 | yrs | 0.08-1.1 | 0.11-2.2 |
| 3-6 | yrs | 0.12-1.6 | 0.18-2.4 |
| 6-11 | yrs | 0.22-2.8 | 0.41-4.5 |
| 11-13 | yrs | 0.28-3.7 | 0.99-6.8 |
| 13-15 | yrs | 0.9 -5.6 | 1.2 -5.9 |
| 15-18 | yrs | 0.91-3.1 | 0.71-4.1 |
| 18-64 | yrs | 0.34-1.9 | 0.45-2.2 |

*Most growth hormone deficient subjects have values
<0.25 U/ml.

Ref: Nichols Institute Reference Laboratories

        b)   Insulin (fasting): 13±5 µU/ml (mean ± SD)
        c)   Hemoglobin A$_1$C: 3.9-7.7%
        d)   Prolactin: <25 ng/ml

II. Sexual Development

    A.   The Sexual Genotype: When genitalia are ambiguous, a
buccal smear is not recommended due to significant
difficulty in interpretation. A karyotype is preferred
as it is much more accurate. It generally takes two
weeks. If a result is needed more quickly,
Y-fluorescence can be done within 3 days.

    B.   The Sexual Phenotype
        1)   Penile Standards for Newborn Males
            Length is measured from the pubic ramus to the tip

of the glans while traction is applied along the length of the phallus to the point of increased resistance.

Mean: 3.5 cm (3rd-97th percentile: 2.8-4.2 cm)
- at ages 0-5 months, a penile length less than 2.5 std. dev. below the mean (i.e. <1.9 cm) is abnormal.
- premature ranges are published in Feldman and Smith (see below).

Ref: Feldman KW, and Smith DW. J Pediatr 1975; 86:395-398. Lee PA, et al. Johns Hopkins Medical Journal 1980; 146:156-163.

2) Clitoral Standards for Newborn Females

Width is measured with the labia majora spread and redundant prepuce skin retracted.

Mean ± 1 SEM:  0-6 months  3.72 ± 0.25 mm
               6-12 months  3.94 ± 0.25 mm

From 27 weeks of gestation to term, the clitoral breadth does not change. However, in proportion to body weight, premature infants have a larger clitoral body than term infants.

Ref: Riley RJ, Rosenbloom AL. J Pediatr 1980; 96:918-919.

3) Tanner Staging of Secondary Sex Characteristics
Breast development (mean age ± SD)
   I. Pre-adolescent with elevation of papilla only.
  II. Breast bud stage with elevation of breast and papilla as small mound and enlargement of areolar diameter. (11.15 ± 1.10)
 III. Further enlargement and elevation of breast and areola, with no separation of their contours. (12.15 ± 1.09)
  IV. Projection of areola and papilla to form a secondary mound above the level of the breast. (13.11 ± 1.15)
   V. Mature stage with projection of papilla only, due to recession of the areola to the general contour of the breast. (Stages IV and V are not distinct in some.) (15.33 ± 1.74)
Genital development (male)
   I. Pre-adolescent with testes, scrotum, and penis approximately the same size and proportion as in early childhood.
  II. Enlargement of scrotum and of testes. The skin of the scrotum reddens and changes in texture. There is little or no enlargement of the penis at this stage. (11.64 ± 1.07)

III. Enlargement of penis, which occurs at first mainly in length. Further growth of testes and scrotum. (12.85 ± 1.04)

IV. Increased size of penis with growth in breadth and development of glans. Further enlargement of testes and scrotum and increased darkening of scrotal skin. (13.77 ± 1.02)

V. Genitalia adult in size and shape. (14.92 ± 1.10)

Pubic hair: male and female (mean age ± SD)

I. Pre-adolescent. The vellus over the pubes is no further developed than that over the abdominal wall, i.e. no pubic hair.

II. Sparse growth of long, slightly pigmented downy hair, straight or only slightly curled, appearing chiefly at the base of the penis or along the labia. (Male: 13.44 ± 1.09; Female: 11.69 ± 1.21)

III. Considerably darker, coarser and more curled. The hair spreads sparsely over the junction of the pubes. (Male: 13.9 ± 1.04; Female: 12.36 ± 1.10)

IV. Hair now resembles adult in type, but the area covered by it is still considerably smaller than in the adult. No spread to the medial surface of thighs. (Male: 14.36 ± 1.08; Female: 12.95 ± 1.06)

V. Adult in quantity and type with distribution of the horizontal pattern. (Male: 15.18 ± 1.07; Female: 14.41 ± 1.12)

VI. Spread up the linea alba - "male escutcheon."

Ref: Tanner JM. Growth at Adolescence, 2nd Edition. Oxford: Blackwell 1962: p. 32-7; Kaye R, Oski FA, Barness LA. Core Textbook of Pediatrics. Philadelphia: J.B. Jippincott 1978; 262-8. as adapted from Marshall WA, Tanner JM. Archives Dis Childhood 1969; 44:291-303.

## Mean Ages of Pubertal Events (±SD) in American Adolescents

| Male | | Female | |
|---|---|---|---|
| Gynecomastia | 13.2±0.8 | Peak height velocity | 12.5±1.5 |
| Voice break | 13.5±1.0 | Peak weight gain | 12.4±1.4 |
| Peak height velocity | 13.8±1.1 | Axillary hair | 13.1±0.8 |
| Peak weight velocity | 13.9±0.9 | Acne | 13.2±0.5 |
| Axillary hair | 14.0±1.1 | Menarche | 13.3±1.3 |
| Acne | 14.3±0.8 | Regular menses | 13.9±1.0 |

Ref: Lee PA. J Adolesc Health Care 1980; 1:26-29.

C. Tests and Procedures
  1. Vaginal Smear
     A test for estrogenization of vaginal mucosa is useful in evaluating precocious puberty.
     Method:1) In children, a good specimen is difficult to obtain because the specimen is easily contaminated by cells from the introitus, perineum, or examiner's fingers. A sterile cotton swab, dipped in normal saline with the excess fluid expressed, is carefully inserted beyond the introitus, moved laterally and withdrawn.
     2) Spread the vaginal secretions on a clean glass slide. A few drops of saline are added to make a wet mount. Methylene blue may be used to stain the nuclei, but an unstained prep can also be read. To make a permanent slide place in 95% ethanol fixative and send to the cytopathology lab.

     Interpetation: 1) Low estrogen states – predominance of round or oval parabasal cells with thick cytoplasm and vesicular nuclei displaying chromatin detail comprising 1/3 of the total cell area.
     2) High estrogen states – predominance of polygonal squamous cells with small pyknotic nuclei.
     3) Intermediate cells with squame-like cytoplasm and nuclei with a reticular chromatin pattern may be variably present, but will predominate in high cortisol or progestin states.

Ref: Frost JK, in Novak E, Novak ER, Woodruff JD (eds). Novak's Gynecologic and Obstetric Pathology 8th ed. Philadelphia: WB Saunders 1979:689-781.

  2. Dexamethasone suppression test in the work-up of premature adrenarche or precocious puberty.
     The source of androgen excess is frequently not obvious; therefore adrenal gland suppression with oral dexamethasone may be necessary.

| Day | 1 | 2 | 3 | 4 | 5 | 6 |
|---|---|---|---|---|---|---|
| Urinary 17-KS | X | X | | | X | X |
| Urinary 17-OHCS | X | X | | | | X |
| Urinary pregnanetriol | X | | | | | X |
| Dexamethasone 1.25 mg per M²/day divided Q6h | | | X | X | X | X |

     Interpretation: Increased, but suppressible, urinary 17-KS and pregnanetriol confirm the diagnosis of CAH. Incomplete suppression of 17-KS, but complete suppression of pregnanetriol, suggests that the patient has already entered into puberty. Markedly increased, nonsuppressible 17-KS suggest the presence of an androgen-producing tumor, most likely adrenal in origin.

Ref: Bacon GE, et al. Pediatric Endocrinology, 2nd Edition. Chicago: Year Book Medical Publishers, 1982, 209.

3. Gonadotropin releasing hormone stimulation test
Measures pituitary LH and FSH reserve. Helpful in the differential diagnosis of precocious sexual development.
Method: Inject LHRH 2.5 mcg/kg IV bolus (adult dose = 100 mcg) and collect samples at -15, 0, 15, 30, 45, 60, 90 and 120 mintues.
Interpretation: A pubertal or adult response shows an LH response in the adult range within 30 minutes. Normal prepubertal children should show no or minimal response.

Ref: Bacon GE, et al. Pediatric Endocrinology, 2nd Edition, 1982; 205; Kelch RP, et al. J Clin Endocrinol Metab 1975; 40:53-61. Ayerst Laboratories Synthetic LHRH Product Information, 1983.

4. HCG stimulation test of Leydig cell function.
Method: Inject HCG (human chorionic gonadotropin) 3000 U/M$^2$ (minimum 1000 U, maximum 5000 U) IM on days 1-5 and measure serum testosterone on days 0 and 6.
Interpretation: A normal response is a rise in serum testosterone and androstenedione to adult levels. This procedure may be used as the first week of the following test.

5. HCG stimulation to induce descent of cryptorchid testes
Method: Inject HCG 3000 U/M$^2$ (minimum 1000 U; maximum 5000 U) IM two or three times per week for six weeks. Examine the patient and measure serum testosterone at the end of the third and sixth weeks. The response to this regimen is quite variable. The best time to use it is controversial.

Ref: Lee PA, et al. Johns Hopkins Medical Journal, 1980; 146:159; Garagorri, et al. J Pediatr 1982; 101:923-7. Lee PA, Personal Communication, 1986.

III. Growth

    A.   Methods of Adult Height Prediction
        1)   Bayley-Pinneau Method: uses Greulich and Pyle bone age.
        2)   RWT Method: uses Greulich and Pyle bone age and midparental heights.

Ref: Roche A, et al. Monogr Paediatr 1975; 3:1-114; Himes JH, et al. Monogr Paediatr 1981;13:1-88; Roche A, Pediatrics 1975; 56:1026.

        3)   TW-2 Method: uses Tanner-Whitehouse bone age.

Ref: Tanner JM, et al. Assessment of Skeletal Maturity and Prediction of Adult Height (TW-2 Method). New York: Academic Press,1975.

    B.   Tests for Growth Hormone (GH)
        At many points during the day, GH is low. Therefore, provocative tests are necessary to document deficiency. Diagnosis requires two abnormal stimulation tests (not screening tests).
        1)   Screening tests
           a)   Sleep specimen
           Most subjects will have a rise in GH 45-60 minutes after the onset of nocturnal sleep. A single value >10 ng/ml rules out GH deficiency.
           b)   Exercise test
           80% or more of normal persons will release significant amounts of GH after vigorous exercise. Fast the patient for at least 4 hours and draw a baseline GH sample. Exercise the patient for 20 minutes (steady jogging). Obtain a second GH sample immediately. Values >10 ng/ml rule out GH deficiency.
           c)   Somatomedin C determination requires EDTA chelated blood. It may be drawn at anytime during the day. SM-C may be useful in detecting patients with quantitative or qualitative deficiencies in growth hormone not picked up by standard provocative tests. It correlates with chronologic age, bone age, and pubertal stage, but the correlation is not excellent. (e.g. the levels of SM-C in young normal children may overlap with those seen in hypopituitarism.)
           Normal: see p. 86.

Ref: Eisenstein E, et al. Pediatrics 1978; 62:526; Cacciari E, et al. J Pediatr 1985; 106:891-4; Reiter E. Compr Ther 1983; 9(2):45-55.

2) Stimulation tests
GH >10 ng/ml effectively rules out GH deficiency.
(Note that some labs use 7 ng/ml as the cut-off for
normal/abnormal rather than 10.) Values between
5-10 ng/ml are equivocal and may indicate partial
deficiency. Results less than 5 ng/ml are definitely
abnormal. A diagnosis of GH deficiency diagnosis
requires two abnormal chemical stimulation tests.

a) Arginine-insulin tolerance test (AITT)
Patient should be fasting. Draw baseline GH.
Infuse 0.5 g/kg arginine HCl (not to exceed 20 g)
IV over 30 minutes. Sample GH at 15, 30, 45, 60,
and 90 minutes. At 90 minutes, give 0.1 U/kg
insulin (diluted to 1 U/ml) rapidly via IV push.
Collect GH and glucose samples at 20, 30, 45, and
60 minutes. As each sample is collected, centrifuge
and separate serum. Observe the patient
continuously for hypoglycemia. $D_{50}W$ should be by
the bedside and IV access established. A valid test
requires either clinical or chemical ($\geq 50\%$ drop in
glucose) hypoglycemia.

Ref: Bacon GE, et al. Pediatric Endocrinology, 2nd Edition.
Chicago: Year Book Medical Publishers 1982; 85-6.

b) L-dopa stimulation test
Give L-dopa orally (125 mg, <15 kg; 250 mg, 15-30
kg; 500 mg, >30 kg) to fasting patient. Collect GH
samples at 0, 20, 40, 60, 90, and 120 minutes.

Ref: Weldon VV, et al. J Pediatr 1975; 87:540-4.

c) Glucagon stimulation test
Patient should be fasting. Draw baseline GH. Give
0.1 mg/kg glucagon IM. Sample GH at 15, 30, 45,
60, 90, 120, 150, and 180 minutes. Reactive
hypoglycemia is possible.

Ref: Vanderschueren-Lodeweyckx M, et al. J Pediatr 1974;
85:182-7.

d) Clonidine stimulation test
The patient should be fasting. Give 5
micrograms/kg (~120 mcg/M²) of clonidine orally.
Give 250 mcg for weights >50 kg. Draw blood (1cc
serum equivalents) at 0,60,75,90, and 120 minutes.
Side effects: dry mouth, drowsiness, hypotension.
Check BP regularly. Keep the patient in bed to
avoid falls.

Ref: Gil-Ad J, et al. Lancet 1979; 2:278-80; and as adopted
from Lanes R, et al. Am J Dis Child 1985; 139:87-8.

IV. Tests of Adrenal and Pituitary Function (normal values p 84)

A. Urinary 17-hydroxycorticosteroids (17-OHCS)
This measures approximately 1/3 of end products of metabolism of cortisol. Collect a 24 hour urine specimen. Refrigerate during collection and process immediately (17-OHCS are destroyed at room temperature).
Interpretation:
- Decreased in inanition states (anorexia nervosa); pituitary disorders involving ACTH; Addison's disease; administration of synthetic, potent corticosteroids (prednisone, dexamethasone, triamcinolone); 21-hydroxylase deficiency; liver disease; hypothyroidism; newborn period (due to decreased glucuronidation).
- Increased in Cushing's syndrome; ACTH, cortisone, cortisol therapy; medical or surgical stress; obesity (occasionally), hyperthyroidism; and 11-hydroxylase deficiency.

B. Urinary 17-ketosteroids (17-KS)
This measures some end products of androgen metabolism. Collect and refrigerate 24 hour urine specimen.
Interpretation:
- Increased in adrenal hyperplasia, (in congential adrenal hyperplasia it may take one to two weeks for 17-KS to rise above the normally high newborn levels. Other signs of CAH would be hyponatremia, hyperkalemia, high 17-OH progesterone, and high androstenedione), virilizing adrenal tumors, Cushing's syndrome, exogenous ACTH, cortisone, androgens (except methyltestosterone), stressful illness (burns, radiation illness, etc.), androgen-producing gonadal tumors.
- Decreased in Addison's disease, anorexia nervosa, panhypopituitarism.

C. Plasma corticosteroids
Collect heparinized blood and separate plasma immediately. Measure cortisol (corticosterone and 11-deoxycortisol may sometimes be needed).
Interpretation:
Abnormal values occur in the same disorders as for abnormal 17-OHCS; however, usually normal in anorexia nervosa, liver disease, hypo- and hyperthyroidism, and obesity. Elevated levels by protein binding assay occur during pregnancy and during estrogen administration.

D. Plasma 17-OH Progesterone (17-OHP)
Collect heparinized blood and separate plasma immediately. Measures precursor which is elevated with certain adrenal enzyme deficiency states (21-and 11-hydroxylase deficiency).

E.   Adrenal Capacity Test
     1)   IM ACTH test
     Measures maximal capacity of adrenal to produce cortisol.
     Procedure:
     Days 1 and 2 collect baseline 24 hour urine for
     17-OHCS. Days 3, 4, and 5 administer 20 USP U/M$^2$
     Acthargel every 8 hours. Collect 24 hour urines on
     days 5 and 6 for 17-OHCS.
     a)   Normal
          Urinary 17-OHCS = 85±15 mg/M$^2$/24h.
     b)   Abnormal
          Lack of response in Addison's disease; subnormal in
          adrenal hyperplasia; hyperresponse at times in
          Cushing's syndrome.
     2)   IV ACTH test
     Procedure:
     Give ACTH (Cortrosyn) IV bolus (0.1 mg, <1 year; 0.15
     mg, 1-5 years; 0.25 mg, >5 years). Draw serum cortisol
     at 0, 30, 60, 90, and 120 minutes. A shorter test (30
     minutes) may be as reliable.
     a)   Normal
          Plasma cortisol 32±4 mcg/dl by 2 hours (or >20
          mcg/dl or 10 mcg/dl increment). In patients whose
          adrenals have been suppressed for more than one
          month, the IV test is usually not prolonged enough
          to produce adrenal reactivation.
     b)   Abnormal
          A lack of response in the presence of Cushing's
          syndrome is characteristic of adrenal carcinoma. A
          normal response does not rule out carcinoma. A
          hyperresponse is indicative of bilateral adrenal
          hyperplasia. A normal response does not rule out
          hyperplasia. Lack of response is suggestive but not
          diagnostic of primary adrenal disease.

Ref: Migeon CJ. In: Collu R, et al. (eds). Pediatric
Endocrinology. New York: Raven Press, 1981; 475; Bacon
GE, et al. Pediatric Endocrinology, 2nd Edition. Chicago:
Year Book 1982; 170.

F.   Pituitary ACTH Capacity (Metyrapone) Test
     Metyrapone inhibits 11-hydroxylase in the adrenal and
     blocks cortisol production. With increased ACTH,
     11-deoxy precursors of cortisol accumulate and are
     excreted as 17-OHCS.
     Procedure:
     Collect 24 hour urine for 17-OHCS on days 1 and 2. On
     day 3 give metyrapone orally 300 mg/M$^2$ (max. dose =
     750 mg) Q4h x 24h (6 doses) (1800 mg/M$^2$/day) and con-
     tinue urine collection. Day 4 is the final 24 hour urine.

1) Normal

Urinary 17-OHCS increase to >9 mg/M$^2$/24h on day 3 or 4. This test may be modified by giving a single midnight dose of metyrapone IV (35 mg/kg, max. 1 gram). Cortisol is measured in an 8 AM sample and 17 OHCS in 24 hour urine collection. Normally a many-fold rise in 17-deoxycortisol and a precipitous drop in cortisol are seen.

2) Abnormal

Little or no increase in urinary 17-OHCS is seen with pituitary ACTH deficiency, hypothalamic tumors, and pharmacologic doses of steroids.

CAUTION - In patients with reduced adrenal secretory capacity, the drug may cause acute adrenal insufficiency. Precede this test by an adrenal capacity ACTH test in these persons.

Ref: Migeon CJ In: Collu R, et al. (eds). Pediatric Endocrinology. New York: Raven Press 1981; 475.

G. Insulin-Induced Hypoglycemia

During AITT for growth hormone, plasma cortisol can be measured at 0 and 60 minutes. Normally plasma cortisol increases by 10 mcg/dl and the maximum level is >20 mcg/dl.

H. Pituitary Dexamethasone Suppression Test

Dexamethasone, a synthetic corticoid, suppresses the secretion of ACTH by the normal pituitary. This decreases endogenous production of cortisol and, hence, also the excretion of 17-OHCS. Dexamethasone is not excreted as 17-OHCS.

Procedure:

Collect 24 hour urine for 17-OHCS on days 1 and 2. Administer dexamethasone 1.25 mg/100 lbs/day po divided Q6h on days 3, 4, and 5 followed by dexamethasone 3.75 mg/100 lbs/day po divided Q6h on days 6, 7, and 8. Collect 24 hour urines on days 1, 2, 4, 5, 7, and 8 for 17-OHCS.

1) Normal: and in obesity.

By day 5, urinary 17-OHCS have fallen to <2 mg/24h.

2) Abnormal:

Cushing's syndrome of any cause, by day 5, 17-OHCS are >2 mg/24h. Cushing's syndrome secondary to adrenal hyperplasia, by day 8, 17-OHCS are <2 mg/ 24h unless hyperplasia is secondary to ectopic ACTH production (lung, mediastinal tumor, etc). Cushing's syndrome due to adrenocortical carcinoma, by day 8, 17-OHCS are >2 mg/24h. In certain hypothalamic tumors, no suppression is possible.

Ref: Bacon GE, et al. Pediatric Endocrinology, 2nd Edition. Chicago: Year Book 1982; 170.

I. **Overnight Screening Dexamethasone Suppression Test**
Dexamethasone, 1 mg is given at 11 P.M. At 8-9 A.M., on the following day, a fasting serum cortisol level is drawn. Normally or in obesity, the serum cortisol should fall below 10 mg%.

J. **Water Deprivation Test**
Useful for the diagnosis of diabetes insipidus. Requires careful supervision since dehydration and hypernatremia may occur.
1) Procedure:
Begin the test in the morning after a 24 hour period of adequate hydration and stable weight. Fluids are restricted for 7 hours. Have the patient empty his bladder and obtain a baseline weight. Urinary specific gravity and volume as well as body weight are measured hourly. Serum sodium is measured every 2 hours. Urine and serum osmolality are measured every 2 hours. Hematocrit and BUN also may be obtained at these times but are not critical. Subjects must be carefully observed to assure that fluids are not ingested during the test. The test should be terminated if weight loss approaches 5%.
2) Interpretation:
Normal individuals who are water deprived will concentrate their urine between 500 and 1400 mOsm/L and plasma osmolality will range between 288 and 291 mOsm/L. In normal children and those with psychogenic DI, urinary specific gravity rises to at least 1.010 and usually greater. The urinary: plasma osmolality ratio exceeds 2. Urine volume decreases significantly, and there should be no appreciable weight loss. Specific gravity remains below 1.005 in patients with ADH-deficient or nephrogenic DI. Urine osmolality remains below 150 mOsm/L, and there should be no significant reduction of urine volume. A weight loss up to 5% usually occurs. At the end of the test, a serum osmolality >290 mOsm/L, Na >150 mEq/L and a rise of BUN and hematocrit provide evidence that the patient did not receive water.

K. **Vasopressin Test**
1) Procedure:
The test is preceded by a 24 hour control period during which intake, output, and urinary specific gravity are measured while the patient receives fluids ad lib. (It may also follow the above water

deprivation test.) The bladder is emptied and aqueous vasopressin is administered, 0.3 ml/M$^2$ SC. (Note that aqueous vasopressin contains 20 U/ml, whereas vasopressin tannate in oil contains 5 U/ml). Intake is monitored, and urinary output and specific gravity are determined every 30 to 60 minutes. A response should occur in 4 to 6 hours. If there is no effect after 6 hours, the test is repeated using 0.6 ml/M$^2$.

2) Interpretation:
Patients with ADH-deficient DI concentrate their urine (to 1.010 and usually greater) and also demonstrate a reduction of urine volume and decreased fluid intake. Patients with nephrogenic DI have no significant change in intake, urine volume, or specific gravity. Constant intake associated with decreased output and increased specific gravity suggests psychogenic DI.

Note: Use of the intranasally administered vasopressin is not recommended for this test.

Ref: sections F-J above. Bacon GE, et al. Pediatric Endocrinology, 2nd Edition. Chicago, Year Book 1982; 258-9.

V. Adrenal and Pituitary Function

   A. Pathway of Steroid Hormone Synthesis

| Mineralocorticoids | Glucocorticoids | Androgens |
|---|---|---|
| | CHOLESTEROL | |
| | ↓ 20,22 desmolase | |
| | Δ-5-PREGNENOLONE ——————————— | |
| | ↓ 3,β-ol-dehydrogenase | ↓ 17-hydroxylase |
| | | 17-OH-PREGNENOLONE |
| | PROGESTERONE | ↓ |
| | ↓ 17-hydroxylase | DEHYDROEPIANDROSTERONE |
| | 17-OH-PROGESTERONE | ↓ 3,β-ol-dehydrogenase |
| ↓ 21-hydroxylase | ↓ 21-hydroxylase | ANDROSTENEDIONE |
| 11-DESOXYCORTICOSTERONE | 11-DESOXYCORTISOL | ↓ |
| ↓ 11-hydroxylase | ↓ 11-hydroxylase | TESTOSTERONE |
| CORTICOSTERONE | CORTISOL | |
| ↓ 18 "oxidation" defect | | |
| ALDOSTERONE | | |

Ref: Bacon GE, et al. Pediatric Endocrinology, 2nd Edition. Chicago: Year Book Medical Publishers, Inc., 1982, 153.

VI. Thyroid Function

A. Screening for Congenital Hypothyroidism
1) The first blood-soaked paper sample is obtained at 3-7 days of life. If total T4(TT4) is less than the absolute standard or lower than 2 standard deviations below the day's mean, a TSH-RIA is run.
2) A second sample is obtained at 14-28 days of life. Approximately 15% of congenital hypothyroidism cases are detected only on this second screening.

Ref: Panney S, Div of Hereditary Disorders, Maryland State Department of Health and Mental Hygiene, Personal Communication, 1986.

B. Thyroid Scan
Useful for assessing thyroidal clearance, for localizing ectopic thyroid tissue, and for structure-function studies of the thyroid such as localization of hyperfunctioning and nonfunctioning thyroid nodules and delineation of the irregular thyroidal iodine kinetics and abnormal distribution of isotope frequently associated with chronic lymphocytic (Hashimoto's) thyroiditis. In the newborn infant, it can differentiate athyreotic or ectopic hypothyroidism from other causes of decreased thyroid function. This information could be important in genetic counseling, as athyreosis or ectopic thyroid tissue usually occurs sporadically, whereas hypofunction due to impaired biosynthesis of thyroid implies an inherited defect. Sensitivity, specificity, convenience, and safety considerations indicate that $^{99M}$Technetium-pertechnetate is preferable to the iodide isotopes (e.g., $^{123}$I and $^{131}$I).

Ref: Heyman S, et al. J Pediatr 1982; 101:571-4, Bauman RA, et al. J Pediatr 1976; 89:268; Fisher DA. J Pediatr 1973; 82:1-9.

C. Technetium Uptake
Measures uptake of technetium by thyroid gland. Uptake is measured only for the first 20 minutes. Normal: 0.24-3.4%.

D. Pituitary TSH Reserve Test
No rise in TSH in the face of a high $T_4$ is confirmatory of hyperthyroidism. No rise in TSH in the face of a low $T_4$ and low TSH suggests pituitary dysfunction.
1) Method
Blood samples for determination of TSH are drawn at -15, 0, +30, and +60 minutes. Synthetic TRH is given IV over 15 to 30 seconds starting at time

zero. The recommended dose of TRH is 7 mcg/kg, although this is not absolutely necessary. Side effects include nausea, a sensation of facial flushing, the urge to urinate, and occasionally vomiting. These effects last from several seconds to two minutes, but they occur in almost all patients. Monitor BP and pulse throughout.

2) Interpretation:

The absolute values for TSH responses vary considerably between laboratories and are affected somewhat by the patient's age and sex. Although the pattern for TSH release also must be considered, a maximal rise in serum TSH of between 5 and 25 mcU/ml is considered normal in most labs.

Ref: Bacon GE, et al. Pediatric Endocrinology, 2nd Edition:135.

VII. Pancreatic Endocrine Function

A. Oral Glucose Tolerance Test (OGTT)
   1. Pre-test Preparation: Calorically adequate diet required for three days prior to the test, consisting of 50% of total calories as carbohydrate.

NOTE: Delay test 2 weeks after period of illness. Discontinue all hyper- or hypoglycemic agents (salicylates, diuretics, oral contraceptives, phenytoin, etc.).

B. Test
   1. Administer 1.75 gm/kg (max 100 gm) of glucose orally after a 12 hour fast allowing up to 5 minutes for ingestion. Mix glucose with water and lemon juice as a 20% dilution. Quiet activity is permissible during the OGTT.

   2. Draw blood samples at 0, 30, 60, 120, 180 and 240 minutes. Analyze urine samples for sugar at 0, 60 and 120 minutes.

C. Interpretation
   (Venous plasma using autoanalyzer ferricyanide method).
   1. Upper limits of normal: Fasting      110 mg%
                                60 min     160 mg%
                               120 min     140 mg%
                               180 min     130 mg%
                               240 min     115 mg%
   2. Two values greater than the above norms or one value above 200 mg% in the absence of overt diabetes mellitus is evidence of chemical diabetes mellitus.

Ref: Rosenbloom A. Metabolism 1973; 22:301.

VIII. <u>Endocrine Emergencies and Treatment</u>

    A. <u>Diabetic Ketoacidosis (DKA)</u>
       1) <u>Evaluation</u>
          a) New or known diabetic? Usual insulin regimen? Last insulin dose? Any infection or other inciting event?
          b) Quick history and physical examination.
       2) <u>Baseline Studies</u>
          a) <u>Fluids</u>
          Normal saline or Ringer's lactate at 20 ml/kg/hr for 1-2 hours. Then 1/2 normal saline + $K^+$ and/or $D_5W$ as appropriate (see below) (1/2 normal saline alone is hypotonic), calculated to replace deficit plus maintenance and on-going losses over 24 hours (usually 10% dehydrated). See fluid and electrolyte table, page 234, for estimated deficits.
          b) <u>Insulin</u>
          Insulin drip is preferred since it allows constant control. There is also less risk of hypoglycemia and too rapid decrease of the serum glucose concentration (hence may lessen risk of cerebral edema).
          - 0.1 unit/kg regular insulin IV bolus to saturate insulin receptors.
          - Follow with continuous drip 0.1 U/kg/hr regular insulin piggybacked in IV line (50 units insulin/250 ml normal saline).
          c) <u>Glucose</u>
          Measure dextrosticks or chemstrips hourly. Rate of glucose fall should be between 80-100 mg/dl/hr. Increase insulin to 0.14-0.20 U/kg if glucose falls at < 50 mg/dl/hr. If glucose drops too rapidly (> 100 mg/dl/hr) continue insulin infusion (0.1 U/kg/hr) and add $D_5W$ to IV. Also, as glucose approaches 250-300 mg/dl, add $D_5W$ to IV.
          d) <u>Electrolytes</u>
             - Potassium:
             Patients with DKA are potassium depleted. Give patients maintenance plus deficit over 24 hours. A general guide is to give 40 meq/L if initial $K^+$ is < normal. Give no $K^+$ initially if $K^+$ is elevated or patient is not making urine.
            - Phosphate:
             $PO_4$ is depleted in DKA and will drop further with insulin therapy. $PO_4$ encourages better oxygenation of tissues. Replace $K^+$, 1/2 as KCl and 1/2 as $K_2PO_4$ for the first 8 hours, then all as KCl. However, let caution be your guide as too much $PO_4$ will cause decreased Ca and tetany.

- Bicarbonate
  This is not administered unless pH is <7.10 and/or $HCO_3^-$ <5. If necessary to give $NaHCO_3$, administer 2 meq/kg IV over 30-60 minutes or add to the first bottle of 1/2 normal saline.

e) Miscellaneous
   Follow vital signs, dextrosticks Q1-2h, glucose, pH, $pCO_2$, electrolytes Q3-4h, EKG periodically to follow $K^+$.

3. Further Insulin Management (see chart, p. 216)
   a) When blood pH >7.3, and ketosis has cleared, discontinue insulin drip, and start "sliding" scale. This is usually in a dosage of 0.1-0.25 units/kg regular insulin to be given subcutaneously Q6-8h.

   b) The next day, 1/2-2/3 of the previous day's total insulin dose is given as an intermediate acting form (NPH, Lente) with further regular insulin coverage at approximately 0.1 U/kg according to blood glucose concentration measured before each meal. The usual time required to stabilize the insulin dosage is 3-5 days. Usual daily maintenance dose in children: 0.5 - 1.0 units/kg/24h; adolescents during growth spurt: 0.8-1.2 units/kg/24h.

Ref: Plotnick, L and Kritzler, R: In: Fosarelli P, (ed) Therapeutic Shorts. Johns Hopkins Hospital Pediatric Outpatient Dept., 1986; Sperling MA: Pediatric Clin North Am 1979; 26:149-69.

B. Preparation for Surgery in Hyperthyroid Patients
   Ideally, the patient will be euthyroid at the time of operation. Propylthiouracil can be given at 5 mg/kg/24h divided Q8h (or 150-300 mg/24h for 6-10 yr old or 300-400 mg/24h for >10 yr old) or methimazole at 1/10th the PTU dosages. Lugol's solution, 5 qtts/24h PO should be given for 10 to 14 days before surgery. However, if surgery is required emergently before a euthyroid status is achieved, beta-blockage alone to control symptoms is adequate. Give propranolol 2.5 mg/kg/24h to start (may be increased to 10 mg/kg/24h max., as needed, to control symptoms) PO divided Q6-8h (unless contraindicated i.e.: asthma, congestive heart failure). Adult dose = 80 mg PO Q8h. The dose on the morning of surgery should not be omitted. It should also be continued for 5 days after surgery.

Ref:  Buckingham BA, et al. Am J Dis Child 1981; 135:112-7, Feek CM, et al. New Engl J Med 1980; 302:883-5; Bacon GE, et al. Pediatric Endocrinology, 2nd Edition. Chicago: Year Book 1982; 128.

C.  **Addisonian Crisis** (acute adrenal failure)
Use D5.9NS to support blood pressure and blood sugar. Give hydrocortisone as an IV bolus of 4 times the daily maintenance dose (i.e. $4 \times 12.5$ mg/M$^2$ or 50 mg/M$^2$), followed by hydrocortisone, 50-100 mg/M$^2$/day divided Q4-6° or preferably as a continuous drip. Mineralocorticoid is given either as deoxycortisone acetate (DOCA) 1.0-2.0 mg Q day IM or as 9-α-fluorocortisol (Florinef), 0.05-0.15 mg Q day PO, as tolerated.

# DEVELOPMENT

I. Since development takes place in an orderly and sequential manner, the phenomena of developmental delay, dissociation, and deviancy are important in the detection of developmental disabilities.

Delay refers to a performance significantly below average in a given area of skill. A developmental quotient below 70 constitutes such a delay.

Dissociation refers to a substantial difference in the rate of development between two areas of skill. Examples are the cognitive-motor differences in some children with mental retardation or cerebal palsy.

Deviancy refers to nonsequential development within a given area of skill. For example, the development of hand preference at 12 months is a departure from the normal sequence, and may be related to difficulty with the other extremity.

A child's rate of development is reflected in the developmental quotient (DQ):

$$DQ = (\text{developmental age} \div \text{chronological age}) \times 100$$

Two separate developmental assessments are more predictive than a single assessment. It is essential that testing be performed in all areas of development. Language remains the best predictor of future intellectual endowment and should serve as the common denominator comparing its rate of development with the other areas which include gross motor, problem solving, adaptive and social skills.

Ref: Caputo AJ, et al. Orth Clin North Am 1981; 12:3-22.

II. Levels of Retardation (Based on Wechsler Scales)

| Degree of Mental Retardation | Measured Intelligence Quotient | Expected Mental Age as an Adult (yrs) |
|---|---|---|
| "Dull Normal" | 80-90 | - |
| "Borderline" | 70-79 | - |
| Mild (Educable) | 55-69 | 9-11 |
| Moderate (Trainable) | 40-54 | 5-8 |
| Severe | 25-39 | 3-5 |
| Profound | Below 25 | Below 3 |

III. DEVELOPMENTAL MILESTONES/LANGUAGE SKILLS

| AGE | GROSS MOTOR | VISUAL MOTOR | LANGUAGE | SOCIAL |
|---|---|---|---|---|
| 1 mo | Raises head slightly from prone, makes crawling movements, lifts chin up | Has tight grasp, follows to midline | Alerts to sound (e.g. by blinking, moving, startling) | Regards face |
| 2 mos | Holds head in midline, lifts chest off table | No longer clenches fist tightly, follows object past midline | Smiles after being stroked or talked to | Recognizes parent |
| 3 mos | Supports on forearms in prone, holds head up steadily | Holds hands open at rest, follows in circular fashion | Coos (produces long vowel sounds in musical fashion) | Reaches for familiar people or objects, anticipates feeding |
| 4-5 mos | Rolls front to back, back to front, sits well when propped, supports on wrists and shifts weight | Moves arms in unison to grasp, touches cube placed on table | Orients to voice 5 mos - orients to bell (localizes lat-, erally) says "ah-goo," razzes | Enjoys looking around environment |
| 6 mos | Sits well unsupported, puts feet in mouth in supine position | Reaches with either hand, transfers, uses raking grasp | Babbles 7 mos - orients to bell (localizes indirectly) 8 mos - "dada/mama" indiscriminately | Recognizes strangers |
| 9 mos | Creeps, crawls, cruises, pulls to stand, pivots when sitting | Uses pincer grasp, probes with fore-finger, holds bottle, fingerfeeds | Understands "no", waves bye-bye 10 mos - "dada/mama" discriminately; orients to bell (directly) 11 mos - one word other than "dada/mama" | Starts to explore environment plays pat-a-cake |

III. DEVELOPMENTAL MILESTONES/LANGUAGE SKILLS (continued)

| AGE | GROSS MOTOR | VISUAL MOTOR | LANGUAGE | SOCIAL |
|---|---|---|---|---|
| 12 mos | Walks alone | Throws objects, lets go of toys, hand release, uses mature pincer grasp | Follows one-step command with gesture, uses two words other than "dada/mama" 14 mos uses three words | Imitates actions, comes when called, cooperates with dressing |
| 15 mos | Creeps upstairs, walks backwards | Builds tower of 2 blocks in imitation of examiner, scribbles in imitation | Follows one-step command without gesture, uses 4-6 words and immature jargoning (runs several unintelligible words together) | |
| 18 mos | Runs, throws toy from standing without falling | Turns 2-3 pages at a time, fills spoon and feeds himself | Knows 7-20 words, knows one body part, uses mature jargoning (includes intelligible words in jargoning) | Copies parent in tasks (e.g. sweeping, dusting), plays in company of other children |
| 21 mos | Squats in play, goes up steps | Builds tower of 5 blocks, drinks well from cup | Points to 3 body parts, uses two-word combinations, has 20 word vocabulary | Asks to have food and to go to toilet |
| 24 mos | Walks up and down steps without help | Turns pages one at a time, removes shoes, pants, etc., imitates stroke | Uses 50 words, two-word sentences, uses pronouns, (I, you, me) inappropriately, points to 5 body parts, understands 2 step command | Parallel play |

## III. DEVELOPMENTAL MILESTONES/LANGUAGE SKILLS (continued)

| AGE | GROSS MOTOR | VISUAL MOTOR | LANGUAGE | SOCIAL |
|---|---|---|---|---|
| 30 mos | Jumps with both feet off floor, throws ball overhand | Unbuttons, holds pencil in adult fashion, differentiates horizontal and vertical line | Uses pronouns (I, you, me) appropriately, understands concept of "one", repeats 2 digits forward | Tells first and last names when asked, gets himself drink without help |
| 3 yrs | Pedals tricycle, can alternate feet when going up steps | Dresses and undresses partially, dries hands if reminded, draws a circle | Uses 3 word sentences, uses plurals, past tense. Knows all pronouns. Minimum 250 words, understands concept of "two" | Group play, shares toys, takes turns, plays well with others, knows full name, age, sex |
| 4 yrs | Hops, skips, alternates feet going downstairs | Buttons clothing fully, catches ball | Knows colors, says song or poem from memory, asks questions | Tells "tall tales", plays cooperatively with a group of children |
| 5 yrs | Skips, alternating feet, jumps over low obstacles | Ties shoes, spreads with knife | Prints first name, asks what a word means | Plays competitive games, abides by rules, likes to help in household tasks |

Ref: Capute AJ, Biehl RF. Pediatr Clin North Am 1973; 20:3-25; Capute AJ, Accardo PJ. Clin Pediatr 1978; 17:847-853; Capute AJ, et al. Am J Dis Child 1986; 140:694-8. Capute AJ, et al. Devel Med Child Neurol 1986; 28:762-71.

108

# GESELL FIGURES

**15 MOS.** IMITATES SCRIBBLE

**18 MOS.** SCRIBBLES SPONTANEOUSLY

**2 YRS.** IMITATES STROKE

**2½ YRS.** DIFFERENTIATES HORIZONTAL AND VERTICAL LINE

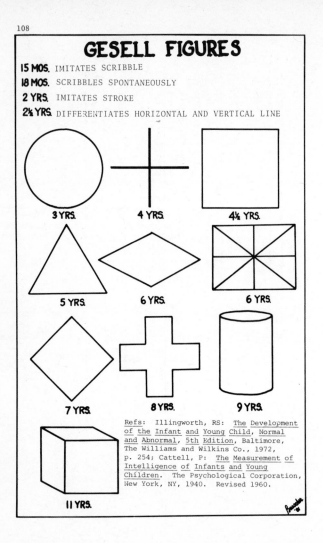

3 YRS.    4 YRS.    4½ YRS.

5 YRS.    6 YRS.    6 YRS.

7 YRS.    8 YRS.    9 YRS.

Refs: Illingworth, RS: The Development of the Infant and Young Child, Normal and Abnormal, 5th Edition, Baltimore, The Williams and Wilkins Co., 1972, p. 254; Cattell, P: The Measurement of Intelligence of Infants and Young Children. The Psychological Corporation, New York, NY, 1940. Revised 1960.

11 YRS.

IV. Visual-motor.

The Goodenough-Harris draw a person (below) and Gesell figures (p. 108) are presented as two screening tests which focus on visual-motor skills and problem solving abilities. For both it is important to observe _how_ the pictures are drawn as well as the final product.

Goodenough-Harris Draw-a-Person Test: Procedure - The child is supplied with a pencil (preferably a No. 2 with eraser) and a sheet of blank paper and instructed to "Draw a person; draw the best person you can." Encouragement may be supplied if needed, i.e., "Draw a whole person", however, under no condition should the examiner suggest specific supplementation or changes.

Scoring and norms: The child receives one point for each detail present (see the following guide).

1. Head present
2. Legs present
3. Arms present

TRUNK
4. Present
5. Length greater than breadth
6. Shoulders

ARMS LEGS
7. Attached to trunk
8. At correct point

NECK
9. Present
10. Outline of neck continuous with head, trunk, or both.

FACE
11. Eyes
12. Nose
13. Mouth
14. 12 & 13 in two dimensions
15. Nostrils

HAIR
16. Present
17. On more than circumference non-transparent

CLOTHING
18. Present
19. Two articles; non-transparent
20. Entire drawing non-transparent (sleeves & trousers)
21. Four Articles
22. Costume complete

FINGERS
23. Present
24. Correct number
25. Two dimension; length > breadth
26. Thumb opposition
27. Hand distinct from fingers and arm

JOINTS
    28. Elbow, shoulder or both
    29. Knee, hip, or both
PROPORTION
    30. Head: 1/10 to 1/2 of trunk area
    31. Arms: Approx. same length as trunk
    32. Legs: 1-2 times trunk length;
        width less than trunk width
    33. Feet: 1/10 to 1/3 leg length
    34. Arms and legs in two dimensions
    35. Heel
MOTOR COORDINATION
    36. Lines firm and well connected
    37. Firmly drawn with correct joining
    38. Head outline
    39. Trunk outline
    40. Outline of arms and legs
    41. Features
EARS
    42. Present
    43. Correct position and proportion
EYE DETAIL
    44. Brow or lashes
    45. Pupil
    46. Proportion
    47. Glance directed front in profile drawing
CHIN
    48. Present; forehead
    49. Projection
PROFILE
    50. Not more than one error
    51. Correct

Goodenough Age Norms

| AGE | POINTS |
| --- | --- |
| 3 | 2 |
| 4 | 6 |
| 5 | 10 |
| 6 | 14 |
| 7 | 18 |
| 8 | 22 |
| 9 | 26 |
| 10 | 30 |
| 11 | 34 |
| 12 | 38 |
| 13 | 42 |

Ref: Taylor E. Psychological appraisal of children with cerebral defects. Harvard Univ. Press, 1961.

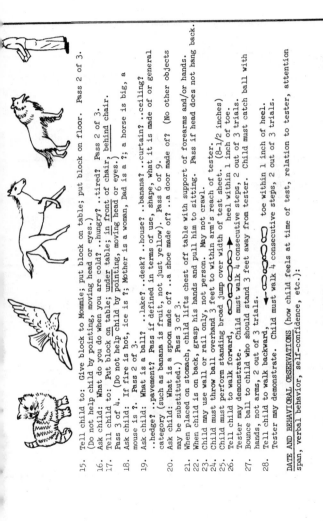

15. Tell child to: Give block to Mommie; put block on table; put block on floor. Pass 2 of 3.
    (Do not help child by pointing, moving head or eyes.)

16. Ask child: What do you do when you are cold? ..hungry? ..tired? Pass 2 of 3.

17. Tell child to: Put block on table; under table; in front of chair, behind chair.
    Pass 3 of 4. (Do not help child by pointing, moving head or eyes.)

18. Ask child: If fire is hot, ice is ?; Mother is a woman, Dad is a ?; a horse is big, a
    mouse is ?. Pass 2 of 3.

19. Ask child: What is a ball? ..desk? ..house? ..banana? ..curtain? ..ceiling?
    ..hedge? ..pavement? Pass if defined in terms of use, shape, what it is made or or general
    category (such as banana is fruit, not just yellow). Pass 6 of 9.

20. Ask child: What is a spoon made of? ..a shoe made of? ..a door made of? (No other objects
    may be substituted.) Pass 3 of 3.

21. When placed on stomach, child lifts chest off table with support of forearms and/or hands.

22. When child is on back, grasp his hands and pull him to sitting. Pass if head does not hang back.

23. Child may use wall or rail only, not person. May not crawl.

24. Child must throw ball overhand 3 feet to within arm's reach of tester.

25. Child must perform standing broad jump over width of test sheet. (8-1/2 inches)

26. Tell child to walk forward, [diagram] heel within 1 inch of toe.
    Tester may demonstrate. Child must walk 4 consecutive steps, 2 out of 3 trials.

27. Bounce ball to child who should stand 3 feet away from tester. Child must catch ball with
    hands, not arms, 2 out of 3 trials.

28. Tell child to walk backward, [diagram] toe within 1 inch of heel.
    Tester may demonstrate. Child must walk 4 consecutive steps, 2 out of 3 trials.

DATE AND BEHAVIORAL OBSERVATIONS (how child feels at time of test, relation to tester, attention
span, verbal behavior, self-confidence, etc.):

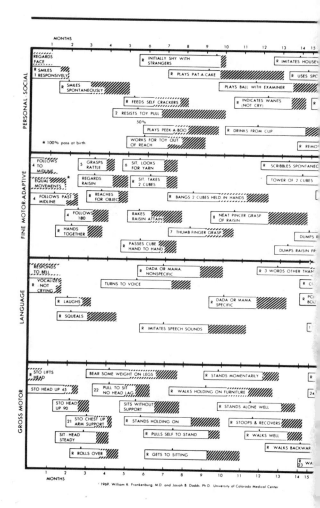

Denver Developmental Screening Test

MONTHS
1 2 3 4 5 6 7 8 9 10 11 12 13 14 15

PERSONAL-SOCIAL

REGARDS FACE
R SMILES RESPONSIVELY
R SMILES SPONTANEOUSLY
* 100% pass at birth
R INITIALLY SHY WITH STRANGERS
R PLAYS PAT A CAKE
R IMITATES HOUSEW
R USES SPC
PLAYS BALL WITH EXAMINER
R FEEDS SELF CRACKERS
R INDICATES WANTS (NOT CRY)
R
2 RESISTS TOY PULL
50%
PLAYS PEEK A BOO
R DRINKS FROM CUP
WORKS FOR TOY OUT OF REACH
R REMOV

FINE MOTOR-ADAPTIVE

FOLLOWS TO MIDLINE
EQUAL MOVEMENTS
4 FOLLOWS PAST MIDLINE
4 FOLLOWS 180
R HANDS TOGETHER
5 GRASPS RATTLE
6 SIT. LOOKS FOR YARN
REGARDS RAISIN
R REACHES FOR OBJEC
3 SIT. TAKES 2 CUBES
R SCRIBBLES SPONTANEO
TOWER OF 2 CUBES
R BANGS 2 CUBES HELD IN HANDS
RAKES RAISIN ATTAIN
8 NEAT PINCER GRASP OF RAISIN
7 THUMB FINGER GRASP
R PASSES CUBE HAND TO HAND
DUMPS R
DUMPS RAISIN FR

LANGUAGE

RESPONDS TO BELL
VOCALIZES R NOT CRYING
R LAUGHS
R SQUEALS
R DADA OR MAMA NONSPECIFIC
TURNS TO VOICE
R 3 WORDS OTHER THAN
R CO
R DADA OR MAMA SPECIFIC
R PO BOL
R IMITATES SPEECH SOUNDS
1

GROSS MOTOR

STO LIFTS HEAD
STO HEAD UP 45
STO HEAD UP 90
STO CHEST UP 21 ARM SUPPORT
SIT HEAD STEADY
R ROLLS OVER
BEAR SOME WEIGHT ON LEGS
22 PULL TO SIT NO HEAD LAG
SITS WITHOUT SUPPORT
R STANDS HOLDING ON
R PULLS SELF TO STAND
R GETS TO SITTING
R STANDS MOMENTARILY
R WALKS HOLDING ON FURNITURE
R STANDS ALONE WELL
R STOOPS & RECOVERS
R WALKS WELL
R WALKS BACKWAR
R 23 WA
24
R

1 2 3 4 5 6 7 8 9 10 11 12 13 14 15
MONTHS

1969. William K. Frankenburg, M.D. and Josiah B. Dodds, Ph.D. University of Colorado Medical Center

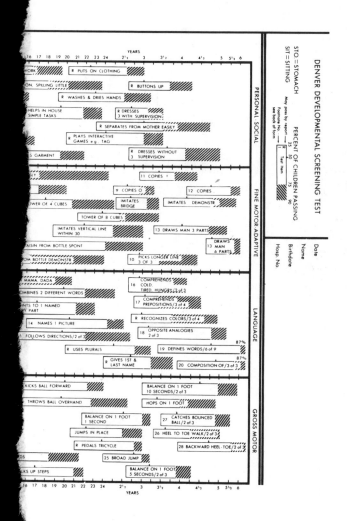

DENVER DEVELOPMENTAL SCREENING TEST

STO = STOMACH
SIT = SITTING

PERCENT OF CHILDREN PASSING
25  50  75  90

May pass by report
Footnote No.
see back of form

R — Test Item

Name
Date
Birthdate
Hosp No

**PERCENT OF CHILDREN PASSING**

YEARS
16 17 18 19 20 21 22 23 24   2½   3   3½   4   4½   5   5½   6

**PERSONAL-SOCIAL**

WORK | R PUTS ON CLOTHING
ON, SPILLING LITTLE | R BUTTONS UP
R WASHES & DRIES HANDS
HELPS IN HOUSE SIMPLE TASKS | R DRESSES 3 WITH SUPERVISION
R SEPARATES FROM MOTHER EASILY
PLAYS INTERACTIVE GAMES e.g. TAG
S GARMENT | R DRESSES WITHOUT 3 SUPERVISION

**FINE MOTOR-ADAPTIVE**

11 COPIES +
9 COPIES O | 12 COPIES
IMITATES BRIDGE | IMITATES DEMONSTR
OWER OF 4 CUBES
TOWER OF 8 CUBES
IMITATES VERTICAL LINE WITHIN 30 | 13 DRAWS MAN 3 PARTS
AISIN FROM BOTTLE SPONT | DRAWS 13 MAN 6 PARTS
ROM BOTTLE DEMONSTR | 10 PICKS LONGER LINE 3 of 3

**LANGUAGE**

MAMA, DADA | 16 COMPREHENDS COLD, TIRED, HUNGRY 2 of 3
OMBINES 2 DIFFERENT WORDS | 17 COMPREHENDS PREPOSITIONS/3 of 4
INTS TO 1 NAMED Y PART | R RECOGNIZES COLORS/3 of 4
14 NAMES 1 PICTURE
FOLLOWS DIRECTIONS/2 of 3 | 18 OPPOSITE ANALOGIES 2 of 3
R USES PLURALS | 19 DEFINES WORDS/6 of 9  87%
GIVES 1ST & LAST NAME | 20 COMPOSITION OF/3 of 3  87%

**GROSS MOTOR**

KICKS BALL FORWARD | BALANCE ON 1 FOOT 10 SECONDS/2 of 3
THROWS BALL OVERHAND | HOPS ON 1 FOOT
BALANCE ON 1 FOOT 1 SECOND | 27 CATCHES BOUNCED BALL/2 of 3
JUMPS IN PLACE | 26 HEEL TO TOE WALK/2 of 3
R PEDALS TRICYCLE | 28 BACKWARD HEEL-TOE/2 of 3
DS | 25 BROAD JUMP
ALKS UP STEPS | BALANCE ON 1 FOOT 5 SECONDS/2 of 3

YEARS
16 17 18 19 20 21 22 23 24   2½   3   3½   4   4½   5   5½   6

112

DATE

NAME

BIRTHDATE

HOSP. NO.

DIRECTIONS

1. Try to get child to smile by smiling, talking or waving to him. Do not touch him.
2. When child is playing with toy, pull it away from him. Pass if he resists.
3. Child does not have to be able to tie shoes or button in the back.
4. Move yarn slowly in an arc from one side to the other, about 6" above child's face.
   Pass if eyes follow 90° to midline. (Past midline; 180°)
5. Pass if child grasps rattle when it is touched to the backs or tips of fingers.
6. Pass if child continues to look where yarn disappeared or tries to see where it went. Yarn should be dropped quickly from sight from tester's hand without arm movement.
7. Pass if child picks up raisin with any part of thumb and a finger.
8. Pass if child picks up raisin with the ends of thumb and index finger using an over hand approach.

9. Pass any enclosed form. Fail continuous round motions.

10. Which line is longer? (Not bigger.) Turn paper upside down and repeat. (3/3 or 5/6)

11. Pass any crossing lines.

12. Have child copy first. If failed, demonstrate.

When giving items 9, 11 and 12, do not name the forms. Do not demonstrate 9 and 11.

13. When scoring, each pair (2 arms, 2 legs, etc.) counts as one part.

V. Primitive Reflexes

These are conveniently divided into:

a) intrauterine/birth reflexes: appear late in gestation, are present at birth, and are suppressed by 6 months

b) late infant reflexes: appear following suppression of the birth reflexes. These are the postural reactions which precede voluntary motor function.

| Reflex | Present by (months) | Gone by (months) |
|---|---|---|
| **A. Intrauterine - Birth Reflexes:** | | |
| Palmar grasp | birth | 4 |
| Plantar grasp | birth | 9 |
| Automatic stepping | birth | 2 |
| Crossed extension | birth | 2 |
| Galant | birth | 2 |
| Moro | birth | 3-6 |
| Tonic neck - asymmetric | birth | 4 |
| symmetric | 5 mos | 8 |
| Lower extremity placing | 1 day | – |
| Upper extremity placing | 3 mos | – |
| Downward thrust | 3 mos | – |
| **B. Late Infant Reflexes:** | | |
| Landau | 3 | 12-24 |
| (extension of head, trunk, legs in prone) | | |
| Derotational righting | 4 | – |
| **C. Other Postural Reflexes:** | | |
| Anterior propping | 6 | – |
| Lateral propping | 8 | – |
| Posterior propping | 10 | – |

Adapted in part from: Milani-Comparetti A, Gidoni EA. Dev Med Child Neurol 1967; 9:631; Caldute AJ. Pediatr Ann 1986; 15:217.

# RADIOLOGIC PROCEDURES

1. Protection from Radiation
   In order to avoid inadvertent irradiation of a fetus or
   embryo, elective diagnostic roentgenograms of the abdomen,
   pelvis, hips, and upper thighs of girls who have menstrual
   periods should be made only during the first 10 days of the
   menstrual cycle. This policy does not apply to girls who
   have an intra-uterine device or who have been on birth
   control pills for more than one month. If a girl is or could
   be pregnant, the physician should either: 1) write on the
   requisition that the examination is necessary despite the
   known or possible pregnancy or 2) schedule the examination
   at a later date.

2. Use of Bisacodyl (Dulcolax)

   A. Contraindications
      Acute surgical abdomen, acute ulcerative colitis.

   B. Tablets
      Bisacodyl acts directly on the colonic mucosa to produce
      peristalsis in the colon. It is enteric coated and tablets
      must be swallowed whole; they must not be chewed or
      crushed. Use suppositories unless you are certain that
      the child can swallow the tablets whole. They should
      not be taken within 1 hour of antacids or milk. Dose:
      below 40 kg: 1 tablet h.s.; above 40 kg: 2 tablets h.s.

   C. Suppositories
      May be used at any age; for infants and children under
      10 kg use one-half suppository. If the first suppository
      does not produce a good bowel movement within 45 min-
      utes, administer a second suppository.

3. Sedation
   Patient motion commonly degrades the quality of pediatric
   imaging examinations. Gentle handling and (occasionally)
   physical restraints usually are all that are needed for
   successful studies. Sedation is often required, particularly
   for children under 4 years of age having CT examinations of
   the head and body. Several drug combinations for pediatric
   sedation appear on page 219.

4. X-Ray Examinations

   A. Upper Gastrointestinal Series
      1) Patient <18 months: NPO for 3 hours before the
         study.

    2)    Patient 18 months and older:

        a)    Clear liquids only after supper. No carbonated beverages on day of study.

        b)    Bisacodyl pill(s) or suppositories (see Section 2B) the evening before the examination.

        c)    Nothing by mouth for 4 hours before the examination.

B.   Contrast Enema

   1)    Infants <18 months: Liquid diet starting evening before the study. No carbonated beverages.

   2)    18 months and older

        a)    Liquid diet for 24 hours before study. No carbonated beverages.

     *b)    Bisacodyl pill(s) or suppository (see Section 2B) the evening before the examination.

     *c)    Bisacodyl suppository the morning of the study.

     *d)    Patients 10 years and older: lukewarm tap water enemas until clear the morning of the examination.

*Omit steps b, c, and d when evaluation is for active colitis, acute surgical abdomen, or possible Hirschsprung disease.

   3)    Air contrast barium enema (over 18 months of age)

        a)    Clear liquid diet 24 hours before study. No carbonated beverages.

        b)    Bisacodyl pill(s) or suppository (see Section 2B) the evening before the examination.

        c)    Lukewarm tap water enemas until clear-- i.e., no stool in the water. This usually takes 2 enemas.

        d)    Bisacodyl enema (Fleet Bisacodyl Prep) will be given in radiology 1 hour before the examination.

C.   Intravenous Urogram (IVP)

(Note: An ultrasound exam of the kidneys frequently can substitute for an IVP.)

All patients should be normally hydrated, but have an empty stomach. Notation must be made on requisition of previous drug reactions and allergies. The examination usually will not be done if the child has a history of allergy to iodine or a previous severe reaction to a contrast agent. The hospital requires that one of the child's parents or the legal guardian reads and signs the special consent form for administration of intravenous contrast agents.

    1)    Infants <18 months should be kept NPO before the exam for the same length of time as the usual interval between feedings.

    2)    18 months or older:

        a)    Bisacodyl pill(s) or suppository (see Section 2B) the night before the examination.

        b)    Nothing by mouth 4 hours before examination.

D.    <u>Voiding Cystourethrogram</u> (VCUG)
No preparation is required.

E.    <u>Gallbladder</u>

    1)    The first examination should be with ultrasound.

    2)    In those rare cases when a cholecystogram is indicated, consult a pediatric radiologist for special instructions.

[The pediatric dose of ipodate (Orografin) is 0.5 gm (one tablet) for each 10 kg of body weight, not to exceed 3.0 gm (six tablets). <u>Never administer more than the recommended dose</u>. If a repeat dose is given within 48 hours, use only 1/2 the above dose. <u>Contraindications</u>: renal or hepatic failure.]

F.    <u>Head and Body Computed Tomography</u> (CT)

    1)    Oral and/or intravenous contrast agents may be necessary, depending upon the specific examination and the information required. (Only intravenous contrast for Head CT scans). No intravenous contrast is given if there is an allergy to iodine or history of severe reaction to a contrast agent. The hospital requires that a special consent form for administration of intravenous contrast agents be signed by one parent or the legal guardian.

    2)    Infants should be kept NPO 3 to 4 hours if possible. The meal before the exam should be held for all children.

5.    <u>Ultrasound Examination</u>

A.    <u>Important Note</u>
Sound waves do not penetrate bone, gas, or barium. Thus, sonograms should be obtained before any barium contrast studies.

B.    <u>Preparation</u>

    1)    Pelvis and lower abdomen:
Full bladder necessary. Patients should be well hydrated with oral or intravenous fluids and should not void (if possible) for 1-3 hours before exam.

    2)    Liver, gallbladder, and biliary tree:
        a)    Infants: NPO 3-4 hours (if possible) before exam.
        b)    Children: NPO 6-12 hours before exam.

6. Nuclear Medicine Examinations

The general rules about radiation protection stated in section 1 apply for all nuclear studies.

Most procedures do not require patient preparation. Consultation with the nuclear medicine physician is encouraged before a study is performed or ordered. Selected studies are discussed below:

A. Bone Imaging

This study is typically positive for osteomyelitis before radiographic changes become evident. A flow study should be ordered for suspected infection. Bone scans are sensitive for metastatic disease. Bone scanning is performed with Technetium (Tc99m) methylene diphosphonate (MDP) while bone marrow imaging uses Tc99m sulfur colloid. See note under Gallium-67 Imaging below.

B. Gallium - 67 Imaging

Gallium-67 is very useful for detecting occult abscesses and tumors in children. This is mediated via binding to transferrin, lactoferrin and intracellular lysosomes. Because Gallium-67 is excreted in part through the colon, a standard barium enema preparation regimen (see Section 4B) should be given with a tap water enema just before sending the patient to nuclear medicine. It is not necessary to keep children NPO. Images are usually obtained at 24, 48, and 72 or 96 hours after injection.
NOTE: Gallium interferes with the detection of technetium for as long as 2 weeks. When both technetium and gallium scans are indicated, perform the technetium scan first (injections for the 2 scans may be made on the same day).

C. Cerebral Imaging

    1)    Early encephalitis, especially herpes simplex, may be discovered by brain scan well before abnormalities can be detected by CT.
    2)    Brain death. Cerebral flow imaging may be helpful in assessing the presence or absence of cerebral perfusion.

D. GI Studies

    1)    Acutely traumatized child: Liver-spleen scans to detect hematomas or lacerations.
    2)    Gastroesophageal reflux.
    3)    Hepatobiliary function - using 99mTc-IDA.

4) Biliary atresia.
5) Meckel's scans: Do before barium studies, since barium interferes with the study.

E. GU Studies
   1) DTPA for renal function and GFR determinations.
   2) DMSA provides evaluation of relative cortical function and added information about renal structure.
   3) Glucoheptonate is an alternate renal radiotracer.
   4) Scrotal imaging is an excellent tool for differentiating testicular torsion from epididymitis.

F. Nuclear Cardiology
   Thallium (perfusion) and gated blood pool studies (MUGA) for ventricular function are the studies performed in young patients. The latter may be useful in following oncology patients receiving cardiotoxic drugs or the evaluation of congenital heart disease. In addition, lung scans may be used to evaluate lung perfusion and the patency of surgically created shunts in patients with congenital heart disease.

G. Miscellaneous Studies and Considerations
   Nuclear medicine is well suited to follow pathophysiological processes; WBC studies for infection, MIBG for pheochromocytoma, PET scanning for CNS problems. Again, consultation should be sought with a Nuclear Medicine physician for appropriate studies.

   Ref: Kirchner PT (ed.). In: Nuclear Medicine Review Syllabus. Society of Nuclear Medicine, New York, 1980.

7. Recommendations for Specific X-ray Procedures

   A. Comparison Radiographs of Limbs
      Comparison views of the normal limb are valuable for:
      1) Suspected osteomyelitis or pyarthrosis.
      2) Suspected knee or ankle effusion.
      3) Possible elbow fracture. A relative large number of ossification centers appear at various times, which may be confusing.
      4) Occasionally helpful to identify or rule out subtle fractures in other sites.

      Ref: Merten DF, et al. Pediatrics 1980; 65:646.

   B. Magnetic Resonance Imaging (MRI)

      Like ultrasonography, MRI does not utilize ionizing radiation. This technique is still in a formative stage; however, MRI is being used to evaluate the following areas:

1) CNS - MRI is better than CT scanning for evaluating the posterior fossa, brainstem, and spinal cord. It is also excellent at evaluating demyelinating disorders because of its ability to differentiate between white and gray matter. MRI, however, does not reveal calcifications which are characteristic in some neoplasms.

2) MEDIASTINUM - MRI is more sensitive than CT for evaluating mediastinal lymphadenopathy.

3) CARDIAC - Flowing blood does not produce a magnetic signal. Thus, MRI provides excellent contrast between blood and myocardium.

4) SKELETAL - MRI is useful in evaluating avascular necrosis of the femoral head and in detecting early signs of osteomyelitis. MRI can also detect extension of bone tumors and marrow replacement by leukemic infiltrates.

NOTE: The magnetic field of the MRI interferes with ferromagnetic devices: ventilators cannot be used in the MRI room, and patients with pacemakers or recently implanted surgical clips should be excluded. Nonetheless, most surgical implantable hardware or prosthetic devices are non-ferrous. Thus, containment of such objects in a patient should not be a contraindication for a MRI scan. If there are doubts, consultation should be sought from a knowledgeable radiologist.

Ref: Kulkarni MV, et al. Pediatr Clin North Am 1985; 32:1509.

PART II

FORMULARY

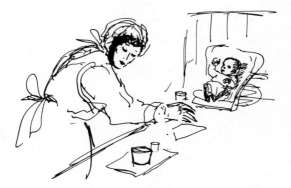

aaron sophen

## DRUG INDEX

DRUG DOSES

| DRUG | HOW SUPPLIED | DOSE AND ROUTE | REMARKS |
|---|---|---|---|
| Acetaminophen (Many trade names) | Tabs: 80, 325, 500<br>Syrup: 160 mg/5 ml<br>Supp: 120, 125, 130, 300, 325, 500, 600, 650 mg<br>Drops: 80 mg/0.8 ml<br>Elixir: 160 mg/5 ml<br>Liquid: 50 mg/15 ml | 0-3mo: 40 mg/dose<br>4-11mo: 80 mg/dose<br>12-24mo: 120 mg/dose<br>2-3yr: 160 mg/dose<br>4-5yr: 240 mg/dose<br>6-8yr: 320 mg/dose<br>9-10yr: 400 mg/dose<br>11-12yr: 480 mg/dose<br>Alternate: 5-10 mg/kg/dose give 4-5 x daily<br>Adult: 300-650 mg Q4h<br>Max. dose: 1000 mg QID | T1/2 - 1-3 hrs. Contraindicated in patients with known G6PD deficiency. Overdose may cause hepatotoxicity, often delayed. See p 247 for management of acetaminophen toxicity. |
| Acetazolamide (Diamox) | Tabs: 125, 250 mg<br>Vials (sodium): 500 mg/5 ml<br>Caps (Sustained Release): 500 mg | Diuretic:<br>Child: 5 mg/kg/dose QD-QOD (PO or IV)<br>Adult: 250-375 mg/dose QD-QOD (PO or IV)<br>Glaucoma:<br>Child: 20-40 mg/kg/day÷Q6h IM or IV; 8-30 mg/kg/day ÷Q6-8h PO.<br>Adult: 1000 mg/day÷Q6h PO; for rapid decrease in pressure give 500 mg/dose IV.<br>Seizures: 8-30 mg/kg/day÷Q6-12h PO. Max: 1 gm/day÷Q6-12h PO.<br>Medical Management of Hydrocephalus: see p 266. | Renal excretion. T1/2 is 4-10h. Paresthesias, polyuria, drowsiness, gastrointestinal irritation (vomiting, diarrhea), transient hypokalemia, reduced urate excretion, and acidosis may occur with long-term therapy; alkalinize urine. IM injection may be painful and should be avoided. |

129

| | | | |
|---|---|---|---|
| Acetylcysteine (Mucomyst) | Vials: (10% or 20%) 4 ml, 10 ml, 30 ml | Nebulizer: 3-5 ml of 20% solution (diluted with equal vol. of $H_2O$ or sterile saline), or 6-10 ml of 10% solution. Administer TID-QID<br>Meconium ileus:<br>5-30 ml given 3-6x/day PO or PR. Usual dose: 10 ml QID<br>For acetaminophen poisoning: See p 247. | May induce bronchospasm, stomatitis, rhinorrhea, and nausea. |
| ACTH (Corticotropin, Acthar) | 1 unit = 1 mg<br>Aqueous (Injection): 25, 40 U/vial<br>Gel: 40, 80 U/ml (1 & 5 ml vials) | Aqueous: 1.6 U/kg/day IV, IM, or SC Q6-8h<br>Gel: 0.8 U/kg/day Q12-24h<br>Infantile spasms: Many regimens exist.<br>Gel: 25-80 U/day (usually 40 U/day) IM or Q24-72h. Gradually taper after 4 wks. | Contraindicated in acute psychoses, CHF, Cushing's disease, Tb, peptic ulcer, ocular herpes, fungal infections, recent surgery, sensitivity to pork. IV administration for diagnostic purposes only. |
| Acyclovir | Vial: 500 mg/10 ml<br>Ointment: 5% (15 gm)<br>Capsules: 200 mg | Herpes simplex virus:<br>Newborns: 30 mg/kg/day÷Q8h IV<br>Children (<12 yrs): 750 mg/$M^2$/day÷Q8h IV; give over one hour.<br>Adults: 15 mg/kg/day÷Q8h IV; give over one hour.<br>Genital HSV: 200 mg PO Q4h x5 doses/day. Treat 10 days for initial genital HSV infection, 5 days for recurrences.<br>Suppression: 200 mg PO TID for max. 6 months<br>Varicella Zoster: 1500 mg/$M^2$/day÷Q8h IV. | Can cause renal impairment; adequate hydration essential to prevent renal tubular crystallization. Encephalopathic reactions have been reported. Dose alterations necessary in preterm infants and in patients with reduced creatinine clearance. |

| Drug | Supply | Dose | Comments |
|---|---|---|---|
| Albumin, human serum (normal serum albumin) | Injection (vials): 5% (5 gm/dl; 180 mEq Na/L); 25% (25 gm/dl; 150 mEq Na/L) 5%: 20, 50, 100 ml bottles 25%: 50, 250, 500 ml bottles | Hypoproteinemia: 0.5-1 gm/kg/ dose IV. Repeat Q1-2 days as calculated to replace on-going losses. Hypovolemia: 0.5-1 gm/kg/dose IV, repeated PRN, Max. dose: 6 gm/kg/day | Contraindicated in severe anemia or CHF. Use with caution in hypervolemia. Allergic reactions are unusual but may occur. Caution: 25% concentration contraindicated in preterm infants due to risk of IVH. |
| Albuterol (Proventil, Ventolin) | Tabs: 2, 4 mg Aerosol inhaler: 90 mcg/dose 200 doses/inhaler Elixir: 2 mg/5 ml Solution for nebulization: 5 mg/ml (Also available in unit doses of 2.5 mg in 3 ml of NS) | Children: 2-5 yr: 0.1 mg/kg/ dose÷Q8h PO up to 12 mg/day 6-11 yr: 2 mg/dose PO TID or Max. dose: 24 mg/day > 12 yrs and adults: Initial: 2-4 mg/dose PO TID or QID Max. dose: 8 mg PO QID Inhalations: 1-2 puffs Q4-6h Nebulization: 0.01-0.03 ml/kg (1 ml max.) in 2 cc NS TID-QID | May cause tachycardia, tremor, nervousness, GI symptoms, and headaches. |
| Allopurinol (Zyloprim) | Tabs: 100, 300 mg | <6 yr: 150 mg/day÷Q8h 6-10yr: 300 mg/day÷Q8h >10yr: 100-200 mg/day÷Q8h Alternative: 10 mg/kg/day ÷Q8h. Max. dose: 800 mg/day | Maintain alkaline urine flow. Decrease dosage with renal insufficiency. Rash, neuritis, hepatotoxicity and GI disturbances may occur. Follow serum uric acid levels. |

| | | | |
|---|---|---|---|
| Aluminum Hydroxide (AmphoJel AlternaGel) (and many other brands) | Caps: 475, 500 mg Gel susp.: 320 mg/5 ml (360 ml bottle) Tablets: 300, 600 mg Gel liquid: 600 mg/5 ml (150, 360 ml bottle) | Peptic Ulcer: Child: 5-12 ml PO Q3-6h or 1 and 3h PC and HS Adult: 15-45 ml PO Q3-6h or 1 and 3h PC and HS Prophylaxis of GI Bleeding: Infant: 2-5 ml/dose Q1-2h per NG tube Child: 5-12 ml/dose Q1-2h per NG tube Adult: 30-60 ml/dose Q1h per NG tube Hyperphosphatemia: 50-150 mg/kg/day÷Q4-6h | May cause constipation, phosphorus depletion. Inhibits gastric emptying. Interferes with absorption of several drugs. 10 ml neutralizes 13 mEq acid. 5 ml contains <0.3 mEq Na. Titrate dose to desired clinical response. |
| Aluminum Hydroxide with magnesium hydroxide (Maalox and many other brands with varying concentration) | Tabs: 400, 800 mg Susp: 180, 360 ml bottles | Same as for $Al(OH)_3$ | Limit to 80 ml suspension daily. 5 ml ≈ 400 mg tab. Magnesium containing antacids have a laxative effect. May cause hypokalemia. Use with caution in renal failure. |

| | | | |
|---|---|---|---|
| Amantadine (Symmetrel) | Cap: 100 mg<br>Susp: 50 mg/5 ml | <u>Children:</u><br>1-9 yrs: 4-8 mg/kg/day÷BID or TID. Do not exceed 150 mg/day<br>9-12 yrs: 200 mg/day÷Q12h<br>Adults: 200 mg/day÷QD or BID<br>Prophylaxis - continue until 90 days past exposure; for continuing exposure give Influenza A vaccine and continue for 2-3 wks. If vaccine not available continue for 90 days.<br>Symptomatic - continue for 24-48 hrs after disappearance of symptoms. | May cause depression, CHF, orthostatic hypotension, and urinary retention. Adjust dose in renal failure. |
| Amikacin Sulfate (Amikin) | Injection: 50 mg/ml (2 ml vial); 250 mg/ml (2, 4 ml vials) | Neonates:<br><7 days:<br><28 wks: 7.5 mg/kg/dose Q24h<br>28-34 wks: 7.5 mg/kg/dose Q18h<br>term: 7.5 mg/kg/dose Q12h<br>>7 days:<br><28 wks: 7.5 mg/kg/dose Q18h<br>28-34 wks: 7.5 mg/kg/dose Q12h<br>term: 7.5 mg/kg/dose Q8h<br>Children and Adults: 15 mg/kg/day ÷ Q8h.<br>Max. dose: 1.5 gm/day<br>Infusion rate:<br>Infant: 1-2 h<br>Children and Adults: 30-60 min | Ototoxicity, nephrotoxicity, rash, fever, eosinophilia, and headache may occur. Monitor levels. Therapeutic levels: peaks between 25-30 mg/L; troughs 5-8 mg/L. Adjust dose with renal impairment. |

| | | |
|---|---|---|
| Aminocaproic acid (Amicar) | Injection: 250 mg/ml<br>Tablets: 500 mg<br>Syrup: 250 mg/ml | IV: 100 mg/kg (or 3 gm/M²<br>x 1 hr) then 1 gm/M²/hr.<br>Max: 18 gm/M²/day<br>PO: 100 mg/kg/dose÷Q6-8h | Inhibits fibrinolysis via<br>inhibition of plasminogen<br>activators and antiplasmin<br>activity. Hypercoagulation<br>may be produced when given<br>in conjunction with oral<br>contraceptives. May cause<br>nausea, diarrhea, malaise,<br>weakness. |
| Aminophylline | Injection (IV):<br>25 mg/ml (79%<br>theophylline)<br>Liquid (oral): 105<br>mg/5 ml (Somophyllin)<br>(86% theophylline)<br>Tablets: 100, 200 mg<br>(79% theophylline) | Loading: 6 mg/kg IV over<br>20 min. (each 1 mg/kg dose<br>raises the serum theophylline<br>concentration 2 mg/L)<br>Maintenance (continuous IV drip):<br>0.2 mg/kg/hr<br>Neonates: 0.2 mg/kg/hr<br>1mo-1yr: 0.2-0.9 mg/kg/hr<br>1-9 yr: 1.0 mg/kg/hr<br>9-16 yr and young adult<br>smokers: 0.8 mg/kg/hr<br>Adults, non-smokers:<br>0.5 mg/kg/hr.<br>PO: Infants: see theophylline<br>1-9 yrs: 20 mg/kg/day÷Q6h<br>9-16 yrs: 16 mg/kg/day÷Q6h<br>Adults: 12 mg/kg/day÷Q6h | Monitoring serum levels is<br>essential especially in in-<br>fants and young children.<br>Side effects: restlessness,<br>GI upset, arrhythmias. See<br>Theophylline preparations,<br>page 215.<br>Therapeutic level: for<br>asthma, 10-20 mg/L; for<br>neonatal apnea, 6-13 mg/L. |

| Drug | Forms | Dosage | Comments |
|---|---|---|---|
| Amiodarone HCl (Cordarone) | Tabs: 200 mg | Children*: 10 mg/kg/day÷Q12h PO x 7-10 days then reduce to 5 mg/kg/day if effective. Max. dose: 15 mg/kg/day for 3-4 weeks. Adults: Loading dose: 800-1600 mg/day for 1-3 weeks Maintenance: 600-800 mg/day x 1 month - then 200-400 gm/day * Not FDA approved for children. | Long half life. Inhibits alpha and beta receptors. Asymptomatic corneal micro-deposits. Alters hepatic enzymes, thyroid function. Pulmonary fibrosis has been reported in adults. May cause worsening of pre-existing arrhythmias with bradycardia and AV block. Anorexia, nausea, vomiting, dizziness, paresthesias. Increases digoxin and quinidine levels. |
| Ammonium Chloride | Tabs: 300, 500 mg; 1 gm Caps: 300, 500 mg Solns./Syrup: 500 mg/5 ml Injection: 0.4 mEq/ml (2.14%); 4.0 mEq/ml (21.4%); 5.0 mEq/ml (26.75%) | Urinary acidification: Child: 75 mg/kg/dose Q6h PO or IV. Max. dose: 2-6 gm/day Adult: 1.5 gm/dose IV Q6h. Max. dose: 6 gm/day IV or 8-12 gm/day PO (QID) Injection: Dilute to concen-tration not >0.4 mEq/ml. Infusion not to exceed 50 mg/kg/hr or 1 mEq/kg/hr | May produce acidosis; do not use in hepatic or renal insuf-ficiency; use with caution in infants. May cause GI irri-tation. |
| Amoxicillin (Amoxil, Larotid, Amoxil, Wymox, Trimox, Utimox, Amcill) | Chewable tabs: 125 mg Caps: 250, 500 mg Drops: 50 mg/ml (15 ml) Susp: 125, 250 mg/5 ml (80, 100, 150 ml) | Child: 20-40 mg/kg/day÷Q8h PO Adult: 250-500 mg/dose÷Q8h PO Gonorrhea (acute uncomplicated): 3 gm as single PO dose with 1 gm probenicid | Renal elimination. Achieves serum levels about twice those achieved with equal dose of ampicillin. Less GI effects, but otherwise similar to ampicillin. |

| | | |
|---|---|---|
| Amoxicillin - clavulanic acid (Augmentin) | Susp: 125 and 250 mg/ 5 ml (31.25 and 62.5 mg clavulanate) Tabs: 125 & 250 mg chewable | Child: 20-40 mg/kg/day as amoxicillin÷Q8h PO Adult: 250-500 mg/dose Q8h PO | Beta lactamase inhibitor extends the activity of amoxicillin to include beta-lactamase producing strains of H. Flu, B. catarrhalis, some S. aureus. Causes more diarrhea than amoxicillin. |
| Amphotericin B (Fungizone) | Injection: 50 mg vials Cream: 3% Lotion: 3% | Topical: apply BID-QID IV: (mix with D5W to concentration 0.1 mg/ml, pH >4.2) Infuse over 6-12 hr Test dose: 0.1 mg/kg/day IV up to max. 1 mg/dose. Initial dose: 0.25 mg/kg/day Increase to 1 mg/kg/day as tolerated by increments of 0.125-0.25 mg/kg/daily or QOD. Max. dose: 1.5 mg/kg/day. Alternate day dose: 1.5 mg/kg/ day QOD | Fever, chills, nausea, vomiting are common side effects. May premedicate with acetaminophen and diphenhydramine 30 min before and 4 hrs after infusion. Hydrocortisone 10-20 mg added to bottle also helps prevent immediate adverse reactions. Monitor renal, hepatic, electrolyte, and hematologic status closely. Hypercalciuria, RTA, renal failure, acute hepatic failure, and phlebitis may occur. |

| Ampicillin (Omnipen, Polycillin, Principen) | Caps: 250, 500 mg; Injection: 125, 250, 500 mg; 1, 2, 4 gm; Drops: 100 mg/ml; Susp: 125, 250 mg and 500 mg/5 ml | Neonates:<br>_<7 days:_ 50-100 mg/kg/day ÷ Q12h IM or IV<br>_>7 days:_ 100-200 mg/kg/day ÷ Q8h IM or IV<br>Mild-moderate infections:<br>50-100 mg/kg/day ÷ Q6h PO, IM, or IV (max: 2-4 gm/day)<br>Severe infections:<br>200-400 mg/kg/day ÷ Q4-6h IM or IV (max: 12 gm/day)<br>Uncomplicated gonorrhea:<br>3.5 gm PO with 1 gm probenicid PO. | Same side effects as penicillin, with cross-reactivity. Rash commonly seen at 5-10 days. May cause interstitial nephritis. |
|---|---|---|---|
| Aspirin (ASA) | Tabs: 65, 75, 200, 300, 325, 500, 600, 650 mg; Tabs (chewable): 65, 81 mg; Caps: 325 mg; Supp: 60, 65, 130, 150, 195, 200, 300, 325, 600 mg and 1.2 gm | Antipyretic: 10-15 mg/kg/dose Q4h up to total 60-80 mg/kg/day (max. dose: 3.6 gm/day) Q4h<br>Antirheumatic: 100 mg/kg/day PO÷Q4h | Use with caution in platelet and bleeding disorders. Follow serum levels when used as antirheumatic. May cause GI upset, allergic reactions, hepatotoxicity. For management of overdose see p 245.<br>Therapeutic levels:<br>20-100 mg/L antipyretic/analgesic<br>100-300 mg/L antiinflammatory |

| | | | |
|---|---|---|---|
| Atropine Sulfate | Tabs: 0.3, 0.4, 0.6 mg<br>Injection: 0.1, 0.3, 0.4, 0.5, 0.6, 0.8, 1.0, 1.2, 2 mg/ml<br>Vials: 0.3, 0.4, 0.5, 0.6, 1.0 mg/ml | General dose recommendation:<br>Child: 0.01 mg/kg/dose PO, SC, IV (max: 0.4 mg/dose); may repeat Q4-6h<br>Adult: 0.5 mg/dose<br>Cardiopulmonary resuscitation:<br>0.01-0.03 mg/kg/dose IV Q2-5 min. x 2-3 PRN. Min. dose: 0.1 mg. Max. dose: 1.0 mg for children and 2.0 mg/dose for adults.<br>Nebulized: 0.05 mg/kg/dose in 2.5 ml NSS (min: 0.25 mg; max: 1 mg) | Dry mouth, blurred vision, fever, tachycardia, constipation, urinary retention, CNS signs (dizziness, hallucinations, restlessness). Contraindicated in glaucoma. Caution with use in asthma. May give via endotracheal tube. |
| Beclomethasone (Vanceril, Beclovent) | Aerosol: 17 gm dispenser,200 metered doses; 42 mcg/dose | Inhalant:<br>6-12 yr: 1-2 inhalations Q6-8h; max: 10 inhalations/day<br>>12 yr: 2 inhalations Q6-8h; max: 20 inhalations/day<br>(1 inhalation = 42 mcg) | Rinse mouth and gargle with water after inhalation; may cause thrush. No systemic affects with doses <1 mg/day. Wean cautiously off steroids once inhalant is used. Not recommended for children <6 yrs. |
| Bethanechol (Urecholine and other brand names) | Tabs: 5, 10, 25, 50 mg<br>Injection: 5 mg/ml | Oral: 0.6 mg/kg/day ÷ Q6-8h PO<br>SC: Use 1/3-1/4 of oral dose<br>For gastroesophageal reflux:<br>2.9 mg/M²/dose Q8h PO<br>Adults: 10-50 mg PO Q6-12h | Contraindicated in asthma, GI, or GU obstruction, peptic ulcer. May cause hypotension, nausea, bronchospasm, salivation, flushing. Atropine is antidote. |
| Bisacodyl (Dulcolax and various other names) | Tabs: 5 mg<br>Supp: 10 mg | Oral: 0.3 mg/kg/dose, 6h before desired effect.<br>Adult: 10-15 mg<br>Rectal:<br><2 yr: 5 mg<br>>2 yr: 10 mg; usually effective within 15-60 min. | Do not chew tablets; do not give within 1 hr of antacids or milk. |

| Drug | Preparation | Dosage | Comments |
|------|-------------|--------|----------|
| Bretylium (Bretylol) | Amp: 50 mg/ml | Not approved for children. >12 yr: 5-10 mg/kg/dose IV over 10-30 min. 5-10 mg/kg/dose Q1-2h IM OR IV if arrhythmia persists on maintenance dose. Maintenance dose: 5-10 mg/kg/dose. Infuse over 10 min Q6h or constant infusion of 1 - 2 mg/min. | For treatment of life-threatening ventricular arrhythmias. Often causes hypotension. May cause transient hypertension or PVC. Adjust dose in renal failure. May be useful in ventricular fibrillation unresponsive to standard therapy. |
| Calcitriol (1,25-dihydroxy-cholecalciferol, Rocaltrol) | Caps: 0.25, 0.50 μg | Children: Dose not established; suggested doses range 0.01-0.05 mcg/kg/day; some with hepatic osteodystrophy may require more. Titrate increments Q2-4 wks based on clinical response. Adults: Initial: 0.25 mcg/day Increment: 0.25 mcg/day Q2-4 wks | Most potent vitamin D metabolite available. Monitor serum calcium and phosphorus. Avoid concomitant use of Mg-containing antacids. Discontinue if hypercalcemia occurs. |
| Calcium chloride (27% calcium) | Solution: 100 mg/ml (10%) (1.36 mEq Ca++/ml); 13.6 mEq Ca++/gm salt (73 mg salt/mEq Ca++) | Infant/Child: 200-300 mg/kg/day PO as 2% soln ÷ Q6h Adult: 4-8 gm/day PO QID For Cardiac Arrest: Infant/Child: 20 mg/kg/dose (0.2 ml/kg/dose) IV Q 10 min. Adult: 250-500 mg/dose (2.5-5 ml/dose) IV Q 10 min. Do not exceed 1 ml/min with IV infusion. | May cause GI irritation, phlebitis. Use intravenously with extreme caution. Acidifying effect; give only 2-3 days, then change to another Ca salt. For hyperkalemia, hypocalcemia or hypermagnesemia in arrest setting. |

| Drug | Preparations | Dosage | Remarks |
|---|---|---|---|
| Calcium Glubionate (Neocalglucon) (6% calcium) | Syrup: 1.8 gm/5 ml (5.6 mEq Ca++/5 ml; 115 mg Ca/5 ml) | Maintenance: Infant/Child: 600-2000 mg/kg/day PO QID (max. dose: 9 gm/day) Neonatal hypocalcemia: 1200 mg/kg/day PO Q4-6h Adult: 6-18 gm/day QID | Administer before meals for best absorption. Absorption inhibited by high phosphate load. High osmotic load of syrup (20% sucrose) may cause diarrhea. |
| Calcium Gluconate (9.4% calcium) | Tabs: 500, 650, 1000 mg Solution (10%): 100 mg/ml (0.45 mEq Ca/ml; 224 mg salt/mEq Ca+) | Maintenance: IV: 200-500 mg/kg/day or 100 mg/kg/dose slowly PO: Infants: 400-800 mg/kg/day ÷Q6h Child: 200-500 mg/kg/day ÷Q6h Adult: 5-15 gm/day÷Q6h IV or PO, not IM For Cardiac Arrest: Infants and Children: 100 mg/kg/dose IV Q10 min. Adults: 10 ml/dose IV Q10 min. | If given IV, watch for bradycardia, hypotension, extravasation. May produce arrhythmias in digitalized patients. Precipitates with bicarbonate. Tissue necrosis may result from infiltrates. Do not use scalp veins. |
| Calcium Lactate (13% calcium) | Tabs: 325, 650 mg (6.5 mEq Ca/gm salt; 154 mg salt/mEq Ca++) | Infant/Child: 400-500 mg/kg/day PO÷Q4-8h Adult: 1.5-3 gm PO TID | Give with meals. Tablets do not dissolve in milk. |
| Captopril (Capoten) | Tabs: 12.5, 25, 50, 100 mg | Neonates: 0.1-0.4 mg/kg/dose PO Q6-24h. Infants: 0.5-0.6 mg/kg/day÷Q6-12h PO Children: 25 mg/day÷Q12h. Adolescents and Adults: Initial: 25 mg PO TID and then increase weekly if necessary by 25 mg/dose to max. of 450 mg/day. | Adjust with renal failure. May cause rash, proteinuria, neutropenia, hypotension, or diminution of taste perception. Known to decrease aldosterone and increase renin production. |

| Drug | Supplied | Dosage | Comments |
|---|---|---|---|
| Carbamazepine (Tegretol) | Tabs: 200 mg | Under 6 yrs:<br>Initial: 10 mg/kg/day PO QD or BID or 100 mg/dose BID<br>Increment: up to 20 mg/kg/day<br>6-12 yr old:<br>Initial: 10 mg/kg/day PO QD or BID or 100 mg/dose BID<br>Increment: 100 mg/day at intervals of 1 day (÷ TID or QID) until best response<br>Maintenance: 20-30 mg/kg/day PO TID or QID<br>Max. dose: 1000 mg/day<br>Adolescent & Adult:<br>Initial: 200 mg BID<br>Increment: 200 mg/day at intervals of 1 day using TID or QID schedule until best response.<br>Maintenance: 600-1200 mg/day TID or QID<br>Max. 12-15 yr: 1000 mg/day<br>Adult: 1200 mg/day | Obtain pretreatment CBC. Monitor for hematologic, hepatic toxicity. Many potential side effects, including; neuritis, drowsiness, dizziness, tinnitus, diplopia, urinary retention, nausea.<br>Therapeutic blood levels: 4-12 mg/L. |
| Carbenicillin disodium (Geopen, Pyopen) | Injection: 1, 2, 5, 10 gm vials<br>Tabs: 382 mg | Neonates:<br>Initial: 100 mg/kg/dose<br>Maintenance:<br><2 kg: 225 mg/kg/day÷Q8h x 7 days, then 400 mg/kg/day÷Q6h<br>>2 kg: 300 mg/kg/day x 3 days, then 400 mg/kg/day÷Q6h<br>Parenteral (IM or IV) for Children/Adult: UTI - 50-200 mg/kg/day Q4-6h<br>Severe infection - 400-500 mg/kg/day Q4-6h;<br>Max. dose: 40 gm/day | May cause anaphylaxis, platelet destruction. Unpredictable interaction with gentamicin. Give through separate IV tubing. May lead to urinary K⁺ loss. Adjust dose with renal failure. Use with caution in patients with penicillin allergies. (1 gm carbenicillin = 4.7 mEq Na). |

| Drug | Forms | Dosing | Comments |
|---|---|---|---|
| Cefaclor (Ceclor) (2nd generation) | Caps: 250, 500 mg Susp: 125, 250 mg/ 5 ml in 75 and 150 ml bottles | Infant and Child: 20-40 mg/kg/day÷Q8h PO Max. dose: 1 gm/day Adult: 250-500 mg/dose Q8h PO Max. dose: 4 gm/day | Not recommended for < 1 mo. Use with caution in penicillin allergic patient or in presence of renal impairment. |
| Cefadroxil (Duricef, Ultracef) (2nd generation) | Susp: 125, 250 mg/5ml Caps: 1 gm Tabs: 500 mg | Infant and Child: 30 mg/kg/day ÷Q12h PO Adult: 1-2 gm/day÷Q12-24h PO | See cephalexin. |
| Cefamandole (Mandol) (2nd generation) | Injection: 0.5, 1 2, 10 gm vials | Child: 50-150 mg/kg/day÷Q4-8h IM or IV Adult: 1.5-6 gm/day÷Q4-8h IM or IV Max. dose: 12 gm/day | Not recommended in patients <1 mo. Use with caution in penicillin-allergic patients or in renal impairment. 1 gm cefamandole = 3.3 mEq Na. Associated with hemostatic abnormalities. |
| Cefazolin (Ancef, Kefzol) (1st generation) | Injection: 0.25, 0.5, 1, 5, 10 gm vials | Infant & Child: 25-100 mg/kg/ day÷Q6-8h IV or IM Adult: 750 mg-6 gm/day÷Q6-8h Max. dose: 12 gm/day | See cephalexin. Use with caution in renal impairment or in penicillin-allergic patients. May cause phlebitis, hematologic abnormalities. Not recommended in patients <1 mo. |
| Cefoperazone (Cefobid) (3rd generation) | Injection: 1, 2 gm vials | Infant and Child: 25-100 mg/kg/ day÷Q12h IM or IV Adult: 2-4 gm/day÷Q12h IM or IV Max. dose: 12/gm/day | Use with caution in penicillin allergic patients or in renal failure. |

| Drug | Injection | Dosing | Comments |
|---|---|---|---|
| Cefotaxime (Claforan) (3rd generation) | Injection: 0.5, 1, 2, 10 gm vials | Neonate: 0-1 wk: 50-100 mg/kg/day ÷Q12h IV or IM; 1-4 wk: 75-150 mg/kg/day ÷Q8h IV or IM; Infant and Child: (<50 kg): 50-180 mg/kg/day÷Q4-6h IV or IM. Adult: (>50 kg): 2-12 gm/day ÷Q6-8h IV or IM | Use with caution in penicillin-allergic patients or in presence of renal impairment. |
| Cefoxitin (Mefoxin) (2nd generation) | Injection: 1, 2 gm vials | Infant and Child: 80-160 mg/kg/day÷Q4-6h IM or IV; Adult: 3-8 gm/day÷Q6-8h IM or IV. Max. 12 gm/day | Use with caution in penicillin-allergic patients or in presence of renal impairment. |
| Ceftazidime (Fortaz) (3rd generation) | Injection: .5, 1, 2, 6 gm vials | Neonate: 60 mg/kg/day÷Q12h IV; Infant and Child: 90-150 mg/kg/day÷Q8h IV; CF: 300 mg/kg/day÷Q6h IV; Adult: 2-6 gm/day÷Q8-12h IV/IM | Use with caution in penicillin allergic patients or in presence of renal impairment. |
| Ceftizoxime (Cefizox) (3rd generation) | Injection: 1, 2 gm vials | Infant and Child: 150-200 mg/kg/day÷Q6-8h IV/IM; Adult: 2-12 gm/day÷Q8-12h IV. Max. dose: 12 gm/day | Use with caution in penicillin allergic patients or in presence of renal impairment. |
| Ceftriaxone (Rocephin) (3rd generation) | Injection: .25, .5, 1, 2, 10 gm vials | Infant and Child: 50 mg/kg/day ÷Q24h IM or IV; Meningitis: 75 mg/kg/dose x 1 then 100 mg/kg/day÷Q12h IV; N. gonorrhea: 125 mg/dose x 1; Adult: 1-2 gm/day÷Q12h IV or IM; Max. dose: 4 gm/day; N. gonorrhea: 250 mg/dose x 1 | Use with caution in penicillin allergic patients or in presence of renal impairment. |

| | | | |
|---|---|---|---|
| Cefuroxime (Zinacef)<br><br>(2nd generation) | Injection: 750 mg and 1.5 gm vials | Neonates: 10 mg/kg/day÷Q12h IM IV<br>Infants and Child: 50-100 mg/kg/day÷Q6-8h IV or IM<br>Meningitis: 200-240 mg/kg/day ÷Q6-8h IV<br>Adults: 2.5-4.5 gm/day IM or IV Q8h<br>Max: 9 gm/day | Use with caution in penicillin-allergic patients or in presence of renal impairment. |
| Cephalexin (Keflex)<br><br>(1st generation) | Tabs: 1000 mg<br>Caps: 250, 500 mg<br>Susp: 125, 250 mg/5 ml<br>Drops: 100 mg/ml | Infant and Child: 25-100 mg/kg/day÷Q6-12h PO<br>Adult: 1 gm/day÷Q6-12h PO<br>Max. dose: 4 gm/day | Some cross-reactivity with penicillins. GI disturbance frequent. Use with caution in renal insufficiency. |
| Cephalothin (Keflin)<br><br>(1st generation) | Injection: 1, 2 gm vials | Infant and Child: 80-160 mg/kg/day÷Q4-6h IV or deep IM<br>Max. dose: 12 gm/day<br>Adults: 2-6 gm/day÷Q4-6h | See cephalexin. May cause phlebitis. |
| Cephradine (Velosef, Anspor)<br><br>(1st generation) | Susp: 125 and 250 mg/5 ml<br>Caps: 250 and 500 mg<br>Injection: 0.25, 0.5, 1, 2, 4 gm vials | Child: PO: 25-100 mg/kg/day ÷Q6-12h<br>IM or IV: 50-100 mg/kg/day÷Q6h<br>Adult: PO: 1 gm/day÷Q6-12h<br>IV: 2-4 gm/day÷Q6h<br>Max. dose: 8 gm/day | See cephalexin. |
| Charcoal activated | See p 243. | | |

| | | | |
|---|---|---|---|
| Chloral Hydrate (Noctec, Aqua-choral) | Caps: 250, 500 mg/ Syrup: 250, 500 mg/ 5 ml Supp: 325, 500, 650 mg | Children: Sedative: 25 mg/kg/dose Q8h PO or rectally Hypnotic: 50-75 mg/kg/dose PO or rectally Adult: Sedative: 250 mg/dose TID PO or rectally Hypnotic: 500 mg to 2 gm/dose PO or rectally | Irritating to mucous membranes; may cause laryngospasm if aspirated. Avoid large doses in severe cardiac disease. GI irritation. Contraindicated in hepatic or renal impairment. Caution in conjunction with furosemide and anticoagulants. |
| Chloramphenicol (Chloromycetin) | Caps: 250 mg Susp: 150 mg/5 ml Vials: 1 gm (100 mg/ml) Otic soln: 0.5% Ophthal soln: 0.16, 0.25, 0.5% Ophthal ointment: 1% Topical cream: 1% | Loading dose (all ages): 20 mg/kg IV or PO Maintenance: <7 days: 10 mg/kg/day÷Q12-24h 1-3 wks: 20 mg/kg/day÷Q8-12h >3 wks: 30 mg/kg/day÷Q6-12h Infants, children, adults: 50-100 mg/kg/day÷Q6h IV or PO *NOTE: Initiate maintenance therapy for neonates<7 days of age at 24 hrs after loading dose. Max. dose: 2 gm/day | Dose recommendations are guidelines for therapy; monitoring of blood levels is essential in neonates and infants. Drug is poorly absorbed IM. Follow hematologic status for dose-related or idiosyncratic marrow suppression. Check levels in face of hepatic or renal dysfunction. Concomitant administration of rifampin may lower serum levels. Therapeutic levels: 15-20 mg/L. |
| Chlorothiazide (Diuril) | Tabs: 250, 500 mg Susp: 250 mg/5 ml Vials: 500 mg (20 ml) | <6 mos: 20-30 mg/kg/day÷Q12h PO >6 mos: 20 mg/kg/day÷Q12h PO Adults: 250-500 mg/dose QD or intermittently. Max. dose: 2 gm/day | Use with caution in liver and severe renal disease. May cause hyperbilirubinemia, hypokalemia, alkalosis, hyperglycemia, hyperuricemia. |

| Drug | Preparations | Dosage | Comments |
|---|---|---|---|
| Chlorpheniramine Maleate (various trade names) | Injection: 10mg/ml<br>Tablets: 4 mg<br>Timed release capsules and tablets 8, 12 mg<br>Syrup: 2 mg/5ml | 2-6 yrs: 1 mg/dose Q4-6h PO<br>6-12 yrs: 2 mg/dose Q4-6h PO<br>Max. dose: 12 mg/day<br>Adults and Adolescents:<br>4 mg/dose Q4-6h PO<br>Max. dose: 24 mg/day<br>Anaphylaxis:<br>0.0875 mg/kg/dose up to 20 mg/dose IV<br>Extended dose: 8-12 mg/day ÷Q12h PO | May cause drowsiness, sedation, or disturbed coordination. Young children may be paradoxically excited. |
| Chlorpromazine (Thorazine, Promapan, Chloramend) | Tabs: 10, 25, 50, 100, 200 mg<br>Spansules: 30, 75, 150, 200, 300 mg<br>Syrup: 10 mg/5 ml<br>Supp: 25, 100 mg<br>Oral Conc: 30, 100 mg/ml<br>Injection: 25 mg/ml (1 and 2 ml vials) | IM or IV: 0.5 mg/kg/dose or 2 mg/kg/day÷Q6-8h<br>PO: 0.5 mg/kg/dose Q4-6h<br>Rectal: 1 mg/kg/dose Q6-8h<br>Max. dose: <5 yrs: 40 mg/day<br>5-12 yrs: 75 mg/day | Adverse effects include drowsiness, jaundice, lowered seizure threshold, extrapyramidal symptoms, hypotension, arrhythmias, agranulocytosis. May potentiate effects of narcotics, sedatives, other drugs. Monitor BP closely. |
| Cholestyramine (Questran, Cumid) | Powder: 9 gm packets<br>Tins: 378 gm (4 gms of active ingredient Anhydrous Cholestyramine in 9 gms Questran Powder) | Children: 240 mg/kg/day cholestyramine ÷ TID. Give PO as slurry in water, juice, etc.<br>Adult: 4 gm TID | May cause constipation, diarrhea, vomiting, vitamin deficiencies (A, D, E, K), alter absorption of other drugs. Give other oral medications 1 hr before or 4-6 hrs after cholestyramine doses. Hyperchloremic acidosis may occur with prolonged use. |
| Cimetidine (Tagamet) | Tabs: 200, 300 mg<br>Vials: 150 mg/ml (2, 8 vials),<br>Syrup: 300 mg/5 ml | Children: 20-40 mg/kg/day ÷Q6h PO/IV<br>Max. dose: 2400 mg/day<br>Adults: 300 mg/dose QID | Use with caution in all patients. Diarrhea, rash, myalgia, neutropenia, gynecomastia, dizziness may occur. |

| Drug | Preparations | Dosage | Comments |
|---|---|---|---|
| Citrate Mixtures, Oral | Each ml contains:<br><br>(mEq)  Na K Citrate<br>Polycitra  1  1  2<br>Polycitra K  0  2  2<br><br>Bicitra  1  0  1<br>(Shohl's) | Children: 5-15 ml/dose Q6-8h PO; or 2-3 mEq/kg/day÷Q6-8h<br>Adult: 15-30 ml PO Q6-8h<br>Dilute dose in water. | Adjust dose to maintain desired urine pH. 1 mEq of citrate is equivalent to 1 mEq HCO₃. Use with caution in patients already receiving potassium supplements. |
| Clindamycin (Cleocin) | Caps: 75, 150 mg<br>Oral liquid: 75 mg/ 5 ml<br>Injection: 150 mg/ml | Children: 8-25 mg/kg/day ÷ Q6-8h PO. 15-40 mg/kg/day ÷ Q6-8h IM or IV.<br>Adults: 150-450 mg Q6h PO; 600-2700 mg/day÷Q6-12h IM or IV.<br>Max. dose: 4.8 gm/day | Not indicated in meningitis. Use with caution in infants and neonates, in hepatic or renal insufficiency. Colitis may occur up to several wks after cessation of therapy, but is generally uncommon in pediatric patients. |
| Clonazepam (Klonopin) | Tabs: 0.5, 1.0 and 2.0 mg | Children: Up to 10 yr or 30 kg: Initial: 0.01-0.03 mg/kg/day ÷Q8h PO<br>Increments: not >0.25-0.5 mg Q3 days, up to maximum maintenance dose of 0.1-0.2 mg/kg/day ÷ Q8h<br>Adult:<br>Initial: 1.5 mg/day TID<br>Increment: 0.5-1 mg Q3 days<br>Max. dose: 20 mg/day | CNS depression, drowsiness and ataxia common. May cause behavioral changes, and other CNS symptoms; increased bronchial secretions. GI, CV, GU, and hematopoietic toxicity may occur. Use with caution in renal impairment. |
| Clotrimazole (Lotrimin, Mycelex) | Cream: 1%<br>Solution: 1%<br>Vaginal tabs: 100 mg<br>Vaginal cream: 1%<br>Oral troche: 10 mg | Topical: apply to skin BID<br>Vaginal Candidiasis: 1 tab in vagina daily x 7 days<br>Thrush: Dissolve one in the mouth TID. | May cause erythema, blister-ing, or urticaria where applied. |

| | | | |
|---|---|---|---|
| Cloxacillin (Tegopen, Cloxapen) | Caps: 250, 500 mg; Oral Sol'n: 125 mg/5 ml | <20kg: 50-100 mg/kg/day ÷ Q6h PO; >20kg: 1-2 gm/day ÷ Q6h PO. Max. dose: 4 gm/day | Same side effects as other penicillins. Give on an empty stomach. |
| Codeine | Tabs (sulfate): 15, 30, 60 mg; Amp (phosphate): 30, 60 mg/ml | Analgesic: <u>Children:</u> 0.5-1.0 mg/kg/dose Q4-6h IV or PO; Adults: 30-60 mg/dose Q4-6h IV or PO. Antitussive: <u>Children:</u> 0.25-0.5 mg/kg/dose Q4h to max. of 30 mg/day; Adults: 15-30 mg/dose Q4-6h | CNS and respiratory depression. Constipation, cramping. May be habit forming. For analgesia, use with acetaminophen orally. |
| Cortisone Acetate | Tabs: 5, 10, 25 mg; Vials: 25, 50 mg/ml | Physiologic replacement: See pages 217-218. Stress: 2-4 x physiologic replacement dose | IM slowly absorbed over several days. |
| Co-trimoxazole (TMP-SMX, Bactrim, Septra) | Tabs (reg. strength): 80 mg TMP/400 mg SMZ; Tabs (double strength): 160 mg TMP/800 mg SMZ; Susp: 40 mg TMP/200 mg SMZ per 5 ml; Injectable: 16 mg TMP/ml and 80 mg SMZ/ml | Doses based on TMP component. Minor infections (PO or IV): < 40 kg: 8-10 mg/kg/day÷Q12h > 40 kg: 320 mg/day÷Q12h UTI prophylaxis: 2 mg/kg/day QD. Severe infections & pneumocystis carinii pneumonitis (PO or IV): 20 mg/kg/day÷Q6-8h Pneumocystis prophylaxis: 10 mg/kg/day÷Q12h | Available as a fixed combination of sulfamethoxazole 5 mg to each 1 mg of trimethoprim. Doses are expressed as the trimethoprim component. Reduce dosage in renal impairment. Monitor hematologic status. For other comments, see sulfisoxazole. |

| Drug | Preparations | Dosage | Comments |
|---|---|---|---|
| Cromolyn (Intal, Nasalcrom, Opticrom) | Caps: 20 mg (for inhalation via "spinhaler") Ampule: 20 mg/2 ml (for nebulization) Nasal solu: 4% (13ml) Opthalmic Solln: 4% (10ml) Aerosol inhaler: 800 mcg/spray 200 doses/inhaler | Inhalant: 20 mg Q6h (for adults and children >5 yrs) Nebulization: One ampule (2ml) Q6-8h (adults and children > 2 yrs old) TID-QID Nasal: One spray each nostril TID-QID Ophthalmic: 1-2 drops OU Q4-6h Aerosol inhaler: 2 puffs QID | Not for acute asthmatic attack. Allow 2-4 wks for adequate trial. May cause rash, cough, bronchospasm, nasal congestion. Not recommended in children <5 yrs or in patients with renal or hepatic dysfunction. |
| Crotamiton (Eurax) | Cream (10%): 60 gm Lotion (10%): 60 ml | Massage into skin of whole body from chin down, with particular attention to folds and creases; reapply 24 hrs later. Cleansing bath should be taken 48 hrs after last application. | Change clothing and bed linens. Clean immediately after treatment. Do not apply to raw or weeping skin. Avoid eyes and mouth. |
| Cyclopentolate/phenylephrine-HCl (Cyclomydril) | Solution: 0.2% cyclopentolate/1% phenylephrine | One drop OU Q5-10min up to 3 times | For the production of mydriasis. |
| Cyclosporine (Sandimmune) | Injection: 50 mg/ml Oral solu: 100 mg/ml (50 ml bottles) | Oral: 15 mg/kg/day as a single dose 4-12 hrs pre-transplant. Give the same dose daily x 1-2 weeks post transplant then reduce by 5%/wk to 5-10 mg/kg/day. IV: 5-6 mg/kg as a single dose 4-12 hrs pre-transplant. Give slowly over 2-6 hrs. Continue the same dose daily post-transplant until the patient can take the oral solution. | Water insoluble and administered in castor oil/ethanol PO or ethanol IV. Peak after PO dose ~ 4 hrs, plasma half-life 14 hrs. Dose dependent nephrotoxicity and hepatotoxicity. Administration with steroids but not other immunosuppressives is allowable. Follow serum levels. |

| Drug | Preparation | Dosage | Comments |
|---|---|---|---|
| Cyproheptadine (Periactin) | Tabs: 4 mg<br>Syrup: 2 mg / 5 ml | 0.25-0.5 mg/kg/day÷Q6-8h PO. Max. total dose:<br>0.5 mg/kg/day<br>Adult: 4-20 mg/day TID | Contraindicated in neonates. Use with caution in asthma. Anticholinergic (atropine-like) effects. |
| Dantrolene (Dantrium) | Cap: 25, 50, 100 mg<br>IV: 0.32 mg/ml in 70 ml vials | Chronic spasticity:<br>Children (>5 yrs):<br>Initial: 0.5 mg/kg PO BID, then give 0.5 mg/kg PO TID or QID and increase by 0.5 mg/kg up to 3 mg/kg QID - do not exceed 100 mg PO QID<br>Adults:<br>Initial: 25 mg PO QD, then give 25 mg PO 2-4 x day and increase by 25 mg increments up to 100 mg PO QID if necessary. See package insert for use with malignant hyperthermia.<br>Malignant hyperthermia:<br>Prevention: 4-8 mg/kg/day ÷ Q6-8h x 2 days prior to surgery<br>Treatment: 1 mg/kg IV, repeat PRN up to a max. cumulative dose of 10 mg/kg. | Contraindicated in active hepatic disease. Monitor transaminases for hepatotoxicity. May cause change in sensorium, weakness, and diarrhea. A decrease in spasticity sufficient to allow daily function not otherwise attainable should be therapeutic goal. Discontinue if benefits are not evident in 45 days. |
| Deferoxamine (Desferal) | Injection: 500 mg | Iron poisoning: see page 250. | |

| | | | |
|---|---|---|---|
| Desmopressin Acetate (DDAVP) | Nasal solution: 100 mcg/ml (in 2.5 ml vial with applicator) Injection: 4 mcg/ml | > 3 mos - 12 yrs: 5-30 mcg/day as 1-2 doses intranasally Adults: 10-40 mcg/day in 2-3 doses. Titrate dose to achieve control of excessive thirst and urination. Max. adult dose: 40 mcg/day | Injection may be used SQ or IV at approx. 10% of intra-nasal dose. Adjust fluid intake to decrease risk of water intoxication. Use with caution in hypertension and coronary artery disease. Duration of effect is 8-12 hrs. |
| Desoxycortico-sterone (DOCA, Percorten) | Injection: 5 mg/ml (in oil) Pellets: 125 mg | 1-5 mg/day IM (in oil) as single dose, or implant 1 pellet Q8-12 mos for each 0.5 mg of daily IM dose | (See pages 217-18.) 1 mg DOCA = 0.1 mg 9α-fluoro-cortisol. IM preferred route. Use pellets only after IM dose is well established. |
| Dexamethasone (Decadron and other brand names) | Tabs: 0.25, 0.5, 0.75, 1.5, 4 mg Vials: 4, 10, 24 mg/ml Oral liquid: 0.5 mg/5 ml Inhalation: 0.143% (0.084 mg/metered dose) | Increased intracranial pressure: Initial dose: 0.5-1.5 mg/kg IV or IM (Adult dose: 10mg) Maintenance: 0.2-0.5 mg/kg/day÷Q6h IV, IM x 5 d, then taper. (Adult dose: 4 mg Q6h) Airway edema: 0.25-0.5 mg/kg/dose Q6h PRN for croup or beginning 24 hrs before elective extubation, then x 4-6 doses. Anti-emetic: 4-8 mg/M² IV loading dose, then 2-4 mg/M² IV Q6h. | (See pages 217-18.) IM route preferred unless patient is in shock or acutely ill (use IV). Toxicity - same as for prednisone. |

| Dextro-amphetamine (Dexedrine and many other brand names) | Tabs: 5, 10 mg<br>Elixir: 5 mg/5 ml<br>Sustained-release caps: 5, 10, 15 mg | **Attention Deficit Disorder:**<br>Starting dose = 0.15 mg/kg/dose Q AM x 2 weeks. If good response, add the same dose QNoon if needed (short acting preparations).<br>Max. dose: 0.5 mg/kg/dose up to 40 mg/day<br>**Narcolepsy:**<br>6-12 yrs: 5 mg/day; increase by 5 mg/day at weekly intervals (range 5-60 mg)<br>>12 yrs: double above dose (range 5-60 mg) | Use with caution in presence of hypertension or cardio-vascular disease. Not recommended for <3 yr. Interrupt administration occasionally to determine need for continued therapy. Many side effects including insomnia, restlessness, and anorexia. Tolerance develops. (Same guidelines as per methyl-phenidate apply.) |
| Diazepam (Valium) | Tabs: 2, 5, 10 mg<br>Amp: 5 mg/ml (for injection) | **Sedative/muscle relaxant:**<br>**Children:**<br>IM or IV: 0.04-0.2 mg/kg/dose Q2-4h (max. dose: 0.6 mg/kg within an 8 hr period)<br>PO: 0.12-0.8 mg/kg/day÷Q6-8h.<br>**Adults:**<br>IM or IV: 2-10 mg/dose Q3-4h PRN<br>PO: 2-10 mg/dose Q6-8h PRN<br>**Status epilepticus:**<br>1 mo - 5 yr: 0.2-0.5 mg/kg/dose<br>1 mo-5 yr:0.2-0.5 mg/kg/dose IV Q10-30 min. (max. total dose: 5 mg). May repeat in 2-4h PRN.<br>>5 yrs: 1 mg/dose IV Q15-30 min. (max. total dose: 10 mg) May repeat in 2-4h PRN<br>Adults: 5-10 mg/dose IV Q10-15 min (max. total dose: 30 mg) May repeat in 2-4h PRN | Hypotension and respiratory depression may occur. Use with caution in glaucoma. Give with caution and depression. Give undiluted - do not mix with IV fluids. Not recommended for use in neonates. In status epilepticus, diazepam must be followed by long acting anticonvulsants.<br>For management of status epilepticus see p 269. |

| Drug | Forms | Dosing | Comments |
|---|---|---|---|
| Diazoxide (Hyperstat, Proglycem) | Amp: 15 mg/ml (injection)<br>Caps: 50, 100 mg<br>Susp: 50 mg/ml | **Hypertensive crisis:**<br>Children: 3-5 mg/kg IV as bolus injection given as fast as possible. May repeat in 30 min, and Q3-10h PRN.<br>Adults: 1-3 mg/kg up to 150 mg; repeat 5-15 min PRN, then Q4-24h<br>**Hypoglycemia** (due to insulin producing tumors):<br>Newborns and infants: 8-15 mg/kg/day÷Q8-12h PO or IV<br>Children and adults: 3-8 mg/kg/day÷Q8-12h PO or IV (start at lowest dose) | May cause hyponatremia, salt and water retention, GI disturbances, ketoacidosis, hyperuricemia, hypertrichosis and arrhythmias. Monitor BP closely for hypotension. Hyperglycemia occurs in majority of patients. Hypoglycemia should initially be treated with IV glucose; diazoxide should be introduced only if refractory to glucose infusion. |
| Dicloxacillin sodium (Dynapen, and many other brand names) | Caps: 125, 250, 500 mg<br>Oral Susp: 62.5 mg/5 ml | Children (<40 kg): 25-75 mg/kg/day÷Q6h<br>Adults (>40 kg): 125-500 mg/dose Q6h. | Similar toxicity and side effects as with cloxacillin. Give 1-2 hrs before meals. Limited experience in neonates and very young infants. |
| Digoxin | See page 214. | | Therapeutic concentration 0.8-2.0 mcg/L |
| Dihydrotachysterol USP (vitamin $D_3$) | Caps: 0.125 mg<br>Sol'n (in oil):<br>0.25 mg/ml<br>Tabs: 0.125, 0.2, 0.4 mg | **Hypoparathyroidism:**<br>Neonates: 0.05-0.1 mg/day<br>Infants/Young Children: 0.1-0.5 mg/day<br>Older Children/Adults: 0.5-1.0 mg/day<br>**Hypophosphatemic Vit. D-resistant rickets:** 0.25-1.0 mg/day<br>**Nutritional rickets:** 5 mg x 1 dose<br>**Renal osteodystrophy:** 0.6-6 mg/day until healing occurs, then 0.25-0.6 mg/day | Monitor serum Ca++ and $PO_4$. Action faster than that of Vit. D. Titrate dosage with patient response. Oral Ca++ supplementation may be required. 1 mg equiv. to 120,000 units Vit. $D_2$.<br>Activated by 25-hydroxylation in liver; does not require 1-hydroxylation in kidney. |

| Drug | Preparations | Dosage | Remarks |
|---|---|---|---|
| Dimenhydrinate (Dramamine and other brand names) | Tabs: 50 mg<br>Sol'n: 15.0 mg/5 ml<br>Amp: 50 mg/ml (injection)<br>Supp: 100 mg | Children (<12 yr):<br>5 mg/kg/day ÷ Q6h PO, IM, PR<br>Max. dose: 300 mg/day<br>Adult:<br>50-100 mg Q4h PO;<br>100 mg QD-BID PR;<br>50 mg IM PRN | May mask vestibular symptoms. Caution when taken with ototoxic agents. Causes drowsiness. |
| Dimercaprol (B.A.L., British anti-Lewisite) | Injection (in oil): 100 mg/ml (3 ml amp) | Give all injections deep IM<br>Lead poisoning:<br>For symptomatic patients with blood lead 70-100 mcg/100 ml: 333 mg/m²/day x 2-3 days.<br>For encephalopathic patients or with blood level > 100 mcg/100 ml: 500 mg/M²/day ÷Q4h x 3-5 days. | May cause hypertension, tachycardia, GI disturbance, headache, fever (30% of children). (Symptoms are usually relieved by anti-histamines.) Contra-indicated in hepatic or renal insufficiency. Urine must be alkaline. May result in renal toxicity. Use cautiously in patient with G6PD deficiency. Do not use concomitantly with iron. See section on lead poisoning page 251. |
| Diphenhydramine (Benadryl and other brand names) | Caps: 25, 50 mg<br>Tabs: 50 mg<br>Elixir: 12.5 mg/5 ml<br>Injection: 10, 50 mg/ml | Children: 5 mg/kg/day÷Q6h PO or deep IM<br>Adult: 10-50 mg/dose Q6-8h<br>For anaphylaxis or phenothiazine overdose: 1-2 mg/kg IV slowly. Max. total dose: 300 mg/day | Side effects common to anti-histamines. CNS side effects more common than GI disturbances. Contraindicated in infants and neonates. |

| Drug | Preparations | Dosage | Comments |
|------|--------------|--------|----------|
| Disopyramide Phosphate (Norpace) | Caps: 100, 150 mg<br>Extended release caps (CR): 100, 150 mg | < 1 yr: 10-30 mg/kg/day÷Q6h<br>1-4 yr: 10-20 mg/kg/day÷Q6h<br>4-12 yr: 10-15 mg/kg/day÷Q6h<br>12-18 yr: 6-15 mg/kg/day÷Q6h<br>Adult: 150 mg/dose÷Q6h | Modify dose in renal or hepatic failure. May cause decreased cardiac output. Anticholinergic effects may occur. Causes dose related AV block, wide QRS, increased QTc, ventricular dysrhythmias. |
| Dobutamine (Dobutrex) | Injection: 250 mg/20 ml vials | Continuous IV infusion:<br>2.5-15 mcg/kg/min.<br>Max. recommended dose:<br>40 mcg/kg/min<br>To prepare for infusion:<br>$$\frac{6 \times wt(kg) \times \text{desired dose (mcg/kg/min)}}{\text{IV infusion rate (ml/hr)}} =$$<br>mg of drug to be added to 100 ml of IV fluid | Monitor blood pressure and vital signs. TI/2 = 2 min. Contraindicated in IHSS. Side effects of tachycardia hypertension, arrhythmias (PVC's) may occasionally occur (especially at higher infusion rates). Adjust rate and duration of therapy according to patient response. Correct hypovolemic states before use. Increases AV conduction, may precipitate ventricular ectopic activity. |
| Docusate (Colace and many other brand names) | Caps: 50, 100, 120, 240 mg<br>Syrup: 20 mg/5 ml 50 mg/15 ml<br>Tab: 50, 100 mg<br>Drops: 10 mg/1 ml | PO:(take with liquids)<br><3 yr: 10-40 mg/day÷OD-QID<br>3-6 yr: 20-60 mg/day÷QD-QID<br>6-12 yr: 40-120 mg/day÷QD-QID<br>>12 yr: 50-240 mg/day÷QD-QID<br>Rectal:<br>Older children and adults: add 50-100 mg to enema solution | PO requires 1-3 days for notable effect. Incidence of side effects is exceedingly low. |

| Drug | Preparations | Dose | Remarks |
|---|---|---|---|
| Dopamine (Intropin) | Injection: 40 mg/ml; 80 mg/ml (5 ml/vial) | Low dose: 2-5 mcg/kg/min: Increases renal blood flow. Less effect on heart rate and cardiac output. Intermediate doses: 5-15 mcg/kg/min: Increases renal blood flow, heart rate, cardiac contractility, and cardiac output. High doses: >20 mcg/kg/min: Alpha adrenergic effects are prominent. Decreases renal perfusion. To prepare for infusion: Same as for Dobutamine. Max. dose recommended: 20-50 mcg/kg/min. | Monitor vital signs and blood pressure continuously. Correct hypovolemic states. Tachyarrhythmias, ectopic beats, hypertension, vasoconstriction, vomiting may occur. Extravasation may cause tissue necrosis. Use cautiously with phenytoin. |
| Doxycycline (Vibramycin and other brand names) | Caps: 50, 100, 300 mg Tabs: 100 mg Oral soln: (as Calcium salt) 50 mg base/5 ml; (as Monohydrate) 25 mg base/5 ml Injection: 100, 200 mg/vial | Initial: <45 kg - 4.4 mg/kg/day ÷ Q12h PO or IV x 1 day; >45 kg - 200 mg/day ÷ Q12h PO or IV x 1 day Maintenance: <45 kg - 2.2 mg/kg/day ÷Q12-24h PO or IV >45 kg - 100 mg/day ÷Q12-24h PO or IV Max. adult dose: 300 mg/day PID: see p. 220. | Use with caution in hepatic and renal disease. May cause increased intracranial pressure. Use in children <8 yrs may result in tooth enamel hypoplasia and discoloration. May cause GI symptoms, photosensitivity, hemolytic anemia, hypersensitivity reactions. Infuse over 1-4 hrs IV; avoid extravasation. See tetracycline. |

| Drug | Supplied | Use/Dose | Comments |
|---|---|---|---|
| Edrophonium (Tensilon) | Injection: 10 mg/ml (1 ml) | Test for myasthenia gravis (IV): Neonate: 0.1 mg/kg/dose IM or sub-q Infant, child, and adult: 0.2 mg/kg/dose IV. Give 20% of the test dose slowly; if no response in 1 min give 1 mg increments. Max: 5-10 mg. For SVT: 0.1-0.2 mg/kg IV total dose. Give 20% of dose every 2 minutes as needed. | Keep atropine available in syringe and have resuscitation equipment ready. May precipitate cholinergic crisis, arrhythmias, bronchospasm. Hypersensitivity to test dose (fasiculations or intestinal cramping) is indication to delay further administration of the drug. |
| EDTA Calcium disodium | Amp: 200 mg/ml (5 ml) | Lead poisoning: 1-1.5 gm/M²/day, ÷ Q4-12h and given x 3-5 days depending on severity. Do not exceed 7 days duration of administration. Can add procaine (final conc. 0.5%) when giving IM. IM route preferred. For specific instructions in class III and IV lead toxicity: see p 253-4. | May cause renal tubular necrosis. Do not use if anuric. Follow urinalysis and renal function. Monitor EKG continuously when giving IV. Rapid IV infusion may cause sudden increase in intracranial pressure in patients with cerebral edema. May cause zinc deficiency by chelation effect. |
| Enalapril Maleate (Vasotec) | Tablets: 5, 10 and 20 mg | Adult: 5 mg PO QD initially up to 40 mg/day as a single or equally divided dose. | Safety and efficacy in children has not been established. Use only when other measures have been unsuccessful. Reduce dose with renal impairment. |

| | | | |
|---|---|---|---|
| Epinephrine (Adrenalin) | 1:1000 (Aqueous): Amp: 1 mg/ml (1 ml) Vials: 1 mg/ml (30 ml) 1:200 (Sus-phrine): Vials: 5 mg/ml (5 ml) 1:10,000 (Aqueous): Prefilled syringes 10 ml Aerosol (15 ml): each contains 300 metered doses equivalent to 0.16 mg/dose or 0.2 mg/dose of epinephrine. | 1:1000 (Aqueous): 0.01 ml/kg/dose SC (max. single dose 0.3 ml); repeat Q15 min x 3-4 or Q4h PRN 1:200 (Sus-phrine): 0.005 ml/kg/dose SC (max. single dose 0.15 ml); repeat Q8-12h PRN Inhalation: 1-2 puffs during attack. Repeat Q4h PRN. Bradycardia/Hypotension: IV drip: 0.1-1.0 mcg/Kg/min To prepare for infusion, see inside front cover. | May produce arrhythmias, tachycardia, hypertension, headaches, nervousness, nausea, vomiting. Necrosis may occur at site of repeated local injection. May be given via ETT. |
| Epinephrine, Racemic (Vaponefrin, Micronefrin, Asthmanefrin) | Solution: 2.25% | Croup: 0.05 ml/kg/dose diluted to 3 ml with saline. Given via nebulizer PRN, but not more frequently than Q2h. Max. dose: 0.5 ml | "Rebound" common. Tachyarrhythmias, headache, nausea, palpitations reported. |
| Ergocalciferol (Drisdol, Calciferol) Vit. $D_2$ | Caps: 0.62 mg (25,000 IU); 1.25 mg (50,000 IU) Sol'n: 0.25 mg/ml (10,000 IU) Injection: 12.5 mg (500,000 IU)/ml Drops: 8,000 IU/ml (0.2 mg) (200 IU/gtt) 1 mg = 40,000 IU | Maintenance: 400 IU/day Renal osteodystrophy: 25,000-250,000 IU/day until healing occurs, then 10,000-25,000 IU/day Rickets: Vit. D dependent: 5,000-15,000 IU/day Vit. D resistant: 25,000-1,000,000 IU/day Nutritional: 10,000 IU/day x 30 days | Monitor serum $Ca^{++}$, $PO_4$, and alk. phos. Titrate dosage to patient response. Maintain serum $Ca^{++}$ 8.5-10.0 mg/dl, and urinary $Ca^{++}$ <3 mg/kg/day. Watch for symptoms of hypercalcemia. Vit. $D_2$ is activated by 25-hydroxylation in liver and 1-hydroxylation in kidney. |

| Erythromycin Preparations (Erythrocin, Pediamycin, Ilosone, E-Mycin and others) | Erythromycin: Tabs: 250, 500 mg Erythromycin Ethyl Succinate: Susp: 200, 400 mg/ 5 ml Drops: 100 mg/2.5 ml Tabs: 200, 400 mg Erythromycin Lactobionate: Vials: 500, 1000 mg Erythromycin Estolate (Ilosone): Tabs: 500 mg Chewable tabs: 125, 250 mg Drops: 100 mg/ml Caps: 125, 250 mg Susp: 125, 250 mg/5ml Erythromycin Stearate Tabs: 125, 250, 500 mg | Oral: Children: 30-50 mg/kg/day ÷ Q6-8h Adults: 1-4 gm/day ÷ Q6h Parenteral: 10-20 mg/kg/day ÷ Q6h IV Rheumatic fever prophylaxis: 500 mg/day ÷ Q12h PO Max. adult dose: 4 gm/day | Avoid IM route (pain, necrosis). GI side effects common (nausea, vomiting, abdominal cramps). Use with caution in liver disease. Estolate causes cholestatic jaundice, although hepatotoxicity uncommon (<2% of reported cases). May produce elevated digoxin, theophylline, and carbamazepine levels. |
| Erythromycin Ethylsuccinate and Acetyl Sulfisoxazole (Pediazole) | Susp: 200 mg erythro and 600 mg sulfa/5 ml | Otitis media: 50 mg/kg/day (as erythro) and 150 mg/kg/day (as sulfa) ÷ Q6h PO Max. dose: 6 gm sulfisoxazole/ day | See adverse effects of erythromycin and sulfisoxazole. Not recommended in infants <2 mos. |

| | | | |
|---|---|---|---|
| Ethambutol (Myambutol) | Tabs: 100, 400 mg | **Adolescents and adults:** 15-25 mg/kg/day as single PO dose. Not recommended for children <12 yrs. Should be used concurrently with another antituberculosis drug. | May cause optic neuritis, especially with larger doses. Obtain baseline ophthalmologic studies before beginning therapy and then monthly. Follow visual acuity, visual fields, and (green) color vision. Discontinue if any visual deterioration occurs. Monitor uric acid, liver function, heme status and renal function. May cause GI disturbances. Adjust with renal failure. |
| Ethosuximide (Zarontin) | Caps: 250 mg Syrup: 250 mg/5 ml | **Initial:** 3-6 yr: 250 mg/day÷Ω12-24h PO >6 yr: 500 mg/day÷Ω12-24h PO Increase as necessary: 250 mg every 4-7 days Maintenance: 20-30 mg/kg/day Max. dose: 1.5 gm/day | Monitor levels. Use with caution in hepatic and renal disease. Ataxia, anorexia, GI distress are adverse effects; rashes and blood dyscrasias are rare idiosyncratic reactions. May increase frequency of grand mal seizures in patients with mixed type seizures. Therapeutic levels: 40-100 mg/L |
| Fentanyl (Sublimaze) | Injection: 50 mcg/ml in 2, 5, 10, and 20 ml ampules. | 2 mcg/kg/dose IM or IV | Onset of action 1-2 minutes with a peak action about 10 minutes and duration 30-60 minutes. As with other opiates, respiratory depression occurs and may persist beyond the period of analgesia. |

| Drug | Preparations | Dosage | Notes |
|---|---|---|---|
| Flecainide Acetate (Tambocor) | Tabs: 100 mg | Children*: 50-150 mg/$M^2$/day ÷Q12h PO. Adults: 100 mg PO Q12h. May increase dose by 50 mg Q12h every 4 days to maximum of 400 mg/day. *Not FDA approved for children. | Adjust dose in renal failure. May aggravate LV failure, sinus bradycardia, preexisting ventricular arrhythmias. May cause increased PR, QRS interval unrelated to efficacy or adverse effects. May cause AV block, dizziness, blurred vision, dyspnea, nausea, headache. |
| Flunisolide (Nasalide) | Nasal solution: 25 mcg/spray 200 sprays/bottle Aerosol inhaler: 250 mcg/dose 50 dose/inhaler | Nasal solution (for nasal use only): Children: (6-14 yrs): 1 spray per nostril TID or 2 sprays per nostril BID. Adult: max: 8 sprays/day Inhaler: 2 puffs BID | Reduce dose to smallest maintenance dose which will control symptoms. Stop after 3 weeks if no clinical improvement. |
| Fluoride | Solution: 0.5, 2, 4 mg/ml Chewable tabs: 0.25, 0.5, 1.0 mg | Dose (mg/day): Concen. of Fluoride in Drinking Water (ppm)<br><br>Age \| <0.3 \| 0.3-0.7 \| >0.7<br>2 wk-2 yr \| 0.25 \| 0 \| 0<br>2-3 yr \| 0.5 \| 0.25 \| 0<br>3-16 yr \| 1.00 \| 0.50 \| 0 | Acute overdose: GI distress and salivation. Chronic excess use: mottled teeth and bone changes. |
| 9α-Fluoro-cortisol (Florinef) | Tabs: 0.1 mg | 0.05-0.15 mg/day PO Usual dose: 0.1 mg/day | Preferably administered in conjunction with cortisone or hydrocortisone. If elevated BP develops, decrease dose to 0.05 mg/day. 0.1 mg 9α-fluorocortisol = 1 mg DOCA. See page 217. |

| | | | |
|---|---|---|---|
| Flurazepam (Dalmane) | Caps: 15, 30 mg | Adolescents & adults 15-30 mg PO QHS Max. dose: 30 mg | Dizziness, GI symptoms, hematologic abnormalities, hepatic dysfunction. Rarely causes paradoxical hyperactivity. Not recommended for children <15 yrs. |
| Furosemide (Lasix and others) | Tabs: 20, 40, 80 mg Amp: 10 mg/ml Oral liquid: 10 mg/ml | Oral: Infants and Children: 2 mg/kg/dose Q6-8h PRN; may increase by 1-2 mg/kg/dose Adult: 20-80 mg/day QD or BID; may increase 20 or 40 mg up to total of 600 mg/day Parenteral: Infants and Children: 1 mg/kg/dose Q12h IM or IV PRN; may increase by 1 mg/kg/dose Adult: 20-80 mg/dose IM or IV Max. single dose (PO, IM, IV): 6 mg/kg | Ototoxicity may occur in presence of renal disease. Use with caution in hepatic disease. May cause hypokalemia, alkalosis, dehydration, and increased calcium excretion. Prolonged use in premature infants may result in nephrocalcinosis. |
| Gamma Benzene Hexachloride (Kwell, Lindane) | Shampoo: 1% Lotion: 1% Cream: 1% | Shampoo: Use < 30 ml per application Lotion: apply to skin, leave on 12-24 hr, then wash off. Change clothing and bed sheets after starting treatment. Treat family members. NOTE: Second application not usually necessary - may repeat application in 7-10 days if lice persist. | Systemically absorbed. Risk of toxic effects is greater in young children; use other agents in infants, young children, and during pregnancy. Avoid contact with face or mucous membranes. CNS toxicity reported with repeated use. |

| Gentamicin (Garamycin and others) | Vials: 10, 40 mg/ml Ophth ointment: 3 mg/gm Drops: 3 mg/ml Topical ointment: 0.1% Intrathecal amp: 2 mg/ml | Parenteral (IM or IV): Neonates* <7 days: <28 wks: 2.5 mg/kg/dose Q24h 28-34 wks: 2.5 mg/kg/dose Q18h term: 2.5 mg/kg/dose Q12h >7 days: <28 wks: 2.5 mg/kg/dose Q18h 28-34 wks: 2.5 mg/kg/dose Q12h term: 2.5 mg/kg/dose Q8h Children: 5-7 mg/kg/day ÷ Q8h Adults: 3-5 mg/kg/day ÷ Q8h Intrathecal/intraventricular: >3 mos: 1-2 mg daily Adult: 4-8 mg daily Ophth drops: 1-2 gtts Q4h Ophth oint: apply Q6-8h *Neonatal doses are the same for gentamicin, tobramycin, and amikacin. | Monitor levels (peak and trough). Monitor renal status; watch for ototoxicity. Higher than recommended doses may be necessary when based on serum levels. Intrathecal or intraventricular administration is adjunctive to parenteral administration. Arachnoiditis, phlebitis are seen uncommonly. Therapeutic levels: 6-10 mg/L (peak); <2 mg/L (trough). |
| Glucagon HCl (Glucagon) | 10 ml vial with 10 ml diluent (1 mg/ml). | For hypoglycemia: <10 kg: 0.1 mg/kg IM up to 1 mg Q30 min. >10kg: 1 mg/dose IM Q30min | Also noted to have a cardio-stimulatory effect at the high dose even in the presence of beta-blockade. |

| | | | |
|---|---|---|---|
| Glycopyrrolate (Robinul) | Tabs: 1, 2 mg<br>Vials: 0.2 mg/ml | Respiratory antisecretory:<br>Children: 0.004-0.010 mg/kg/dose Q4-8h IV<br>Adults: 0.1-0.2 mg/dose Q4-8h IV. Max. dose: 0.2 mg/dose or 0.8 mg/day<br>Reverse neuromuscular block: 0.2 mg per each mg neostigmine IV<br>Oral: Adult: 1-2 mg BID-TID<br>Children: Dose not established | Atropine-like side effects.<br>Use with caution in hepatic and renal disease, ulcerative colitis, asthma. |
| Griseofulvin Microcrystal-line (Grifulvin V, Grisactin, Fulvicin) | Microsize tabs: 125, 250, 500 mg<br>Caps: 125, 250, 500 mg<br>Susp: 125 mg/5 ml<br>Ultramicrosize tabs: 330 mg = 500 mg microsize | Children >2 yrs: 15-20 mg/kg/day QD PO. Give with milk, eggs, or other fatty foods.<br>Adult: 500 mg/day QD.<br>Decrease dose accordingly if using ultramicrosize.<br>Max. adult dose: 1 gm/day | Monitor hematologic, renal, and hepatic function. Possible cross-reactivity in penicillin-allergic individuals. Contraindicated in porphyria, hepatic disease. Usual treatment period 4-6 wks (for tinea unguum, 4-6 mos). Photosensitivity reactions may occur. |
| Haloperidol (Haldol) | Injection (IM use only):<br>5 mg/ml<br>Tabs: 0.5, 1, 2, 5, and 10 mg<br>Solution: 2 mg/ml | Children 3-12 years:<br>Acute agitation: 0.5-1.0 mg PO<br>Psychosis: 0.05-0.15 mg/kg/day ÷BID or TID PO<br>Tourette's syndrome: 0.05-0.075 mg/kg/day÷BID or TID PO<br>>12 Years:<br>Acute agitation: 2-5 mg IM, PO.<br>Repeat in 1 hour PRN. | Use with caution in patients with cardiac disease because of the risk of hypotension, and in patients with epilepsy since the drug lowers the seizure threshold. Extrapyramidal symptoms can occur. For treatment of toxicity see p 259. |

| Heparin sodium | Injection: 10, 100, 1,000, 5,000, 10,000, 20,000, 40,000 units/ml Repository injection: 20,000 U/ml 120 U = approx. 1 mg | Infants and Children: Initial: 50 U/kg IV bolus Maintenance: 10-25 U/kg/hr as continuous infusion, or 100 U/kg/dose Q4h IV Adults: Initial: 10,000 U IV bolus Maintenance: 5,000-10,000 units Q4h IV intermittently or as constant infusion. | Adjust dose to give clotting time of 20-30 min or PTT of 1½-2½ x control value before dose. Antidote: Protamine sulfate (I mg per 100 U heparin in previous 4 hr) |
|---|---|---|---|
| Hydralazine (Apresoline) | Tabs: 10, 25, 50, 100 mg Amps: 20 mg/ml | Hypertensive crisis: Children: 0.1-0.5 mg/kg/dose IM or IV Q4-6h PRN Adults: 20-40 mg IM or IV Q3-6h PRN Chronic hypertension: Children: 0.75-3 mg/kg/day ÷Q6-12h PO Adults: 10-50 mg/dose PO QID | Use with caution in severe renal and cardiac disease. May cause lupus- and arthritis-like syndromes. CV, neurologic, GI, hematologic, dermatologic reactions may be seen. Follow blood pressure closely. May cause reflex tachycardia. |
| Hydrochloro-thiazide, USP (Esidrix) (Hydrodiuril) | Tabs: 25, 50, 100 mg | Infants and Children: 2-3 mg/kg/day÷Q12h PO Adult: 25-100 mg/day QD or BID Max. adult dose: 200 mg/day | See chlorothiazide. |

| Drug | Formulations | Physiologic replacement & Stress Doses: | |
|---|---|---|---|
| Hydrocortisone (Solu-cortef) | Tabs: 5, 10, 20 mg<br>Oral susp: 2 mg/ml<br>Na Phosphate: Vials:<br>50 mg/ml<br>Na succinate<br>(Solu-Cortef):<br>Vials: 100, 250,<br>500, 1000 mg/ml<br>Acetate (Hydrocertone):<br>Vials: 25, 50 mg/ml | See pages 217-18.<br>Status asthmaticus: Loading:<br>4-8 mg/kg/dose (max. 250 mg)<br>then 8 mg/kg/day ÷ Q6h IV<br>Adult: 100-500 mg/dose Q6h IV. | Na succinate used for IV administration. Na phosphate may be given IM, SQ or IV. A corticosteroid with less mineralocorticoid activity is recommended for prolonged use. |
| Hydroxyzine (Atarax, Vistaril) | Tabs (HCl): 10, 25,<br>50, 100 mg<br>Caps (pamoate): 25,<br>50, 100 mg<br>Syrup (HCl): 10 mg/<br>5 ml<br>Susp (pamoate): 25<br>mg/5 ml<br>Vials (HCl): 25, 50<br>mg/ml | Oral:<br>Children: 2 mg/kg/day ÷ Q6h<br>Adult: 25-100 mg/dose QID<br>Parenteral:<br>Children: 0.5-1.0 mg/kg/dose<br>Q4-6h IM PRN<br>Adult: 25-100 mg/dose IM PRN<br>Max. adult dose: 600 mg/day | May potentiate barbiturates, meperidine and other depressants. May cause dry mouth, drowsiness, tremor, convulsions. |
| Ibuprofen (Motrin) | Tabs: 300, 400,<br>600, and 800 mg | Adults: 400 mg/dose Q4-6h<br>Max. adult dose: 2.4 gm/day<br>Not FDA approved for children | GI distress (lessened with milk), rashes, ocular problems. Inhibits platelet aggregation. Use cautiously in patients with aspirin hypersensitivity. |
| Imipenen - Cilastatin (Primaxin) | Vial: 250, 500 mg | 50 mg/kg/day÷Q6-8h IV.<br>Usual adult dose:<br>250-500 mg Q6h IV<br>Maximum dose: 4 gm/day. | For IV use, give slowly over 30-60 minutes.<br>Adverse effects: pruritis, urticaria, and penicillin allergy. Not approved for children < 12 yrs. |

| | | | | |
|---|---|---|---|---|
| Imipramine (Tofranil) | Tabs: 10, 25, 50 mg<br>Caps: 75, 100, 125, 150 mg<br>Vials: 12.5 mg/ml | | Antidepressant: Not FDA approved for children <12 yr, but recommended doses for children are:<br>Begin with 1.5 mg/kg/day TID and increase Q3-4 days to a max. of 5 mg/kg/day.<br>Adult:<br>Initial: 75-150 mg/day BID;<br>Maintenance: 50-300 mg/day QD at bedtime<br>Max. adult dose: 300 mg/day<br>Enuresis: Not recommended in children < 6 yr<br>Initial: 10-25 mg Q HS<br>Increment: 10-25 mg/dose at 1-2 wk intervals until max. dosage for age or desired effect is achieved. Continue x 2-3 mos, then taper.<br>Max. dose:<br>6-8 yr: 50 mg/day<br>8-10 yr: 60 mg/day<br>10-12 yr: 70 mg/day<br>12-14 yr: 75 mg/day | Minor side effects include: dry mouth, drowsiness, constipation, dizziness. One evening dose may reduce sedation in the first weeks of therapy. Monitor EKG, BP, CBC at start of therapy and with dose changes. Adjust dose downward if PR interval reaches .22 sec, if QRS reaches 130% of baseline, if HR rises above 130/min, or if BP is more than 140/90. Tricyclics may trigger the onset of mania. Therapeutic levels for depression: 125-225 mcg/L |

167

| Drug | Preparations | Dosage | Remarks |
|---|---|---|---|
| Indomethacin (Indocin) | Caps: 25, 50 mg Injection: investigational drug | __Anti-inflammatory:__ > 14 yrs old: 1-3 mg/kg/day ÷TID or QID (max. dose: 100 mg/day. Adults: 50-150 mg/day÷BID-QID. Closure of ductus arteriosus: 0.1-0.25 mg/kg/dose. Repeat at intervals of 12-24 hr up to a total of 3 doses. <br><br> Dose (mg/kg) <br> Age \| 1 \| 2 \| 3 <br> <48 hrs \| 0.2 \| 0.1 \| 0.1 <br> 2-7 days \| 0.2 \| 0.2 \| 0.2 <br> >7 days \| 0.2 \| 0.2 \| 0.25 | In neonates: monitor renal and hepatic function before and during use. May ↓ platelet aggregation. GI disturbances, headache, blood dyscrasias may occur. |
| Insulin | | See insulin preparations. Page 216. | See DKA and subsequent insulin management. Pages 101-102. |
| Ipecac | 7% Syrup: 15 and 30 ml | | See page 243. |
| Iron Dextran (Imferon and others) (2% Fe) | Amp: 2, 5, 10 ml (IM or IV) (contains 50 mg elemental Fe/ml) | Total dose in mg Fe: a) surface area (M²) x 55 x (13.5-Hb in gm%) = mg Fe needed IM or IV OR b) Wt (kg) x 2.5 x (13.5 - pt's Hb in gm%) = mg Fe needed IM or IV. Note: Add 10-50% to above for replenishment of iron stores. Max. IV dose: 2 ml/day. Max. daily dose: <5 kg: 0.5 ml; <10 kg: 1.0 ml; <50 kg: 2.0 ml; >50 kg: 5.0 ml | Oral therapy with iron salts is preferred. Numerous side and adverse effects, including anaphylaxis, fever, myalgias, arthralgias. Use "Z-track" technique for IM administration. Inject test dose (0.5 ml) on first day. Give IV at rate of <1 ml/min. undiluted, up to 2 ml/day. |

| | | Treatment of iron deficiency | |
|---|---|---|---|
| Iron Preparations | Ferrous sulfate (20% Fe): Drops (Fer-in-sol): 75 mg (15 mg Fe)/ 0.6 ml Syrup (Fer-in-sol): 90 mg/5 ml (18 mg Fe/5 ml) Elixir (Feosol): 220 mg (44 mg Fe)/ (5 ml) Caps & Tabs: 200 mg (40 mg Fe), 300 mg (60 mg Fe) Ferrous gluconate (11.6% Fe): Elixir: 300 mg (35 mg Fe)/5 ml Tabs: 320 mg (37 mg Fe) Caps (sustained-release): 435 mg (50 mg Fe) Caps: 325 mg (38 mg Fe) | anemia: 6 mg elemental Fe/kg/day ÷ TID PO Prophylaxis: (single dose or ÷ BID-TID, PO): Preterm infant - 2 mg elemental Fe/kg/day Full-term infant - 1 mg elemental Fe/kg/day Max. prophylactic dose: 15 mg/ day as elemental Fe | Do not use in hemolytic disorders. Less GI irritation when given with meals. Vitamin C 200 mg per 30 mg iron may enhance absorption. Liquid iron preps may stain teeth. Give with dropper or drink through straw. |
| Isoetharine (Bronksol, Bronkometer) | Aerosol (10, 15 ml dispensers): 20 metered doses/ml Each dose 340 mcg isoetharine Solution: 1% (10 mg/ ml) | Aerosol: 1-2 puffs Q3-4h PRN Nebulization: 0.25-0.5 ml 1% solution diluted to 2 ml in NS (1:8-1:4 dilution) Q4h PRN. May be used more frequently with careful monitoring. | Toxicity: nausea, tachycardia, hypertension, anxiety, headache. |

| | | | |
|---|---|---|---|
| Isoniazid (INH) | Tabs: 50, 100, 300 mg<br>Amp: 100 mg/ml<br>Syrup: 50 mg/5 ml | **Therapeutic:**<br>Infants and children: 10-20 mg/kg/day as single dose or ÷ Q12h PO or IM.<br>(max. dose: 300-500 mg/day);<br>Adults: 5 mg/kg/day QD (max. dose: 300 mg/day)<br>**Prophylaxis:**<br>Infants and children:<br>10 mg/kg/day as single daily dose or ÷ Q12h PO<br>(max. dose: 300 mg/day)<br>Adults: 300 mg/day QD | CNS, hepatic side effects may occur with higher doses. Hepatotoxicity is rare in children; follow LFT's q month. Supplemental Pyridoxine (1-2 mg/kg/day) is recommended. |
| Isoproterenol (Isuprel) | **Isoproterenol HCL:**<br>Tabs: 10, 15 mg<br>Solutions (vials):<br>1:400 (2.5 mg/ml)<br>1:200 (5 mg/ml)<br>1:100 (10 mg/ml)<br>Aerosol (15 ml dispensers): 80 mcg, 120 mcg/dose<br>Injection: 200 mcg/ml (1:5000) | **Sublingual:** 5-10 mg/dose Q6-8h<br>PRN (max.: 30 mg/day).<br>Aerosol: 1-2 puffs up to 5 times/day<br>Nebulized solution:<br>Children:0.01 ml/kg/dose<br>(max.: 0.05 ml/dose) diluted with NS to 2 ml.<br>Give Q4h PRN;<br>Adult: 0.25-0.5 ml diluted with NS to 2 ml Q4h PRN.<br>IV: 0.1-1.5 mcg/kg/min.<br>Begin with 0.1 mcg/kg/min. and increase every 5-10 min. by 0.1 mcg/kg/min. until desired effect or heart rate >180 bpm or arrhythmia occurs.<br>Max. dose: 1.5 mcg/kg/min.<br>To prepare for infusion:<br>See inside front cover. | Use with care in CHF, ischemia, or aortic stenosis. May precipitate arrhythmias in combination with epinephrine. Avoid "abuse" of inhaler. Patients with continuous IV infusion should be followed by continuous monitoring for arrhythmias, hypertension, and myocardial ischemia. Not for treatment of asystole or for use in cardiac arrests unless bradycardia is due to heart block. |

| Drug | Forms | Dosage | Adverse effects |
|---|---|---|---|
| Isotretinoin (Accutane) | Caps: 10, 20, 40 mg | Cystic acne: 0.5-1.0 mg/kg/day÷Q12h x 15-20 weeks. | Adverse effects: cheilitis, xerosis, pruritus, epistaxis, hyperlipidemia, elevated ESR, rarely pseudotumor cerebri. |
| Kanamycin (Kantrex) | Caps: 500 mg<br>Vials: 37.5 mg/ml, 250 mg/ml, 333 mg/ml | For IM or IV administration:<br>Neonates: <7 days / >7 days<br>BW <2000 gm: 15 mg/kg/day ÷Q12h / 20 mg/kg/day ÷Q12h<br>BW >2000 gm: 20 mg/kg/day ÷Q12h / 30 mg/kg/day ÷Q8h<br>Infants and children 15-30 mg/kg/day ÷ Q8-12h IM or IV Max. dose: 1.5 gm/day IV<br>Bacterial overgrowth: 50-100 mg/kg/day÷Q6h PO Max: 4 gm QD | Renal, ototoxicity. Administer over 30 min. if IV. Reduce dosage frequency with renal impairment. Therapeutic levels: peak: 25-30 mg/L; trough: <6 mg/L |
| Ketoconazole (Nizoral) | Tabs: 200 mg | Children > 2 yrs: 3.3-6.6 mg/kg/day QD PO<br>Adult: 200-400 mg/day QD PO | Monitor liver functions in long term use. Drugs which decrease gastric acidity will decrease absorption. |
| Lactulose (Cephulac) | Syrup: 10 gm/15 ml | Infant: 2.5-10 ml/day ÷ TID-QID PO<br>Older children, adolescents: 40-90 ml/day÷TID-QID PO<br>Adults: 30-45 ml/dose TID or QID PO | Use with caution in diabetes mellitus. GI discomfort, diarrhea may occur. If initial dose causes diarrhea, reduce immediately. Discontinue drug if diarrhea persists. Goal is 2-3 soft stools per day. |

| Drug | Forms | Dosage | Notes |
|---|---|---|---|
| Levothyroxine (Synthroid) | Tabs: 25, 50, 100, 150, 200, 300, 400 mcg<br>Injection solution: 0.1 mg/ml<br>Vials: 500 mcg/vial | Neonates:<br>PO: 25-50 mcg/day QD;<br>IV: 20-40 mcg/day QD<br>4 wk - 1 yr:<br>PO: 50-75 mcg/day QD (5-6 mcg/kg/day)<br>IV: 40 mcg/day QD<br>Children/Adolescents:<br>PO: Maintenance: 75-200 mcg/day (3-5 mcg/kg/day)<br>Initially give 1/4 of daily maintenance dose. Increase by increments of 1/4 maintenance dose at weekly intervals.<br>IV: 75% of oral dose.<br>Adults:<br>PO:<br>Initially 25-50 mcg/day<br>Increase by 25-50 mcg/day at intervals of 1 month.<br>Maintenance: 100-200 mcg/day (1.4-3 mcg/kg/day).<br>IV: 75% of oral dose QD | Use with caution in patients on anticoagulants. Titrate dosage with clinical status and serum $T_4$ (100 mcg levothyroxine = 65 mg thyroid USP), and TSH |
| Lidocaine (Xylocaine) | Vials: 0.5, 1, 1.5, 2, 4, 5%<br>(1% solution = 10 mg/ml)<br>Cream: 3%<br>Ointment: 2.5, 5%<br>Susp (viscous): 2%<br>Jelly: 2% | Anesthetic: apply or infiltrate locally PRN (max. total dose: 4-5 mg/kg)<br>Anti-arrhythmic: Single bolus 1 mg/kg/dose slowly IV; may repeat Q5-10 min PRN (max. dose: 3-4.5 mg/kg/hr)<br>Continuous infusion (IV):<br>CONTINUED | Topical use facilitates sensitization. Use sparingly orally to minimize aspiration. Side effects: hypotension, seizures, asystole, respiratory arrest. Decrease dose in presence of hepatic or renal failure. Contra- |

| | CONTINUED | | |
|---|---|---|---|
| Lidocaine | Prefilled syringes: 10 mg/ml (1%) 100 mg/5 ml (2%) | Continuous infusion (IV): 20-50 mcg/kg/min To prepare infusion: See inside front cover. | indicated in Stokes-Adams attacks, SA, AV, or intraventricular block. Prolonged (24 hr) infusion may result in toxic accumulation of lidocaine in plasma. Therapeutic levels 1.5-6.0 mg/L. Toxicity occurs at > 7 mg/L. |
| Lorazepam (Ativan) | Tabs: 0.5, 1, 2 mg Injection: 2 mg/ml, 4 mg/ml | IV: 0.03-0.05 mg/kg/dose up to max. of 4 mg Q6h. Adults: 2-6 mg/day÷Q8-12h PO | May cause respiratory depression, especially in combination with other sedatives. |
| Lypressin (Diapid) | Nasal spray: 50 U/ml (2.0 U/spray) (8 ml/dispenser) | Diabetes insipidus: 1-2 sprays into each nostril QID and HS. If patient requires more than 2-3 sprays per dose, increase frequency of doses rather than larger amounts/dose | Titrate dose with thirst, urinary frequency. Coronary vasoconstriction may occur with large doses. |
| Magnesium Citrate | Solution: 300 ml bottles | 4 ml/kg/dose PO Max. dose: 200 ml | Use with caution in renal insufficiency. |
| Magnesium Hydroxide (Milk of Magnesia) | Suspension (USP Magma): 8% Tabs: 325 mg (equivalent to 3.75 ml suspension) | Children: 0.5 ml/kg/dose or 40 mg/kg/dose PO PRN Adults: 15-30 ml/dose | See Mg citrate. |

| | | | |
|---|---|---|---|
| Magnesium Sulfate | Injection: 100 mg/ml (0.8 mEq/ml) (10%) 500 mg/ml (4 mEq/ml) (50%) Oral solution: 50% (Epsom salts) | Cathartic: Child: 0.25 gm/kg/dose PO; Adult: 10-30 gm dose PO Hypomagnesemia: IV or IM: 25-50 mg/kg/dose Q4-6h x 3-4 doses. Repeat PRN; PO: 100-200 mg/kg/day÷QID. Maintenance: 0.25-0.50 mEq/ kg/day or 30-60 mg/kg/day IV to max. dose: 1000 mg/day | When given IV, monitor BP, respirations, and serum level. Calcium gluconate (IV) should be available as antidote. Use with caution in renal insufficiency. |
| Mannitol | Injection: 50, 100, 150, 200, 250 mg/ml (5, 10, 15, 20, 25%) | Anuria, Oliguria: (Test dose) 0.2 gm/kg/dose IV over 3-5 min. If there is no diuresis within 2 hrs, discontinue mannitol. Cerebral edema: Acute Intra- cranial hypertension: 0.25 gm/ kg IV push, repeat Q5 min. PRN (May give furosemide 1 mg/kg concurrently or 5 min. before mannitol.) May in- crease dose gradually to 1 gm/kg/dose if necessary for satisfactory response. Preoperative for Neurosurgery: 1.5-2 gm/kg IV over 30-60 min. | May cause circulatory over- load and electrolyte distur- bances. For hyperosmolar therapy, keep serum osmola- lity at 310-320 mOsm/kg. Caution: may crystallize with concentration > 20%. |

| Drug | Formulations | Dosing | Notes |
|---|---|---|---|
| Mebendazole (Vermox) | Tabs (chewable): 100 mg | Pinworms: 100 mg x 1, repeat in 2 weeks if not cured. Hookworms, Roundworms (Ascaris), Whipworm (Trichuris): 100 mg BID x 3 days | May cause diarrhea and abdominal cramping in cases of massive infection. Use with caution in children <2 yr. |
| Meperidine HCl (Demerol) | Tabs: 50, 100 mg Elixir: 50 mg/ml Vials: 25, 50, 75, and 100 mg/ml | PO, IM, IV and SQ: Children: 1-1.5 mg/kg/dose Q3-4h PRN Adults: 50-100 mg/dose Q3-4h PRN. 75 mg Demerol is equivalent to 10 mg morphine. Max. dose: 100 mg | Contraindicated in cardiac arrhythmias, asthma, increased intracranial pressure. Potentiated by MAO inhibitors, phenothiazines, isoniazid and other CNS-acting agents. Use lower dose if IV. |
| Metaproterenol (Metaprel, Alupent) | Syrup: 10 mg/5 ml Tabs: 10, 20 mg Inhaler: each metered dose = 650 mcg (15 ml containers) approximately 300 doses per inhaler. Inhalant solution: 5% (10 ml bottle) Single dose inhalant solution: 0.6% (2.5 ml) | Inhalation: Aerosol: 1-3 puffs Q3-4h to max. of 12 puffs/day Nebulized solution: Dilute 0.2 - 0.3 ml of 5% soln. in 2.5 ml NS or give 2.5 ml of 0.6% soln. Usual dose Q4-6h and up to Q1h for severe bronchospasm. Oral: <6 yr: (Dose not well-established in this age group) 1.3-2.6 mg/kg/day÷TID or QID 6-9 yr: 10 mg/dose TID-QID >9 yr - Adult: 20 mg/dose TID-QID | Adverse reactions as with other β-adrenergic agents. Excessive use may result in cardiac arrhythmias. |

| | | | |
|---|---|---|---|
| Methadone | Tabs: 5, 10 mg<br>Vials: 10 mg/ml<br>Soln: 1 mg/ml | Children: 0.7 mg/kg/day ÷ Q4-6h PO or SC PRN pain<br>Adults: 2.5-10 mg/dose Q3-4h PRN pain PO, IV, SQ.<br>Detoxification or maintenance: see package insert | Respiratory depression, hypotension. Generally not indicated in children <16 yrs old. |
| Methicillin<br>(Staphcillin) | Vials: 1, 4, 6 gms | Newborn:<br>_<7 days_: 50-100 mg/kg/day ÷Q12h IV, IM<br>_>7 days_: 100-200 mg/kg/day ÷Q6-8h IV, IM<br>Children: 100-400 mg/kg/day ÷Q4-6h IV, IM<br>Adult: 4-12 gm/day÷Q4-6h<br>Max. adult dose: 12 gm/day. | Allergic cross-reactivity with and same toxicity as penicillin. May cause hematuria and nephritis.<br>Contains 2.5 mEq Na/gm. |
| Methimazole<br>(Tapazole) | Tabs: 5, 10 mg | Children:<br>_Initial_: 0.4-0.7 mg/kg/day ÷Q8h<br>Maintenance: 50% initial daily dose ÷ TID<br>Adults:<br>_Initial_: 15-60 mg/day÷TID<br>Maintenance: 5-30 mg/day÷TID | Readily crosses placental membranes. Blood dyscrasias, dermatitis, hepatitis, arthralgia, CNS reactions, hypothyroidism may occur.<br>T1/2 = 6h. |
| Methoxamine hydrochloride<br>(Vasoxyl) | Injection: 20 mg/ml | Children: 0.25 mg/kg/dose IM 0.08 mg/kg/dose slow IV<br>Adults: 5-20 mg/kg/dose IM 3-5 mg/dose IV | May cause sustained excessive BP elevation, headache, nausea. |
| Methsuximide<br>(Celontin) | Caps: 150, 300 mg | _Initial_: 300 mg/day x 1 week<br>Increase by 300 mg/day each wk x 3 wks to max. of 1.2 gms/day given in divided doses.<br>Usual maintenance dose is 10 mg/kg/day. | GI symptoms, blood dyscrasias, CNS symptoms, and behavioral changes may occur. Use with caution in presence of renal or liver disease. Follow LFT's and urinalysis. |

| Methyldopa (Aldomet) | Tabs: 125, 250, 500 mg<br>Amp: 50 mg/ml<br>Susp: 250 mg/5ml | 10 mg/kg/day÷Q6-12h PO; increase PRN at 2 day intervals. Max. dose: 65 mg/kg or 3 gm/day, whichever is less.<br>Hypertensive crisis: 20-40 mg/kg/day÷Q6h IV | Contraindicated in pheochromocytoma and active hepatic disease. Positive direct Coombs, fever, hemolytic disease, leukopenia, sedation, GI disturbance. |
|---|---|---|---|
| Methylene blue | Amp: 10 mg/ml (1%) | Methemoglobinemia: 1-2 mg/kg/dose IV over 5 min. | Use with caution in G6PD deficiency. |
| Methylphenidate (Ritalin) | Tabs: 5, 10, 20 mg<br>Slow release 20 mg (8 hr duration) | Attention Deficit Disorder: Starting dose = 0.3 mg/kg/dose Q AM x 2 weeks. If good response, add the same dose Q Noon if needed.<br>Max. dose: 1 mg/kg/dose, not to exceed 60 mg/day | Need to rule out learning disability, severe emotional disturbance or mental retardation. In high dose, may suppress growth through appetite suppression. May increase BP and HR. May interfere with sleep secondary to rebound overactivity. Contraindicated in glaucoma. Close supervision advised. |
| Methylprednisolone (Medrol, Solu-Medrol, DepoMedrol) | Tabs: 2, 4, 8, 16, 24, 32 mg<br>Injection (IV or IM): Na succinate (Solu-Medrol): 40, 125, 500, 1000 mg vials<br>Injection (IM Repository): 20, 40, 80 mg/ml | Anti-inflammatory/Immunosuppressive: 0.4-1.6 mg/kg/day ÷Q6-12h.<br>Status Asthmaticus: Loading: 1-2 mg/dose x 1. Maintenance: 1.6 mg/kg/day÷Q6h IV<br>Adult: 10-250 mg/dose Q4-6h IM or IV | See pages 217-18. Dose of methylprednisolone = 1/6 of cortisone dose. Repository used mainly for local therapy. Can be used IM for systemic effects as infrequently as Q week. |

177

| Drug | Formulation | Dosage | Comments |
|---|---|---|---|
| Metoclopramide (Reglan) | Tabs: 10 mg<br>Injection: 5 mg/ml<br>Syrup: 1 mg/ml | For GE reflux or GI dysmotility:<br>Children (IV or PO):<br>1-6 yr: 0.1 mg/kg/dose QID<br>6-12 yr: 2.5-9 mg/dose QID<br>Adult (IV or PO): 10 mg/dose<br>Anti-emetic: 1-2 mg/kg/dose Q2-6h IV. | For gastroesophageal reflux, administer 30 min before meals and at bedtime. May cause extrapyramidal sx, esp. at higher doses. Premedicate with diphenhydramine when using as an antiemetic. |
| Metronidazole (Flagyl) | Tabs: 250 mg<br>Vag. supp: 500 mg<br>Injection: 500 mg<br>(not currently approved for children <12) | Amebiasis:<br>Children: 35-50 mg/kg/day TID PO x 10 days.<br>Adults: 750 mg/dose PO TID x 5-10 days.<br>Anaerobic Infection:<br>Loading dose 15 mg/kg IV followed by 7.5 mg/kg/dose Q6h IV or PO to max of 4 gm/day<br>Neonates:<br>Loading dose: 15 mg/kg<br>Maintenance:<br><7 d: 7.5 mg/kg/dose Q12h<br>>7 d: 7.5 mg/kg/dose Q8h<br>Gardnerella vaginalis vaginitis:<br>500 mg PO BID x 7 days<br>Giardiasis:<br>Children: 5 mg/kg/dose PO TID x 10 days<br>Pelvic Inflammatory Disease:<br>1 gm BID PO, IV<br>Trichomonas vaginitis:<br>Children: 5 mg/kg/dose PO TID x 7 days<br>Adults: 250 mg/dose PO TID x 7 days or 2 gm PO x 1. | Nausea, diarrhea, urticaria, leukopenia, vertigo. Candidiasis may worsen. Patients should not ingest alcohol for 24 hr after dose (disulfuram type reaction). Potentiates anticoagulants. IV infusion must be given slowly over 1 hour. |

| Drug | Preparations | Dosage | Comments |
|---|---|---|---|
| Mexiletine HCl (Mexitil) | Caps: 150, 200, 250 mg | Children*: 2-4 mg/kg/dose PO Q8H<br>Adults: 150-300 mg/dose PO Q8h. May increase or decrease by 50-100 mg at intervals of 2-3 days.<br>Max: 1200 mg/day<br>* Not FDA approved for children. | May aggravate preexisting arrhythmias. Anorexia, nausea, vomiting, diarrhea, constipation, dizziness, tremor all can occur. |
| Miconazole (Monistat) | Cream: 2%<br>Lotion: 2%<br>Vaginal cream: 2%<br>Injection: 10 mg/ml | Topical: Apply BID x 2-4 wks<br>Vaginal: 1 applicator - measured dose QHS x 7 days.<br>IV: >1 yr.: 15-40 mg/kg/day÷Q8h, max. of 15 mg/kg/dose<br>Adults: 200-1200 mg/dose Q8h. | Side effects of IV therapy: phlebitis, pruritus, rash, nausea, vomiting, fever, drowsiness, diarrhea, anorexia, and flushes. Decrease in Hct and plt. have been reported. |
| Midazolam (Versed) | Vials: 5 mg/ml | Adult doses:<br>Pre-op sedation: 0.07 - 0.08 mg/kg IM<br>Sedation for procedures:<br>Begin with 0.035 mg/kg IV over two min; repeat as necessary to a max of 0.2 mg/kg. | Pediatric doses not established. Causes respiratory depression as with other benzodiazepines. Lower the dose by 25% when narcotics are given concurrently. |
| Minocycline (Minocin) | Caps: 50, 100 mg PO, IV<br>Syrup: 50 mg/5 ml<br>Vials: 100 mg | Children: (8-12 yrs):<br>Initial: 4 mg/kg/dose x 1<br>Maintenance: 2 mg/kg/day÷Q12h<br>Adolescents/Adults:<br>Initial: 200 mg/dose x 1<br>Maintenance: 100 mg/day÷Q12h | High incidence of vestibular dysfunction. Hepatic metabolism and renal excretion.<br>T1/2 = 18 hrs |

| | | | |
|---|---|---|---|
| Mithramycin (Mithracin) | Vials: 2.5 mg (refrigerate) | IV: has been used in hyper-calcemia associated with malignancies. 25 mcg/kg/dose in 1 L $D_5W$ or NS over 4-8 hrs, QD x 1-4 days. Repeat at weekly intervals if necessary or maintain 1-3 doses weekly. | Bone marrow depression, hemorrhagic diathesis with coagulopathy, cellulitis on extravasation, nausea, vomiting, hypocalcemia, hepatotoxicity, renal toxicity. |
| Morphine sulfate | Elixir: 2, 4 mg/ml Tabs: 10, 15, 30 mg Injection: 8, 10, 15 mg/ml Supp: 5, 10, 20 mg | Analgesia and tetralogy (cyanotic) spells: 0.1-0.2 mg/kg/dose SC, IV or IM. Repeat Q2-4h PRN Adults: PO: 10-30 mg Q4h PRN IV: 4-10 mg Q3h PRN | IM/IV dose equivalent to 6 x PO. Naloxone may be used to reverse effects, especially respiratory depression. |
| Nafcillin (Staphcillin) | Caps: 250 mg Tabs: 500 mg Vials: 250 mg/ml Oral solution: 250 mg/5 ml | Newborn: <7 days: 40 mg/kg/day ÷ Q12h; IV or IM >7 days: 60 mg/kg/day ÷ Q6-8h; IV or IM Older infants and children: 50-100 mg/kg/day÷Q6h PO or 100-200 mg/kg/day÷Q12h IM or ÷Q4h IV. (15-30 min. infusion) Adults: 4-12 gm/day IM Q6h or IV Q4h, PO Q4-6h | Allergic cross-sensitivity with penicillin. Oral route not recommended due to poor absorption. |
| Naloxone (Narcan) | Amp: 0.4 mg/ml (400 ug/ml) Neonatal narcan: 0.02 mg/ml | 5-10 mcg/kg/dose IM or IV. Repeat as necessary Q3-5 min. Adult dose: 0.4 - 2.0 mg/dose Q2-3 min. x 1-3. May give 10 fold higher dose if needed for diagnosis or therapy. | Does not cause respiratory depression. Short duration of action may necessitate multiple doses. For very large ingestions 100-200 mcg/kg have been necessary. |

| | | | |
|---|---|---|---|
| Neomycin Sulfate | Tabs: 500 mg<br>Vials: 500 mg<br>Oral susp: 125 mg/5 ml | <u>Prematures and Newborns:</u><br>50 mg/kg/day÷Q6h PO<br>Infants and Children: 50-100<br>mg/kg/day÷Q6h PO<br>Adult: 50 mg/kg/day÷Q6h PO<br>Hepatic Encephalopathy: Acute:<br>2.5-7 gm/M²/day÷Q6h PO x<br>5-7 days; Chronic: 2.5 gm/M²/<br>day PO QID.<br>Bowel Prep: 90 mg/kg/day Q4h<br>x 3 days | Follow for renal or ototoxi-<br>city. Contraindicated in<br>ulcerative bowel disease or<br>intestinal obstruction. |
| Neostigmine (Prostigmine) | Tabs: 15 mg<br>(bromide)<br>Amp: 0.25, 0.5 mg/ml,<br>1 mg/ml<br>Vials: 1 mg/ml | <u>Myasthenia Gravis:</u><br><u>Test dose:</u><br>  Children: 0.04 mg/kg IM<br>    0.02 mg/kg IV<br>  Adults: 0.02 mg/kg IM<br><u>Treatment:</u><br>  <u>Children:</u><br>    IM, IV, SC: 0.01-0.04 mg/<br>      kg/dose Q2-3h PRN.<br>    PO: 2 mg/kg/day÷Q3-4h<br>  Adults:<br>    IM, IV, SC: 0.5 mg/dose<br>      Q3-4h PRN.<br>    Max: 10 mg/day;<br>    PO: 15 mg/dose Q3-4h<br>    (CONTINUED) | Titrate for each patient, but<br>avoid excessive cholinergic<br>effects. Caution in asthma-<br>tics. Contraindicated in<br>intestinal and urinary<br>obstruction. May cause<br>cholinergic crisis. Keep<br>atropine available. |

| | | | |
|---|---|---|---|
| Neostigmine (Prostigmine) | (CONTINUED) | Reversal of Nondepolarizing Neuromuscular Blocking Agents: Children: 0.07-0.08 mg/kg/dose IV with atropine or glyco-pyrrolate Adults: 0.5-2 mg/dose IV with atropine or glycopyrrolate Max. dose: 2.5 mg/dose | |
| Nifedipine (Procardia) | Caps: 10 mg | Not FDA approved for children The following doses have been used in children: 0.25-0.5 mg/kg/dose Q6-8h PRN PO or sublingual, not to exceed 30 mg/dose or 180 mg/day | May cause severe hypotension, peripheral edema, flushing, tachycardia, headaches, dizziness, nausea, palpitation, syncope. |
| Nitrofurantoin (Furadantin, Macrodantin) | Tabs 50, 100 mg Susp: 25 mg/5 ml Caps: (Macrocrystal) 25, 50, 100 mg Injection: 180 mg vial | Children: 5-7 mg/kg/day÷Q6h PO Prophylaxis: 1-2 mg/kg÷QHS PO Adults: 50-100 mg/dose Q6h PO Max. adult dose 400 mg/day Prophylaxis: 50-100 mg QHS PO | Large range of hypersensitivity reactions. Contraindicated in severe renal disease, G6PD deficiency, and in infants <1 month of age. Dosage may require reduction in prolonged usage (>2 wks). Give with food or milk. |
| Nitroglycerine, intravenous | Injection: 0.8 mg/ml 5 mg/ml | 0.5-20 mcg/kg/min continuous IV infusion To prepare for infusion: see inside front cover | In small doses (1-2 mcg/kg/min) acts mainly on systemic veins and decreases preload. At 3-5 mcg/kg/min acts on systemic arterioles to decrease resistance. Must use polypropylene infusion sets to avoid plastic adsorbing drug. May cause headache, flushing, GI upset, blurred vision, methemoglobinemia. |

| Drug | Preparation | Dose | Comments |
|---|---|---|---|
| Nitroprusside (Nipride) | Vial: 50 mg | Dilute with D₅W and wrap in aluminum foil. Constant infusion: Dissolve 15 mg/kg x wt(kg) in 250 ml D₅W. Then rate in mcg/kg/min = rate in ml/hour. Begin at 1.0 mcg/kg/min. Titrate dose to BP. Range 0.5-10 mcg/kg/min. | Must be monitored with arterial line. Produces profound hypotension, metabolic acidosis and CNS symptoms when overdosed. Monitor thiocyanate levels with long term use (>48 hr). Levels should not exceed 120 mg/L. |
| Nystatin | Tabs: 100,000, 500,000 U. Susp: 100,000 U/ml. Topical powder, oint., cream: 100,000 U/gm. Vag supp: 100,000 U | Premature and Newborn Infants: 400,000 U/day÷Q6-8h PO. Older Infants and Children: 1-2 mil U/day ÷ Q6-8h. Vaginal: 1 supp QHS x 10 d. Topical: Apply BID-QID until 2-3d after infection has cleared. | May produce diarrhea and GI symptoms. |
| Oxacillin | Capsules: 250, 500 mg. Oral Soln: 250 mg/5 ml | PO: Give on empty stomach. Children: 50-100 mg/kg/day÷Q6h. Adults: 500-1000 mg/dose÷Q4-6h. Limited experience in newborns. | Same as methicillin. |
| Oxtriphylline (Choledyl) | Many preparations (64% theophylline). See p 215. | See doses under Theophylline and convert to an equivalent amount of oxtriphylline. (16 mg theophylline = 25 mg oxtriphylline) | Same as theophylline. Therapeutic level: 10-20 mg/L. |
| Pancreatic enzymes, (Pancrease, Viokase, Cotazyme) | Enteric coated microspheres (Pancrease): capsules. Non-enteric coated (Viokase, Cotazyme) Tablets. Powder (Viokase, Cotazyme) | Enteric Coated: 1-2 capsules with meals, and 1 capsule with snacks. Microspheres may be mixed with each feeding for infants. Non-enteric coated: 3-12 tablets or 1-4 tsp. with each meal. Titrate according to patient's needs. | May cause occult GI bleeding, hyperuricemia, and hyperuricosuria with high doses. |

| Drug | Supply | Dosage | Comments |
|---|---|---|---|
| Pancuronium Bromide (Pavulon) | Injection: 1, 2 mg/ml | Neonates: (test dose) Initial: 0.02 mg/kg/dose Maintenance: 0.03-0.09 mg/kg/dose Q1/2-4h PRN >1 mo. - Adult: Initial: 0.04-0.10 mg/kg/dose Maintenance: 0.02-0.10 mg/kg/dose Q30-60 min. Defasciculating dose: 0.006-0.01 mg/kg/dose Individualize dosage according to patient's response. | Must be prepared to intubate within 2 min. of induction. Drug effect accentuated by hypothermia, acidosis, neonatal age, decreased renal function, halothane, succinylcholine, hypokalemia and aminoglycoside antibiotics. May cause tachycardia. |
| Paraldehyde | Amp: 1 gm/ml Oral Solution: 1 gm/ml | Sedative: 0.15 ml (150 mg)/kg/dose PO, IM or PR in equal amount of veg. oil Anticonvulsant: Deep IM: 0.15 ml (150 mg)/kg/dose Q4-6h; PR: 0.3 ml (300 mg)/kg/dose in oil Q4-6h; IV: May infuse continuously at 0.1 to 0.15 ml paraldehyde/kg/h (Dilute to 5% solution in normal saline, max. infusion rate 1 ml/min). | Do not use discolored solution. Avoid plastic equipment. Contraindicated in hepatic or pulmonary disease. Overdose may cause cardiorespiratory depression. IM may give sterile abscesses. IV route requires close monitoring, including EEG at frequent intervals. |
| Paregoric (Camphorated Opium Tincture) | Tincture: 2 mg/5 ml (0.4 mg morphine/ml) | Analgesia: Children: 0.25-0.5 ml/kg/dose PO QD-QID Adults: 5-10 ml PO QD-QID Neonatal Opiate Withdrawal: Initial: 0.2-0.3 ml/dose Q3-4h Increment: 0.05 ml/dose until symptoms abate. Max. dose: 1-2 ml/kg/day or 0.7 ml/kg/dose | Same side effects as morphine (constipation, lethargy). Taper neonatal dose after symptoms are controlled for several days by 10% Q2-3 days. |

184

| Drug | Preparations | Dosage | Remarks |
|---|---|---|---|
| Pemoline (Cylert) | Tabs: 18.75, 37.5, 75 mg<br>Chewable: 37.5 mg | Initial: 37.5 mg Q AM<br>Increments: 18.75 mg/wk<br>Max. dose: 112.5 mg/day<br>Not recommended for children <6 yrs old. | May cause insomnia, anorexia, hypersensitivity; follow liver functions; use with caution in renal disease. Effect may not be seen until 3-4 weeks of therapy. Long term use associated with growth inhibition. |
| Penicillamine (Cuprimine) | Caps: 125, 250 mg<br>Tabs: 250 mg | Lead chelation therapy<br>500 mg/M² /day PO QD<br>See page 253. | Must be in lead free environment, as can increase absorption of lead if present in GI tract. Follow CBC, LFT's and urine. Can cause cataracts. |
| Penicillin G Preparations<br><br>Potassium<br><br><br><br><br><br>Sodium | Injection: 200,000, 500,000 U/vial; 1, 5, 10, 20 million U/vial<br>Oral liquid: 200,000, 400,000 U/5 ml<br>Tabs: 100,000, 200,000, 400,000, 500,000, 800,000 Units<br><br>Injection: 1, 5 million U/vial | Newborn:<br>IV or IM:<br><7 days: 50,000-150,000 U/kg/day ÷ Q12h;<br>>7 days: 75,000-250,000 U/kg/day ÷ Q6-8h<br>Children:<br>IV, IM: 25,000- 500,000 U/kg/day÷Q4-6h<br>PO:<br>Children: 40,000-80,000 U/kg/day÷Q6h<br>Adults: 300,000-1.2 mil U/day÷Q6h<br><br>(CONTINUED) | 1 mg = approx. 1600 U<br>Salt Content:<br>K Salt: 1 million U (625 mg) contains 1.68 mEq K<br><br>Na Salt: 1 million U (625 mg) contains 1.68 mEq Na<br><br>NOTE: Pen. G. must be taken 1/2 hr before or 2 hrs after meals.<br>Side effects: Anaphylaxis, skin rashes, serum sickness. |

## Penicillin Preparations (CONTINUED)

| Drug | Preparations | Dosage |
|---|---|---|
| Benzathine (Bicillin L-A) | Injection: 300,000 and 600,000 U/ml | Newborns: 50,000 U/kg x 1<br>Infants/Young Children: 300,000-600,000 U x 1<br>Older Children (>30 kg): 900,000 U x 1<br>Adults: 1.2 mil. U x 1<br>Rheumatic fever prophylaxis: 600,000 U Q2 wks or 1.2 mil. U Q month |
| Procaine | Injection 300,000, 500,000, 600,000 U/ml | Newborn: 50,000 U/kg/day QD. Avoid use in this age group because of sterile abscesses and procaine toxicity.<br>Children: 100,000-600,000 U/day QD or BID<br>Adults: 600,000-1 mil U/day QD or BID |
| Bicillin C-R | Tubex: 300,000 U Procaine + 300,000 U Benzathine/ml | Acute streptococcal infections 1.2 mil. U x 1 |
| Bicillin C-R 900/300 | Tubex: 900,000 U Benzathine + 300,000 U Procaine/2 ml | |
| Penicillin V Potassium (Pen Vee K, V-Cillin K) | Tabs: 125 mg (200,000 U), 250 mg (400,000 U), 500 mg (800,000 U)<br>Oral Solution: 125, 250 mg/5 ml | Children: 25,000-50,000 U/kg/day÷Q6h PO<br>Rheumatic Fever Prophylaxis: 250 mg (400,000 U)/day ÷Q12h PO |

| | | | |
|---|---|---|---|
| Pentamidine Isethionate (Pentam 300) | Vial: 300 mg | 4 mg/kg/dose Q day IM or IV x 10 days for T. gambiense; x 12-14 day for Pneumocystis carinii. Risks of therapy >14 days are not well defined. | Monitor closely for hypo-glycemia, as well as trans-ient hypotension, tachy-cardia, nausea, vomiting. Mild hepatotoxicity, mild anemia (megaloblastic) and granulocytopenia, renal toxicity are seen. IV in-fusion must be over 10 hr to reduce risk of hypoten-sion. |
| Pentobarbital (Nembutal) | Tabs (prolonged): 100 mg Caps: 30, 50, 100 mg Elixir: 20 mg/5 ml Supp: 30, 60, 120, 200 mg Amp: 50 mg/ml | Sedation: Children: 2-6 mg/kg/dose Adults: 30 mg TID-QID PO To induce coma: Initial: 3-5 mg/kg IV x 1 Maintenance: 2-3.5 mg/kg/dose Q1h as needed | No advantage over phenobar-bital for control of seizures. Adjunct in treatment of increased intracranial pres-sure. May cause drug-related isoelectric EEG. Toxic levels: > 1 mg/L |
| Phenazopyridine (Pyridium) | Tabs: 100, 200 mg | Children 6-12 yr: 100 mg TID until symptoms are controlled Adults: 200 mg TID until symptoms are controlled | Caution in presence of G6PD deficiency, GI problems or renal insufficiency. May cause methemoglobinemia, hemolytic anemia. Colors urine orange. |

| | | |
|---|---|---|
| Phenobarbital (Luminal) | Drops: 16 mg/ml<br>Tabs: 8, 15, 30, 65<br>100 mg<br>Elixir: 20 mg/5 ml<br>Spans: 60, 100 mg<br>Vials: 65 mg/ml,<br>130 mg/ml, 165 mg/ml | Sedation: 2-3 mg/kg/dose PO,<br>IM Q8h PRN. Slower acting<br>barbiturates are preferred.<br>Status epilepticus: See p 269.<br>15-25 mg/kg IV:<br>Max.: 600 mg/day<br>Chronic anticonvulsant:<br>Children: 4-6 mg/kg/day PO÷<br>Q12h - follow levels and<br>correlate to clinical response<br>Adult: 150-250 mg/day÷BID<br>(1-3 mg/kg/day). | IV administration may cause respiratory arrest or hypotension. Contraindicated in hepatic or renal disease and porphyria. T1/2 approximately 96 hours in children. Paradoxical reaction in children (not dose related) may cause hyperactivity, irritability, insomnia. Therapeutic levels: 15-40 mg/L. |
| Phenylephrine (Neo-Synephrine) | Vials: 10 mg/ml (1% solution)<br>Nasal drops: 0.125, 0.25, 0.5, 1%<br>Nasal solution: 0.25, 0.5, 1.0%<br>Ophthalmic solution: 10%<br>Elixir: 5 mg/5 ml | Hypotension:<br>Children:<br>IM or SC: 0.1 mg/kg/dose<br>Q1-2h PRN<br>IV bolus: 5-20 mcg/kg/dose<br>Q10-15 min. PRN<br>IV drip: 0.1-0.5 mcg/kg/min.<br>Adults:<br>IM or SC : 5-10 mg/dose<br>Q1-2h PRN<br>IV bolus: 0.25-1 mg/dose<br>Q10-15 min. PRN<br>IV drip: 1-4 mcg/min (10 mg/ 100 ml saline - adjust dosage rate to desired effect)<br>To prepare for infusion:<br>See inside front cover.<br>CONTINUED | Use cautiously in presence of hypertension, arrhythmias, hyperthyroidism, or hyperglycemia. May cause tremor, insomnia, palpitations. For SVT: dose may be doubled and repeated Q5min until systolic BP is 2 times initial BP. |

188

| | | |
|---|---|---|
| Phenylephrine | CONTINUED | **Paroxysmal supraventricular** <u>Tachycardia:</u> (give IV push)<br>Children: 5-10 mcg/kg/dose<br>Adults: 0.25-0.5 mg/dose<br>**Decongestant:**<br>Oral: 1 mg/kg/day Q4h to max.<br>adult dose of 10 mg/dose or<br>60 mg/day<br>Topical: (give up to 3 days)<br>Infants: 0.125% sol'n Q3-4h<br>Children: 0.25% sol'n Q3-4h<br>Adults: 0.25-1% sol'n Q3-4h | |
| Phenytoin<br>(Dilantin) | Caps: 30, 100 mg<br>Tabs: 50 mg<br>(Infatab)<br>Susp: 30 mg/5 ml<br>(Ped.), 125 mg/5 ml<br>Amps: 50 mg/ml | **Status epilepticus:** See p 269.<br>15-20 mg/kg IV;<br>Max. dose: 1000 mg/day<br>**Maint. for seizure disorders**<br>Infants/Children: 4-7 mg/kg/<br>day÷QD or BID IV or PO<br>Adults: 300-400 mg/day<br>÷QD or BID IV or PO<br>**Anti-arrhythmic:**<br>Children: IV: 2-4 mg/kg over<br>5 min.; PO: 2-5 mg/kg/day<br>Adults: IV: 100 mg Q5min up<br>to total dose: 500 mg,<br>repeat in 2h PRN; PO: 250<br>mg/dose QID x 1 day, then<br>250 mg/dose BID x 2 days,<br>then 300-400 mg/day÷QD-QID | T1/2 is variable (7-42 hrs)<br>and dose dependent. Useful<br>in ventricular tachycardia<br>and digitalis-induced<br>arrhythmias (esp. PAT with<br>block). Not FDA approved for<br>ventricular arrhythmias.<br>Side effects include<br>gingival hyperplasia,<br>hirsutism, dermatitis,<br>blood dyscrasias, ataxia,<br>lymphadenopathy, liver<br>damage, and nystagmus.<br>For seizure disorders,<br>therapeutic levels: 10-<br>20 mg/L. |

| Phosphorus Supplements | (Neutraphos): Per capsule: 250 mg P (14 mEq, 8.1 mM), 7 mEq Na, 7 mEq K (Neutraphos-K): Per capsule: 250 mg P (14 mEq, 8.1 mM), 14 mEq K (Na-P Injection): 94 mg P/ml (3 mM), 4 mEq Na/ml (K-P Injection): 94 mg P/ml (3 mM), 4.4 mEq K/ml | 1-2 gm P/day ÷ QID OR: 2.5 - 15 mg/kg/dose Q6h depending on serum levels (mg/dl): phos. level   dose 0.5-1 mg/dl   7-8 mg/kg < 0.5 mg/dl   15 mg/kg | All can cause GI discomfort and diarrhea. Begin at doses of 0.5-1.0 gm/day and increase slowly. Use of Na salts may aggravate GI symptoms. Injectable forms may also be given PO. |
| Physostigmine Salicylate (Antilirium) | Vial: 1 mg/ml | For antihistamine overdose or anticholinergic poisoning: see page 256-8. | Atropine is the antidote for physostigmine and should always be available. |
| Piperacillin (Pipracil) | Vial: 2, 3, 4 gm/vial | Children >12 yr and adults: 200-300 mg/kg/day ÷ Q4h or Q6h; IV or deep IM | Similar to penicillin. Piperacillin has been used in children < 12 yrs in dosage of 75-100 mg/kg/day. |
| Piperazine (Antepar) | Tabs: 250, 500 mg Syrup: 500 mg/5 ml Wafer: 500 mg | Enterobius vermicularis (pinworm): 65 mg/kg/day to max. of 2.5 g/day QD x 7 days. May repeat in 1 week if necessary. Ascaris lumbricoides (roundworm): 75 mg/kg/day QD x 2 days to max. of 3.5 gm/day. | Contraindicated in epilepsy. Large doses may cause vomiting, urticaria, muscle weakness, blurred vision. |

| | | | |
|---|---|---|---|
| Potassium Iodide (SSKI) | Tab: 300 mg<br>Syrup: 325 mg/5 ml<br>Saturated sol'n<br>(SSKI): 1 gm/ml | For thyrotoxicosis:<br>Children: 200-300 mg/day<br>÷ BID - TID<br>Adults: 300-900 mg/day TID | Contraindicated in pregnancy. GI disturbance, metallic taste, rash, inflammation of salivary glands, headache, lacrimation, rhinitis are symptoms of iodism. |
| Potassium Supplements | Potassium Chloride:<br>(1 gm = 13.3 mEq K)<br>Injection: 2 mEq/ml<br>Powder: 20 mEq/packet<br>Sol'n: 5% (10 mEq/15 ml)<br>10% (20 mEq/15 ml)<br>20% (40 mEq/15 ml)<br>Tab: 4, 8, 10 mEq<br>Potassium Gluconate:<br>(1 gm = 4.3 mEq K)<br>Elixir: 1.56 gm/5 ml<br>(6.66 mEq K/5 ml)<br>Tab: 2, 5mEq<br>Potassium Triplex:<br>Acetate-Bicarbonate-<br>Citrate. Oral Sol'n.<br>500 mg of each salt/5<br>ml. (15 mEq K / 5 ml) | Dose based on clinical requirements. Starting dose should be determined by considering maintenance K losses and desired supplementation. Usual starting dose in diuretic therapy: 1-2 mEq/kg/day. Max. rate of infusion 0.5-1 mEq/kg/hour. | May cause GI disturbances and ulcerations. Monitor serum K$^+$. Hyperkalemia may present with cardiac arrhythmias, cardiac arrest. |
| Prazocin HCl (Minipress) | Caps: 1, 2, 5 mg | Not FDA approved for children. The following doses have been used in children:<br>25-40 mcg/kg/dose Q6h PO<br>Adults: 1 mg BID-TID initially. Increase slowly to 20 mg/day ÷ BID-TID PO | May cause syncope, tachycardia, hypotension, dizziness, headache, drowsiness, fatigue, nausea. |

| Prednisone | Tabs: 1, 2.5, 5, 10, 20, 50 mg<br>Liquid: 5 mg/5 ml | **Physiologic replacement:**<br>4 - 5 mg/M²/day÷BID<br>**Nephrotic Syndrome:**<br><u>Initial:</u> 2 mg/kg/day (max. of 80 mg/day) TID-QID until urine is protein-free x 5 days or for max. of 28 days. If proteinuria persists, dose may be changed to 4 mg/kg/dose QOD for an additional 28 days.<br>Maintenance: 2 mg/kg/dose QOD x 28 days. Then taper over 4-6 weeks.<br>**Asthma:**<br><u>Acute exacerbation:</u> 0.5-1 mg/kg/day up to 20-40 mg/day x 3-5 days.<br>Severe refractory asthma: 5-10 mg/dose QD or 10-30 mg QOD. Attempt to taper and/or wean to aerosol corticosteroid.<br><u>Anti-inflammatory or Immuno-suppressive:</u> 0.5-2 mg/kg/day or 25-60 mg/M²/day Q6-12h | See page 217-18.<br>Methylprednisolone preferable in hepatic disease since prednisone must be converted in the liver to methyl-prednisolone. Long-term, low maintenance doses may be beneficial in relapsing nephrotic syndrome. |

| Primidone (Mysoline) | Tabs: 50, 250 mg<br>Susp: 250 mg/5 ml | <8 yrs:<br>Initial: 125 mg/day QD<br>Increment: 125 mg/day at weekly interval.<br>Maintenance: 10-25 mg/kg/day TID-QID<br>>8 yrs-adult:<br>Initial: 250 mg/day QD<br>Increment: 250 mg/day at weekly intervals.<br>Maintenance: 750-1500 mg/day TID-QID. | Primidone is metabolized to phenobarbital and has the same toxicities. Follow both primidone and phenobarbital levels.<br>Therapeutic level: 8-12 mg/L of primidone or 15-40 mg/L of phenobarbital |
|---|---|---|---|
| Probenecid (Benemid) | Tabs: 0.5 gm | Use with Penicillin.<br><u>Children (2-14 yr):</u> 25 mg/kg starting dose, 40 mg/kg/day ÷ QID<br><u>Adult Dose (>50 kg):</u><br>2 gms probenecid ÷ QID.<br>For gonorrhea Rx -- 1 gm probenecid 30 min before PCN or ampicillin. | Alkalinize urine in gouty patients, use with caution if history of peptic ulcer. Headache, GI symptoms, hypersensitivity, anemia. Contraindicated in children <2 yrs and in patients with renal insufficiency. |
| Procainamide (Pronestyl) | Tabs: 250, 375, 500 mg<br>Tabs (SR): 250, 500 mg<br>Caps: 250, 375, 500 mg<br>Injection: 100, 500 mg/ml | <u>Children:</u><br>IM: 20-30 mg/kg/day÷Q4-6h<br>Max. dose: 4 gm/day.<br>(Peak effect in 1 hr).<br>IV:<br>Loading: 10-15 mg/kg/dose over 30 min.<br>Maintenance: 20-80 mcg/kg/ min. by continuous infusion.<br>Max. dose: 50-60 mg/kg/day<br>PO: 15-50 mg/kg/day Q3-6h<br>Max. dose: 4 gm/day<br>CONTINUED | Contraindicated in myasthenia gravis, complete heart block. May cause lupus-like syndrome, Coombs positivity, thrombocytopenia. Monitor IV use closely with BP's, EKG. QRS widening >0.02 seconds suggest toxicity. May cause arrhythmias, GI complaints, confusion. Therapeutic levels: 4-10 mg/L. |

| | | | |
|---|---|---|---|
| Procainamide | CONTINUED | **Adults:**<br>**IM:**<br>  Loading: 1 gm/dose x 1.<br>  Maintenance: 250 mg/dose Q3h<br>**IV:**<br>  Loading: 1 gm over 30 min<br>  Maintenance: 1-3 mg/min by<br>  continuous infusion<br>PO: 250-500 mg/dose Q3-6h<br>  (usual dose 50 mg/kg/day or<br>  2-4 gm/day) | |
| Prochlorperazine<br>(Compazine) | Tabs: 5, 10, 25 mg<br>Syrup: 5 mg/5 ml<br>Oral concentrate:<br>  10 mg/ml<br>Supp: 2.5, 5, 25 mg<br>Spans: 10, 15, 30,<br>  75 mg<br>Amp: 5 mg/ml | **Children >10 kg or >2 yr:**<br>0.4 mg/kg/day÷Q6-8h PO<br>or PR; 0.2 mg/kg/day÷Q6-8h<br>IM<br>**Adults:**<br>PO: 5-10 mg/dose TID-QID<br>PR: 25 mg BID<br>IM: 5-20 mg/dose Q4-6h.<br>Max. IM dose: 40 mg/day | Toxicity as for other pheno-<br>thiazines. Extrapyramidal<br>reactions, drowsiness may<br>occur. Do not use IV route<br>in children. Do not use in<br>children <10 kg or <2 yr.<br>old |
| Promethazine<br>(Phenergan,<br>Provigan) | Tabs: 12.5, 25,<br>  50 mg<br>Amp: 25, 50 mg/ml<br>Syrup: 6.25 mg/5 ml,<br>  25 mg/5 ml<br>Supp: 12.5, 25, 50<br>  mg | **Antihistaminic:**<br>Children: 0.1 mg/kg/dose<br>Q6h and 0.5 mg/kg/dose Q HS<br>PO, PRN<br>Adults: 12.5 mg TID and<br>QHS<br>**Nausea and Vomiting:**<br>Children: 0.25- 0.5 mg/kg/<br>dose IM, PO, or PR Q4-6h PRN<br>Adults: 12.5-25 mg Q4-6h PRN<br>**Sedative and Preoperative:**<br>Children: 0.5-1 mg/kg/dose<br>Q6h IM PRN<br>Adults: 25-50 mg/dose<br>**Motion Sickness:**<br>Children: 0.5 mg/kg/dose<br>Q12h PO, PRN | Toxicity similar to other<br>phenothiazines (see chlorpro-<br>mazine). |

| Propranolol (Inderal) | Tabs: 10, 20, 40, 80 mg<br>Injection: 1 mg/ml<br>Formulation for oral form (no commercial product available): Final concentration 1 mg/ml. Ten 10 mg tabs crushed and mixed with 200 mg Na Benzoate. Add simple syrup QS to 100 cc. Adjust pH = 5.0 with citric acid. Stable x 2 mo in refrigerator<br>Capsules (extended release): 80, 120, 160 mg | **Arrhythmias:**<br><u>Children:</u> 0.01-0.10 mg/kg/dose, slow IV push; may repeat Q6-8h PRN (max. single dose: 1 mg); 0.5- 4.0 mg/kg/day÷Q6-8h PO (max. daily dose: 60 mg)<br><u>Adults:</u> 1 mg/dose IV repeated Q5 min up to total 5 mg<br>**Tetralogy Spells:** 0.15-0.25 mg/kg/dose IV slowly -- may repeat in 15 min x 1 (max. single dose: 10 mg) then maintenance: 1-2 mg/kg/dose Q6h PO<br>**Thyrotoxicosis:**<br><u>Neonatal:</u> 2 mg/kg/day PO Q6h<br><u>Adolescents and Adults:</u><br>IV: 1-3 mg/dose x 1 over 10 min<br>PO: 10-40 mg Q6h<br>**Hypertension:** Starting dose 0.5-1.0 mg/kg/day ÷ Q6-12h (max. dose: 2 mg/kg/day)<br><u>Adults:</u><br>Initial: 40 mg/dose PO BID;<br>Increment: 10-20 mg/dose at intervals of 3-7 days<br>Max. dose: 320-480 mg/day PO<br>**Migraine Prophylaxis:**<br><35 kg: 10-20 mg PO TID<br>>35kg: 20-40 mg PO TID<br><u>Adults:</u> Initially, 80 mg/day ÷Q6-8h PO. Usual effective dose range: 160-240 mg/day. | Contraindicated in asthma and heart block. Use with caution in presence of obstructive lung disease, heart failure, renal or hepatic disease. May cause hypoglycemia, hypotension, nausea, vomiting, depression, weakness. |

| Drug | Preparations | Dosage | Comments |
|---|---|---|---|
| Propyl-thiouracil (PTU) | Tabs: 50 mg | Children: Initial: 5-7 mg/kg/day ÷Q8h PO or 50-150 mg/day ÷Q8h PO<br>6-10 yrs: 50-150 mg/day ÷Q8h PO<br>>10 yrs: 150-300 mg/day ÷Q8h PO<br>Maintenance: Adjust to patient response. Usually 1/3 - 1/2 the initial dose beginning when the patient is euthyroid.<br>Adults:<br>Initial: 300 mg/day÷Q8h PO.<br>Maintenance: 100-150 mg/day ÷Q8h PO | May cause blood dyscrasias, fever, liver disease, dermatitis, urticaria, malaise, arthralgias. Monitor thyroid function. 100 mg PTU = 10 mg methimazole. |
| Prostaglandin E₁ (PGE, alprostadil, Prostin VR) | Amps: 500 mcg/ml | Neonates:<br>Initial: 0.05 mcg/kg/min<br>Advance to 0.4 mcg/kg/min<br>Maintenance: when increase in pO₂ is noted, decrease immediately to lowest effective dose (e.g. 0.01 mcg/kg/min). | For palliation only. Continuous vital sign monitoring essential. May cause apnea, fever, seizures, flushing, bradycardia, hypotension, and diarrhea. Decreases platelet aggregation. |
| Protamine Sulfate | Amp: 10 mg/ml | Heparin Antidote: 1 mg will neutralize approximately 100 U of heparin. For IV heparin, base dose on amount received in previous 2 hours.<br>Max. dose: 50 mg IV with rate not to exceed 5 mg/min. | Actual dosage depends on route of administration and time elapsed since heparin dose. Can cause hypotension, bradycardia. Rarely heparin rebound has occurred. |
| Pseudoephedrine (Sudafed, Novafed) | Tabs: 30, 60 mg<br>Syrup: 30 mg/5 ml<br>Capsules (sustained release): 60, 120 mg | Children: 4 mg/kg/day ÷Q6h PO<br>Adults: 30-60 mg Q6-8h<br>Sustained release: >12 yrs - adults: 1 cap PO Q12h | Use with caution in hypertension. May cause nervousness, restlessness. |

| Drug | Form | Dosage | Comments |
|---|---|---|---|
| Pyrantel Pamoate (Antiminth) | Susp: 250 mg/5 ml | Ascariasis (roundworm), hookworm, enterobiasis (pinworm): In children and adults: 11 mg/kg as single dose (max. dose: 1 gm). May repeat x 1 in 2 wks. | Nausea, vomiting, anorexia, transient SGOT elevations. Use with caution with pre-existing liver dysfunction. |
| Pyrethrins (A-200 Pyrinate, Pyrinal, Rid) | Available as gel, shampoo and solution, all in combination with piperonyl butoxide | For pediculosis: Apply to hair or body area affected for 10 min., then wash thoroughly; may repeat in 7-10 days. | For topical use only. Avoid eye or facial contact and PO intake. Avoid repeat applications in < 24 hrs. |
| Pyrvinium Pamoate (Povan) | Tabs: 50 mg | Enterobiasis: 5 mg/kg/dose PO as single dose. Repeat in 2 wks. Max. dose: 350 mg | May cause GI symptoms, colors stools red. May stain teeth. Swallow tabs whole. |
| Quinacrine (Atabrine) | Tabs: 100 mg | Giardiasis: 8 mg/kg/day ÷Q8h PO. Give single dose 1st day, 2 doses 2nd day and 8 mg/kg/day in 3 doses after meals on 3rd day x 5 days. Max. dose: 300 mg/day. Tapeworms: 15 mg/kg/day PO ÷ into 2 doses 1 hr apart. Saline purge night before 1st dose and 2 hrs after last dose. Max. dose: 800 mg. | May cause GI disturbances, dermatosis, bone marrow depression, psychosis. May cause temporary yellow color in skin (not jaundice). Use with caution in patients with G6PD deficiency. |

| Drug | Preparations | Dose | Comments |
|---|---|---|---|
| Quinidine | Gluconate:<br>Tabs: 324 mg<br>Vials: 80 mg/ml<br>Sulfate:<br>Tabs: 100, 200, 300 mg<br>Extended Release<br>Tabs: 300 mg<br>Caps: 200, 300 mg<br>Injection: 200 mg/ml | Test Dose: 2 mg/kg PO<br>Therapeutic Dose:<br>Children:<br>IV: not recommended<br>PO: 15-60 mg/kg/day÷Q6h<br>Adults:<br>IM: 400 mg/dose Q4-6h<br>IV: 200-400 mg/dose<br>PO: 100-600 mg/dose Q4-6h.<br>Begin at 200 mg/dose and titrate to desired effect.<br>Therapeutic levels: 2-5 mg/L | Toxicity indicated by increase of QRS interval by >0.02 seconds (skip dose or stop drug). May cause GI symptoms, hypotension, tinnitus, blood dyscrasias. Can cause increase in digoxin levels if these drugs are used concomitantly. When used alone may cause 1:1 conduction in atrial flutter leading to V fib. May get idiosyncratic reaction of V tach with low levels, especially when initiating therapy. |
| Ranitidine (Zantac) | Tabs: 150 mg<br>Vials: 25 mg/ml | Children:<br>PO: 2-4 mg/kg/day ÷ Q12h<br>IV: 1-2 mg/kg/day ÷ Q6-8h<br>Adults: 150 mg PO BID, or 50 mg IV Q6-8h. | Usual adverse reactions include headache and GI disturbance. |
| Ribavirin (Virazole) | Vials for aerosol:<br>6 gm/100 ml | Administer by aerosol 12-18 hrs/day for at least 3 and not more than 7 days.<br>The 6 gm Ribavirin vial is diluted in 300 ml sterile water to a final concentration of 20 mg/ml. | Must be administered with Viratek Small Particle Aerosol Generator. Most effective if begun early in the course of illness, generally in the first 3 days. |

| Drug | Preparations | Dose | Comments |
|---|---|---|---|
| Rifampin (Rimactane, Rifadin) | Caps: 150, 300 mg Liquid: 10 mg/ml (1%) can be made according to directions found in package insert. | Antituberculosis: Children: 10-20 mg/kg/day QD Adults: 600 mg/day QD Meningococcal carriers or meningitis prophylaxis: 0-1 mo: 10 mg/kg/day ÷Q12h x 2 days. > 1 mo: 20 mg/kg/day ÷Q12h x 2 days. Max. dose: 600 mg Q12h H. Flu Carriers or Prophylaxis: 0-1 mo: 10 mg/kg/day QD x 4 d > 1 mo: 20 mg/kg/day QD x 4 d Max. dose: 600 mg/day | Causes red discoloration of body secretions (e.g. urine, saliva, including tears which can permanently stain contact lenses). Also reduces effectiveness of oral contraceptives; recommend alternate methods of birth control. Give 1 hr before or two hrs after meals. Use with caution in liver dysfunction. |
| Scopolamine hydrobromide, USP hyoscine hydrobromide, Transdermscop | Tabs: 400, 600 μg Injection: 0.3, 0.4, 0.5, 0.6, 0.8, 1.0 mg/ml Ophth. Sol'n: 0.25% Transdermal 0.5 mg | 6 mcg/kg/dose PO or SC Transdermal for children >12 yrs over 3 days only | See atropine. Contraindicated in urinary or GI obstruction and glaucoma. Transdermal reported to cause unilateral mydriasis. |
| Secobarbital (Seconal) | Caps: 50, 100 mg Supp: 30, 60, 120, 200 mg Injection: 50 mg/ml Elixir: 22 mg/5 ml Tabs: 50-100 mg Tabs (enteric coated): 50-100 mg | Sedation: Children: 6 mg/kg/day÷Q8h PO Adults: 20-40 mg PO BID-TID or 200-300 mg PO 2-3h pre-operatively | See amobarbital. T1/2 = 20-28 hrs. |
| Selenium Sulfide (Selsun) | 2.5% Solution | Tinea versicolor: apply weekly x 4 weeks to affected areas. Lather and rinse from body areas after 5 min or from face after 10 min. Avoid eyes and genital area. | Local irritation, rare discoloration of hair, hair loss. |

| Sodium Polystyrene Sulfonate (Kayexalate) | Oral powder: 450 gm Susp: 25% in Sorbitol Solution (4.1 mEq Na$^+$/gm) | Children: Practical Exchange Rate: 1 mEq K per 1 gm resin. Calculate dose according to desired exchange Q6h PO or Q2-6h PR. Usual dose: 1 gm/kg/dose Q6h PO or Q2-6h rectally Adults: 15-60 gm PO or 30-60 gm rectally Q6h. | Use cautiously in presence of renal failure. (Na exchanged for K$^+$; may also cause hypomagnesemia and hypocalcemia). Do not administer with antacids or laxatives containing Mg$^{++}$ or Al$^{+++}$. Systemic alkalosis may result. |
|---|---|---|---|
| Spectinomycin (Trobicin) | Vials: 2 mg/5 ml, 4 mg/10 ml | Children: 40 mg/kg x 1 Adults: 2 gm IM as single dose. 4 gm if PCN resistant gonorrhea prevalent. | Not effective for syphilis. Vertigo, malaise, nausea, anorexia, chills, fever, urticaria. |
| Spironolactone (Aldactone) | Tabs: 25 mg | Children: 1.0-3.3 mg/kg/day ÷BID-QID Adults: 25-100 mg/day÷BID-QID Max. dose: 200 mg/day | Contraindicated in acute renal failure. May potentiate ganglionic blocking agents and other antihypertensives. May cause hyperkalemia, GI distress. |
| Streptomycin sulfate | Vials: 500 mg/ml | Premature and Full Term: 20-30 mg/kg/day÷Q12h IM up to 10 days Children: 20-40 mg/kg/day ÷Q8h IM up to 10 days Adults: 15-25 mg/kg/day ÷Q12h IM x 7-10 days, then 1 gm/dose QD Tuberculosis: 20-50 mg/kg/day IM single dose (use higher dose for TB meningitis) Max. dose: 2 gm/day. | Reduce dose in presence of renal insufficiency. Follow auditory status. May cause CNS depression, other neurologic manifestations. |

| | | | |
|---|---|---|---|
| Succinylcholine (Anectine) | Vials: 20, 50, 100 mg/ml | **Neonates and Children:**<br>Initial: 1-2 mg/kg/dose x 1<br>Maintenance: 0.3-0.6 mg/kg at intervals of 5-10 min PRN.<br>**Adults:**<br>Initial:0.6-1.1 mg/kg/dose x 1<br>Maintenance: 0.3-0.6 mg/kg at intervals of 5-10 min PRN;<br>Continuous infusion: not recommended in children.<br>Adults: 0.5-10 mg/min.<br>(average dose 2.5 mg/min).<br>Titrate dose to desired effect. | Premedicate patient with atropine prior to administration. Duration of action: 10 min. Must be able to intubate patient within 1 min. Side effects: bradycardia, hypotension, arrhythmia. Beware of prolonged depression in patients with liver disease, malnutrition, aminoglycoside Rx, hypothermia, hyperkalemia, pseudocholinesterase deficiency. |
| Sucralfate (Carafate) | Tabs: 1 gm | Children: Not approved for children <12 yr.<br>Adults: 1 gm PO QID (1 hr AC and QHS) | May cause constipation. Not approved for children < 12 years old. |
| *Sulfacetamide Sodium (Sulamyd) | Ophth Sol'n: 10%, 15%, 30%<br>Ophth Ointment: 10% | Ribbon of ointment QID and QHS<br>1 - 2 drops Q2-3h | See sulfisoxazole. |
| Sulfadiazine | Tabs: 60, 250, 300, 500 mg<br>Tabs (chewable): 300 mg<br>Susp.: 0.5 gm/5 ml | **Newborn:** Do not use.<br>Children >2 mo old:<br>Loading: 75 mg/kg/dose PO x 1<br>Maintenance: 150 mg/kg/day ÷Q6h PO. Max. dose: 6 gm/day.<br>**Adults:**<br>Loading: 2-4 gm x 1<br>Maintenance: 1 gm Q4-6h.<br>**Malaria:**<br>Children: 100-200 mg/kg/day÷QID to a max. of 2 gm/day x 5 days<br>**Meningococcal prophylaxis:**<br><1 yr: 500 mg QD x 2 days<br>1-12 yr: 500 mg BID x 2 days<br>>12 yr: 1 gm BID x 2 days | May cause crystalluria (keep urine output high and alkaline), fever, rash, hepatitis, vasculitis, bone marrow suppression. Hemolysis in patients with G6PD deficiency. |

201

| Drug | Preparations | Dosage | Comments |
|---|---|---|---|
| Sulfasalazine (Salicylazo-sulfapyridine, Azulfidine) | Tabs: 500 mg; Enteric Coated Tabs: 500 mg; Oral susp: 125 mg/5 ml | Initial: 75-150 mg/kg/day ÷Q3-6h PO; Maintenance: 40 mg/kg/day ÷Q6h PO; Max. adult dose: 6 gm/day | Orange-yellow discoloration of alkaline urine. Severe hypersensitivity reactions, blood dyscrasias, CNS changes, renal damage. Use with caution in G6PD deficiency. |
| Sulfisoxazole (Gantrisin) | Tabs: 500 mg, 1 gm; Susp: 500 mg/5 ml; Syrup: 500 mg/5 ml; Amp: 400 mg/ml; Ophth Sol'n: 40 mg/ml; Ophth ointment: 40 mg/gm | Initial: 75 mg/kg/dose PO, 50 mg/kg/dose IV; Maintenance: 150 mg/kg/day ÷Q4-6h PO; 100 mg/kg/day÷Q6h IV; Maximum: 6 gm/day; Adults: Loading: 2-4 gm x 1; Maintenance: 4-8 gm/day Q4-6h; Otitis Media Prophylaxis: 50-75 mg/kg/day÷BID; Rheumatic Fever Prophylaxis: <30 kg: 500 mg/day PO single dose. >30 kg: 1 gm/day PO single dose. Ophth Sol'n: 2-3 gtts Q4-8h; Ophth Ointment: 1-3 x daily | Contraindicated in infants <2 mos, near-term pregnant or nursing mothers. Use cautiously in presence of renal or liver disease, or G6PD deficiency. Maintain adequate fluid intake. |
| Terbutaline (Brethine, Bricanyl) | Tabs: 2.5, 5 mg; Injection: 1 mg/ml; Inhaler: 200 mcg/metered spray, 300 doses per inhaler, | PO: <12 yr: Initial: 0.05 mg/kg/dose TID, increase as required. Max. dose: 0.10 mg/kg/dose TID or total of 5 mg/day >12 yr – Adults: CONTINUED | Nervousness, tremor, headache, nausea, as with other sympathomimetic agents. |

| | | | |
|---|---|---|---|
| Terbutaline | CONTINUED | | Initial: 2.5 mg/dose TID<br>Maintenance: Usually 5 mg<br>or 0.075 mg/kg/dose TID<br>SC:<br><u>&lt;12 yr</u>: 0.005-0.010 mg/kg/<br>dose, max. of 0.25 mg/dose<br>Q15-20 min. x 2<br><u>&gt;12 yr - Adults</u>: 0.25 mg/dose<br>Q15-30 min. PRN x 1 only.<br>Total of 0.5 mg is not to be<br>exceeded within a 4 hr period.<br><u>Inhaler</u>: 2 inhalations Q4-6 hrs. | |
| Terfenadine<br>(Seldane) | Tabs: 60 mg | <u>Adults and Adolescents</u>:<br>60 mg BID PO | Significantly less sedative<br>effect than other antihista-<br>mines. |
| Tetracycline<br>HCL<br>(many brand<br>names) | Tabs: 250, 500 mg<br>Caps: 100, 250, 500<br>mg<br>Drops: 100 mg/ml<br>(5 mg/gtt)<br>Syrup: 25 mg/ml<br>Vials: 100, 250, 500<br>mg<br>Ophth oint: 1%, 3%<br>Ophth susp: 1% | <u>Older Infants and Children</u>:<br>PO: 25-50 mg/kg/day ÷ Q6h<br>IM: 15-25 mg/kg/day ÷ Q8h<br>12h (not to exceed 250 mg/<br>injection)<br>IV: 10-20 mg/kg/day ÷ Q12h<br><u>Children &gt;40 kg - Adults</u>:<br>PO: 1-2 gm/day÷Q6h<br>IM: 250-300 mg/day÷Q8-12h<br>IV: 250-500 mg/dose Q6-12h,<br>depending on severity of<br>illness<br><u>Chlamydia Genital Infections</u>:<br>500 mg Q6h PO (see p. 220) | Not recommended in patients<br>&lt; 8 yrs due to tooth stain-<br>ing and decreased bone<br>growth. Also not recommend-<br>ed for use in pregnancy due<br>to these effects on the<br>fetus. Give on empty sto-<br>mach. May cause nausea and<br>GI upset.<br>(Max. dose: 2 gm/day) |

| Theophylline | Many preparations See page 215. | **Neonatal apnea**<br>Loading dose: 5 mg/kg/dose PO<br>Maintenance (before levels):<br>Preterm: (<36 wks) 1-2 mg/kg<br>day÷Q8-12h<br>Term: (or >36 wks) up to<br>1 month: 2-4 mg/kg/day<br>÷Q8-12h<br>**Bronchospasm:**<br>Loading dose (PO): 0.8 mg/kg/<br>dose for each 2 mg/L desired<br>increase in theophylline<br>level.<br>Maintenance (PO) (before levels):<br>0-2 mo: 3-6 mg/kg/day÷Q8h<br>2-6 mo: 6-15 mg/kg/day÷Q6h<br>6-12 mo: 15-22 mg/kg/day÷Q6h<br>1-9 yr: 22 mg/kg/day÷Q6h<br>9-12 yr: 20 mg/kg/day÷Q6h<br>12-16 yr: 18 mg/kg/day÷Q6h<br>Adults: 13 mg/kg/day÷Q6h<br>Max: 900 mg/day<br>Divide dosage BID or TID for<br>long-acting preparations. | Drug metabolism varies widely with age, drug formulation and route of administration. Most common side effects and toxicities are nausea, vomiting, anorexia, nervousness, tachycardia and seizures. Serum levels should be monitored. Therapeutic levels:<br>Bronchospasm: 10-20 mg/L<br>Apnea: 7-13 mg/L<br>Note: An alternative dosing regimen for infants less than 1 yr is:<br>Dose (mg/kg/day) =<br>0.2 (age in weeks) + 5.<br>Ref: Hendeles L. pers. comm; 1984. |
| Thiopental sodium (Pentothal) | Injection: 250, 400, 500 mg syringes 0.5, 1 gm vials | **Cerebral edema:** 1.5-3.0 mg/kg/ dose IV Repeat PRN increased intracranial pressure<br>**General anesthesia:**<br>Children: 2 mg/kg x 1 IV<br>Adults: 3-5 mg/kg x 1 IV<br>Maintenance:<br>Children: 1 mg/kg PRN<br>Adults: 50-100 mg PRN | T1/2 is 3-8h in blood, but probably <30 seconds in brain. Toxicity: respiratory depression, hypotension, anaphylaxis, decreased cardiac output. Contraindicated in acute intermittent porphyria. |

| | | | |
|---|---|---|---|
| Thioridazine (Mellaril) | Tabs: 10, 15, 25, 50, 100, 150, 200 mg<br>Concentrate: 30 mg/ml, 100 mg/ml<br>Susp: 5, 20 mg/ml | Children (2-12 yrs): 1.0 mg/kg/day÷Q6-12h, increase gradually.<br>Adult: Initially, 150-300 mg/day÷Q6-12h.<br>Max. dose: 800 mg/day | Drowsiness, extrapyramidal reactions, autonomic symptoms, paradoxical reactions, endocrine disturbances. |
| Ticarcillin (Ticar) | Vials: 1, 3, 6 gm | Neonates (< 2 kg):<br>0-7 d: 150 mg/kg/day÷Q8h, IV<br>> 7 d: 225 mg/kg/day÷Q8h, IV<br>Neonates (> 2 kg):<br>0-7 d: 225 mg/kg/day÷Q8h, IV<br>> 7 d: 300 mg/kg/day÷Q8h, IV<br>Children and Adults:<br>200-300 mg/kg/day÷Q4-6h IV<br>Uncomplicated UTI:<br>50-100 mg/kg/day÷Q6-8h IM or IV. (Use 1 gm Q6h IM or IV in adults).<br>Max. IM dose should not exceed 2 gm/injection. | Each gram contains 5.2 mEq Na. Activity similar to carbenicillin. |

| Drug | Preparations | Dosing | Comments |
|---|---|---|---|
| Ticarcillin/ Clavulanate Potassium (Timentin) | Vials: 3.1 gm (3.0 gm Ticarcillin and 0.1 gm Clavulanate) 3.2 gm (3.0 gm Ticarcillin and 0.2 gm Clavulanate) | Dosing as with Ticarcillin | Activity similar to Ticarcillin except that beta-lactamase inhibitor broadens spectrum to include staph aureus and H. Flu. |
| Tobramycin (Nebcin) | Amp: 20 mg/2 ml, 80 mg/2 ml | Neonates: Tobramycin doses are the same as those for gentamicin. Children: 7.5 mg/kg/day ÷ Q8h Adults: 3-5 mg/kg/day ÷Q8h IV and IM | Ototoxicity, nephrotoxicity. Activity similar to other aminoglycosides. Therapeutic levels: Peak: 6-10 mg/L Trough: <2 mg/L |
| Tolazoline (Priscoline) | Vials: 25 mg/ml | 1-2 mg/kg IV push test dose. Then: 1-2 mg/kg/hr constant IV infusion. Dissolve 50 mg/kg x wt (kg) in 50 ml $D_5W$. Then ml/hr = mg/kg/hr. | Monitor blood pressure, renal status and bone marrow status. GI and pulmonary hemorrhage have been observed. |
| Tolmetin Sodium (Tolectin) | Tabs: 200 mg Caps: 400 mg | Children: Initial: 15 mg/kg/day÷TID Increment: 5 mg/kg/day at 1 week intervals until therapeutic effect or adverse effects are observed. Max. dose: 30 mg/kg/day Adults: Initial: 400 mg TID Maintenance: Titrate to desired effect. Usually, 600-1800 mg/day TID | Not recommended for age <2 yrs. May cause GI irritation or bleeding. |

| | | | |
|---|---|---|---|
| Tolnaftate (Tinactin) | Cream: 1%<br>Sol'n: 1%<br>Powder: 1%<br>Liquid, aerosol: 1%<br>Powder, aerosol: 1% | Apply cream or 1-2 gtts of solution topically BID for 2-6 wks. | Persistent infection may require systemic therapy with griseofulvin. |
| Triamcinolone (Kenalog, Aristocort, Kenacort) | Injection, Repository: 40 mg/ml<br>Injection, intralesional: 5, 25, 40 mg/ml<br>Syrup: 2 mg, 4 mg/ml<br>Tabs: 1, 2, 4, 8, 16 mg<br>Topical preparation: 0.025%, 0.1%, 0.5% | Intralesional injection: 1 mg maximum/site at weekly or less frequent intervals<br>Systemic use: 1/6 of dose recommended for cortisone<br>Topical: Apply to affected areas BID-QID. Use least potent preparation which is effective | See section on Adrenocorticosteroids, page 217-18. |
| Trimethobenzamide HCL (Tigan) | Caps: 100, 250 mg<br>Supp: 100, 200 mg<br>Amp: 100 mg/ml | Children<br>15-40 kg:<br>　Oral: 100-200 mg TID-QID<br>Rectal (not for use in neonates):<br>　<15 kg: 100 mg TID-QID<br>　>15 kg: 100-200 mg TID-QID<br>Injectable not recommended for children<br>Adults:<br>　Oral: 250 mg TID-QID<br>　Rectal: 200 mg TID-QID<br>　Injectable: 200 mg IM TID-QID | CNS disturbances are common in children (extrapyramidal symptoms, drowsiness, confusion, dizziness). |

| | | | |
|---|---|---|---|
| Trimethoprim-Sulfamethoxazole | See Co-Trimoxazole | | |
| Tripelennamine (Pyribenzamine) | Tabs: 25, 50 mg<br>Long-acting tabs: 50, 100 mg<br>Elixir: 37.5 mg/5 ml | Children: 5 mg/kg/day÷Q4-6h PO. Max. dose: 300 mg/day. Adults: Tabs: 25-50 mg Q4-6h. Sustained release tabs: 50-100 mg Q8-12h. Max. dose: 600 mg/day | Drowsiness and other side effects of antihistamines. |
| Valproic Acid (Depakene Depakote) | Syrup: 250 mg/5 ml<br>Caps: 250 mg<br>Enteric coated tabs: 250, 500 mg | Initial: 10-15 mg/kg/day÷ BID PO. Increment: 5-10 mg/kg/day at weekly intervals to max. of 60 mg/kg/day. Maintenance: 30-60 mg/kg/day ÷QD-TID. | GI, liver and hematologic toxicity; weight gain, transient alopecia, pancreatitis. Drug interactions - increases phenobarbital levels by 30-40%. Can cause hyperammonemia. Therapeutic levels: 50-100 mg/L |
| Vancomycin (Vancocin) | Amp: 500 mg/10 ml<br>Oral Sol'n: 500 mg/6 ml | Neonates:<br>< 7 days<br>< 1000 gm: 10 mg/kg Q24h<br>1000-2000 gm: 10 mg/kg Q18h<br>> 2000 gm: 10 mg/kg Q12h<br>> 7 days<br>< 1000 gm: 10 mg/kg Q18h<br>1000-2000 gm: 10 mg/kg Q12h<br>> 2000 gm: 10 mg/kg Q8h<br>Older Infants and Children: CNS infection: 45 mg/kg/day ÷ Q8h IV. Other infections: 30 mg/kg/day÷Q8h IV<br>Adults: 40 mg/kg/day (max. dose: 2 gm/day) ÷Q6h IV<br>Oral dose: 2 gm/1.73 $M^2$/day÷Q6h | Ototoxicity, nephrotoxicity. Causes phlebitis. Therapeutic levels: 10-25 mg/L. Toxic at > 40 mg/L |

| | | |
|---|---|---|
| Vasopressin (Pitressin) | Amp: 20 U/ml (aqueous) <br> Amp: 5 U/ml (tannate in oil) <br> Nose Drops: 50 U/ml (arginine vaso- pressin - Diapid) | Aqueous: 0.5-3 ml/day Q8h SC. <br> Tannate in Oil: 0.25 ml/dose IM Q1-3 days PRN; may increase to 1-2 ml/dose. <br> Nose Drops: 1-2 gtts in each nostril Q4-6h PRN. Titrate dose to achieve control of thirst and urination. | Side effects include tremor, sweating, vertigo, abdominal discomfort, nausea, vomiting urticaria, anaphylaxis. |
| Verapamil (Isoptin, Calan) | Tabs: 80, 120 mg <br> Amps: 2.5 mg/ml | Initial IV dose: administer over 2-3 min. May repeat after 30 minutes. <br> 1-15 yr: 0.1-0.3 mg/kg (usually 2-5 mg) Do not exceed 5 mg <br> Adult: 5-10 mg (0.15 mg/kg) <br> Adult antianginal dose: <br> 80 mg Q6-8h PO <br> Max. dose: 480 mg/day | Indicated for treatment of supraventricular tachyarrhyth- mias. Contraindicated in CHF hypotension, shock, 2nd or 3rd degree AV block and right-to-left shunt. Use only with extreme caution in infants; may cause apnea, severe bradycardia, or hypo- tension. IV beta adrenergic blocking agents should not be administered within a few hours of verapamil as both cause myocardial depression. Use only with continuous ECG monitoring. Have calcium and isoproterenol ready to reverse hypotension or bra- dycardia. |

| Drug | Supplied | Dosage | Comments |
|---|---|---|---|
| Vidarabine (Adenine arabinoside, Ara-A, Vira-A) | Injection: 200 mg/ml<br>Ophth oint: 3% | Herpes simplex virus encephalitis and neonatal HSV infection: 15 mg/kg/day given IV over 12 hrs x 10 days (add to standard IV fluids) Keratoconjunctivitis: Apply ointment to lower conjunctival sac Q3hrs, 5 x/day. Discontinue if not improved in 7 days. | Document HSV infection prior to therapy. Use with caution in renal and hepatic disease. Monitor hepatic and hematologic function. Do not dilute in biologic or colloid fluids. |
| Vitamin $K_1$ (Aqua-Mephyton, Konakion, Phytonadione) | Tabs: 5 mg<br>Amp: 1 mg/0.5 ml (aqueous)<br>Amp: 10 mg/ml (emulsion) | Neonatal hemorrhagic disease: Prophylaxis and treatment:0.5-1.0 mg/dose IM, SC, or IV x 1. Oral anticoagulant overdose: Infants: 1-2 mg/dose Q4-8h IV Children and Adults: 5-10 mg/dose IV Liver disease or Malabsorption: 2.5-25 mg/day PO Vit. K deficiency: Infants and Children: 1-2 mg/dose IV x 1 or 2-5 mg/day PO. Adults: 5-25 mg/day PO | Follow protime. Use with caution in presence of severe hepatic disease. Large doses (>25 mg) in newborn may cause hyperbilirubinemia. IV injection not to exceed 3 mg/$M^2$/min or 5 mg/min. IV doses may be associated with flushing, dizziness, hypotension, anaphylaxis. |

Ref:
1. Package insert for products.
2. Benitz, WE and Tatro, DS: The Pediatric Drug Handbook, Year Book Medical Publishers, Inc., Chicago, IL, 1981.
3. Boyd, JR (editor-in-chief): Facts and Comparisons, J. P. Lippincott Co., St. Louis, MO, 1986.
4. Copyright 1986 PHYSICIANS' DESK REFERENCE, Published by Medical Economics Co., Inc., Oradell, NJ 07649.
5. McEvey G, McQuarrie GM (eds.) Drug Information 86, American Hospital Formulary Service.

CANCER CHEMOTHERAPEUTIC AGENTS

| Drug Class and Name | Primary Clinical Use | Route | Toxicity  A=Acute  D=Delayed  * = Dose limiting side effects |
|---|---|---|---|
| **Alkylating Agents** | | | |
| Busulfan (myleran) | CML, BMT | PO | A: Nausea and vomiting; rare diarrhea. D: Bone marrow depression*; pulmonary infiltrates and fibrosis; hyperpigmentation; gynecomastia; ovarian failure; leukemia. (Note: Dose limitation for BMT: liver failure) |
| Cisplatin (Cis-DDP) | brain, neuroblastoma, germ cell, Wilms, osteosarcoma, bladder, head and neck CA. | IV | A: Nausea and vomiting; fever; hemolytic uremic syndrome; Raynaud's syndrome. D: Renal damage*; bone marrow depression; ototoxicity; hemolysis; hypomagnesemia; peripheral neuropathy; hypocalcemia; hypokalemia. |
| Carmustine (BCNU) | brain, Hodgkins non-Hodgkins | IV | A: Nausea and vomiting; local phlebitis. D: Delayed leukopenia and thrombocytopenia (may be prolonged)*; pulmonary fibrosis (may be irreversible); delayed renal damage; reversible liver damage. |
| Chlorambucil | Hodgkins | PO | D: Bone marrow depression*; pulmonary infiltrates and fibrosis; leukemia; hepatic toxicity; hallucinations. |
| Cyclophosphamide | lymphoma, leukemia, sarcomas, neuroblastoma, some carcinomas | PO  IV | A: Nausea and vomiting. D: Bone marrow depression*; hemorrhagic cystitis; pulmonary infiltrates and fibrosis; hyponatremia; leukemia; bladder cancer. (Note: Dose limitation for BMT: cardiac necrosis) |
| **Antimetabolites** | | | |
| Cytarabine HCl (cytosine arabinoside, Ara-C) | AML, ALL, lymphoma | SC  IM  IV  IT | A: Nausea and vomiting; diarrhea; anaphylaxis; fever; flu-like syndrome. D: Bone marrow depression*; conjunctivitis; megaloblastosis; oral ulceration; hepatic damage; encephalopathy with high doses. |

## Cancer Chemotherapeutic Agents (continued)

| Drug Class and Name | Primary Clinical Use | Route | Toxicity  A=Acute  D=Delayed  * = Dose limiting side effects |
|---|---|---|---|
| Fluorouracil (5-FU) | Head and neck, GI carcinoma | IV | A: Nausea and vomiting; diarrhea, hypersensitivity reaction. D: Oral and GI ulcers; bone marrow depression*; neurological defects, usually cerebellar. |
| Hydroxyurea (Hydrea) | CML, AML | PO | A: Nausea and vomiting; allergic reactions to tartrazine dye. D: Bone marrow depression*; stomatitis. |
| Methotrexate (MTX) | ALL, non-Hodgkins osteosarcoma, metastatic CNS tumors, some brain tumors, various carcinomas | PO IM IV IT | A: Nausea and vomiting; diarrhea; fever; anaphylaxis. D: Oral and gastrointestinal ulceration*, bone marrow depression*; hepatic toxicity including cirrhosis; renal toxicity; pulmonary infiltrates and fibrosis; depigmentation; encephalopathy and anaphylactoid reactions with high doses; osteoporosis. |
| Mercaptopurine (6-MP) | ALL, CML, Histiocytosis X, AML | PO IV | A: Nausea and vomiting; diarrhea. D: Bone marrow depression, cholestasis and rarely hepatic necrosis, oral and intestinal ulcers*; allopurinal may increase overall toxicity. |
| Thioguanine (6-TG) | AML, CML | PO IV | A: Occasional nausea and vomiting. D: Bone marrow depression*, hepatic damage; stomatitis. |

### DNA Binding Agents

| | | | |
|---|---|---|---|
| Bleomycin (Blenoxane) | Hodgkins, non-Hodgkins, germ cell tumors, squamous cell cancer | SC IM IV | A: Nausea and vomiting, fever; anaphylaxis and other allergic reactions; rash. D: Pneumonitis and pulmonary fibrosis*; rash; stomatitis; Raynaud's phenomenon. |
| Dactinomycin (Actinomycin D) | Wilms' tumor, rhabdomyosarcoma, soft tissue sarcomas | IV | A: Nausea and vomiting; diarrhea; local reaction and phlebitis; anaphylactoid reaction. D: Stomatitis; oral ulceration*; bone marrow depression*; folliculitis; dermatitis in previously irradiated areas. |

## Cancer Chemotherapeutic Agents (continued)

| Drug Class and Name | Primary Clinical Use | Route | Toxicity<br>A=Acute  D=Delayed  * = Dose limiting side effects |
|---|---|---|---|
| Daunorubicin (Daunomycin) | ALL<br>AML | IV | A: Nausea and vomiting; red urine (not hematuria); severe local tissue damage and necrosis on extravasation; diarrhea; transient EKG changes; ventricular arrhythmia; anaphylactoid reaction. D: Bone marrow depression*; cardiotoxicity*; (may be irreversible, but may be decreased by weekly schedule); conjunctivitis |
| Doxorubicin (Adriamycin) | ALL, Wilms, rhabdomyosarcoma, neuroblastoma, soft tissue sarcomas, bone tumors. | | A: Nausea and vomiting; diarrhea; red urine (not hematuria); severe local tissue damage and necrosis on extravasation; transient EKG changes; anaphylactoid reaction. D: Bone marrow depression*; cardiotoxicity*; (may be irreversible); stomatitis, anorexia; diarrhea; fever and chills. |
| **Tubulin Binding Agents** | | | |
| Etoposide (VP-16, Vepesid) | Hodgkins, non-Hodgkins, leukemia, neuroblastoma, brain tumors | IV | A: Nausea and vomiting; diarrhea; fever; rash. D: Bone marrow depression*; peripheral neuropathy. |
| Teniposide (VM-26) | Hodgkins, lymphomas, neuroblastoma | IV | A: Nausea and vomiting; diarrhea; phlebitis; anaphylactoid symptoms. D: Bone marrow depression*; peripheral neuropathy. |
| Vinblastine sulfate (Velban) | Hodgkins, Testicular cancer | IV | A: Nausea and vomiting*; local reaction and phlebitis with extravasation. D: Bone marrow depression*; stomatitis; loss of deep tendon reflexes; jaw pain; muscle pain; paralytic ileus; inappropriate ADH secretion. |

Cancer Chemotherapeutic Agents (continued)

| Drug Class and Name | Primary Clinical Use | Route | Toxicity A=Acute D=Delayed * = Dose limiting side effects |
|---|---|---|---|
| Vincristine sulfate (Oncovin) | ALL, lymphomas, solid tumors, breast cancer | IV | A: Local reaction with extravasation. D: Peripheral neuropathy*; alopecia; mild bone marrow depression; constipation; paralytic ileus; inappropriate ADH secretion; hepatic damage; jaw pain. |

Miscellaneous

| Drug Class and Name | Primary Clinical Use | Route | Toxicity A=Acute D=Delayed * = Dose limiting side effects |
|---|---|---|---|
| Asparaginase (Elspar) | ALL, AML, lymphomas | IM IV | A: Nausea and vomiting; fever, chills; headaches; hypersensitivity, anaphylaxis; abdominal pain; hyperglycemia leading to coma. D: CNS depression or hyperexcitability; acute hemorrhagic pancreatitis; coagulation defects; thrombosis; renal damage; hepatic damage. |
| Dacarbazine (DTIC) | Neuroblastoma, soft-tissue sarcoma | IV | A: Nausea and vomiting; diarrhea; anaphylaxis; pain on administration; flu-like syndrome. D: Bone marrow depression*; alopecia; renal impairment; hepatic necrosis; facial flushing, paresthesia; photosensitivity. |
| Leukovorin | | PO IV IM | Useful in preventing methotrexate toxicity. |
| Thiotepa (triethylene-thiophosphoramide) | Meningeal leukemia | IV IT | A: Nausea and vomiting; local pain, D: Bone marrow depression*; menstrual dysfunction; interference with spermatogenesis; pulmonary infiltrates and fibrosis; leukemia. |

Ref: Medical letter, 1985; 27:13-20.

## DIGOXIN

| Age | Oral Dose[1] | |
| --- | --- | --- |
| | Total Digitalizing Dose[2] | Daily Maintenance Dose[3] |
| Premature | 20 mcg/kg | 5 mcg/kg |
| Full term | 30 mcg/kg | 8-10 mcg/kg |
| < 2 yrs | 40-50 mcg/kg | 10-12 mcg/kg |
| 2-10 yrs | 30-40 mcg/kg | 8-10 mcg/kg |
| > 10 yrs | 0.75-1.25 mg | 0.125-0.25 mg |

1) IM or IV dose is 75% of oral dose (except in > 10 yo, IV = PO). Doses above are for congestive heart failure; doses needed in supraventricular tachycardia may be somewhat higher.

2) Given as $\frac{1}{2}$ the digitalizing dose initially, then $\frac{1}{4}$ the digitalizing dose Q8-18h x 2.

3) Given in 2 divided doses per day (except in > 10 yo given as one dose qd).

How Supplied:
  oral: capsules: 50, 100, 200 mcg
                  (100% bioavailable; use IV/IM dose)
        tablets: 150, 250, 500 mcg
        elixir: 50 mcg/ml

  parenteral: 100 and 250 mcg/ml injections

Comments:
Excreted via kidney. Use with caution in renal failure. Contraindicated in patients with ventricular dysrhythmias. May cause AV block or dysrhythmias. In the patient treated with digoxin, cardioversion or calcium infusion may lead to V fib (pretreatment with lidocaine 1 mg/kg IV may prevent this). For signs and treatment of toxicity, see p 249.

Therapeutic Concentration: 0.8 - 2.0 mcg/L

## ORAL THEOPHYLLINE PREPARATIONS

I. <u>Immediate</u> <u>Release</u> (Q6h doses):

   <u>Aminophylline</u>:

| | |
|---|---|
| Aminophylline | Tabs: 100, 200 mg |
| | (79% theophylline) |
| Somophyllin | Liquid: 105 mg/5 ml |
| | (86% theophylline) |

   <u>Oxtriphylline</u> (64% theophylline):

| | |
|---|---|
| Choledyl | Elixir: 100 mg/5ml* |
| | Solution: 50 mg/5 ml |
| | Tabs: 100, 200 mg |

   <u>Theophylline</u>:

| | |
|---|---|
| Elixophyllin | Caps: 100, 200 mg |
| | Elixir: 80 mg/15 ml* |
| Slo-phyllin | Tabs: 100, 200 mg |
| | Syrup: 80 mg/15 ml |
| Somophyllin-T | Caps: 100, 200, 250 mg |
| Theophyl-225 | Tabs: 225 mg |
| Theophylline | Tabs: 100, 200, 300 mg |
| | Elixir: 80 mg/15 ml* |
| | Solution: 80 mg/15 ml |

   *contains 20% alcohol

II. <u>Sustained</u> <u>Release</u> (Q8-12h doses):

   <u>Oxtriphylline</u> (64% theophylline)

      Choledyl SA Tabs: 400, 600 mg

   <u>Theophylline</u>:

      Elixophyllin SR Caps: 125, 250 mg
      Slo-Phyllin Gyrocaps Caps: 60, 125, 250 mg
      Somophyllin-CRT Caps: 100, 200, 250, 300 mg
      Theo-Dur Tabs: 100, 200, 300 mg
      Theo-Dur Sprinkle Caps: 50, 75, 125, 200 mg
      Theophyl-SR Caps: 125, 250 mg
      Theophylline SR Tabs: 100, 200, 300 mg
        (generic)

III. <u>Sustained</u> <u>Release</u> (Q24h doses):

   <u>Theophylline</u>:

| | |
|---|---|
| Theo-24 | Caps: 100, 200, 300 mg |

# INSULIN

(NOTE: See DKA and subsequent insulin management pages 101-102.)

Insulin is currently available as human, purified pork, pork/beef, and beef preparations. The human and more purified preparations produce less subcutaneous atrophy and insulin resistance.

| Type of Insulin | Time and Route of Administration | Time of Onset (HR) | Peak (HR) | Duration of Action (HR) | General Kinetic Category |
|---|---|---|---|---|---|
| Regular | IV (for ketoacidosis 0.1 u/kg bolus, then 0.1 u/kg/hr as continuous ±U infusion; or SQ 15-20 minutes before meals. | 1/2-1 | 2-5 | 5-8 | Rapid Onset and Short Duration |
| *Semi-Lente (Amorphous Zinc) | 1/2-3/4 hr before breakfast; deep SQ, never IV | 1/2-1½ hrs | 5-10 | 12-16 | |
| Lente (combination of 30% semi-lente & 70% ultra-lente) | 1 hr before breakfast; deep SQ; never IV | 1-2½ hrs | 7-15 | 24 | Intermediate Onset and Intermediate Duration |
| *NPH (Neutral-Protamine-Hagedorn) | 1 hr before breakfast SQ | 1-2 hrs | 6-12 | 18-24 | |
| Ultra-lente | 1 hr before breakfast; deep SQ, never IV | 4-8 hrs | 10-30 | 36+ | Delayed Onset and Long Duration |

*Human NPH may have a slightly decreased duration of action as compared to pork-derived NPH and the dose conversion may not be one-to-one.

ADRENOCORTICOSTEROIDS

1. Doses for Physiologic Replacement[1]

   A. Glucocorticoid

      Hydrocortisone (mean ±SD)[2]
         IM or IV: 12 ± 2 mg/$M^2$/day, QD
         PO: twice the IM/IV dose per day, divided TID

      Cortisone Acetate (mean ±SD)[3]
         IM: 15 ± 2.5 mg/$M^2$/day, QD
         PO: twice the IM dose per day, divided TID

      Prednisone
         PO: 4-5 mg/$M^2$/day, divided BID

[1]Stress doses for glucocorticoids are 2-4 x physiologic replacement doses.
[2]In infants with congenital virilizing adrenal hyperlasia (CVAH), one can administer hydrocortisone 37 mg/$M^2$ IM Q3 days.
[3]Dose of cortisone acetate may be reduced 50% for hypopituitarism.

   B. Mineralocorticoid

      Deoxycorticosterone Acetate (DOCA) -
        1.0-2.0 mg/day IM (in oil), single dose

      9α-fluorocortisol (Florinef) -
        0.05-0.15 mg/day PO

2. Equivalent Doses for Same Clinical Effects

| Drug | Glucocorticoid Anti-Inflammatory | Mineralo-corticoid |
|---|---|---|
| Cortisone | 100 mg | 100 mg |
| Hydrocortisone | 80 mg | 80 mg |
| Prednisone | 20 mg | 100 mg |
| Prednisolone | 20 mg | 100 mg |
| Methylprednisolone | 16 mg | no effect |
| Triamcinolone | 16 mg | no effect |
| 9αFluorocortisol | 5 mg | 0.2 mg |
| Dexamethasone | 2 mg | no effect |
| DOCA | no effect | 2 mg |

3. Duration of Action

| | |
|---|---|
| Cortisone acetate: | 6 hr PO; 3 days IM |
| Hydrocortisone: | 4-6 hrs IV (1/2 life 60 min) |
| Triamcinolone: | 8-12 hrs PO |
| Dexamethasone: | 8-12 hrs PO |
| Prednisone: | 6-8 hrs PO |

4. Common Side Effects with Prolonged Usage

   A. Acute Withdrawal: Fever, myalgia, arthralgia, malaise, hypotension, hypoglycemia, shock.

   B. Complications of Prolonged Use: Hypokalemic alkalosis, glycosuria, increased susceptibility to infection, exacerbation of peptic ulcers, myopathy, psychoses, osteoporosis and vertebral compression fractures, thromboembolic phenomena, Cushing's habitus, acne, hirsutism, cataracts, hypertension, and ecchymoses.

5. Some Common Dermatologic Steroid Preparations

   Lowest Potency
      0.25% Hydrocortisone
      0.25% Methylprednisolone acetate (Medrol)
      0.04% Dexamethasone † (Hexadrol)
      0.5% Hydrocortisone
   Low Potency
      0.01% Fluocinolone acetonide† (Synalar, Fluonid)
      0.01% Betamethasone valerate† (Valisone)
      1.0% Hydrocortisone
      0.025% Triamcinolone acetonide†  (Kenalog)
   Intermediate Potency
      0.1% Betamethasone valerate† (Valisone)
      0.025% Fluocinolone acetonide†  (Synalar, Fluonid)
      0.05% Flurandrelonide†  (Cordran)
      2.5% Hydrocortisone
      0.1% Triamcinolone acetonide†  (Kenalog)
   Highest Potency
      0.05% Fluocinomide†  (Lidex)
      0.5% Triamcinolone acetonide†
      0.2% Fluocinolone† (Synalar HP)

   †Fluorinated preparation

   Fluorinated steroids may cause skin atrophy and telangiectasiae with chronic use (>2 wks). Most compounds above are available in creams and ointments. Most are dispensed in 15, 30, and 60 gram tubes (except Betamethasone valerate which is dispensed in 45 gram tubes). One gram of topical cream or ointment covers a 10 cm x 10 cm area. A 30 to 60 gram tube will cover the entire body of an adult one time.

## PEDIATRIC SEDATION

Very little published information is available regarding the relative efficacy and safety of various pediatric sedation regimens used prior to diagnostic or therapeutic outpatient procedures (e.g., CT Scan, EEG, suturing). The following chart outlines several drug combinations which have been used in the Johns Hopkins Hospital Children's Center. Clinical response is variable and close monitoring is mandatory. Refer to the Formulary for further cautions and side effects.

| Drug | Usual Dose | Route | Cardiac Catheterization Acyanotic | Cyanotic |
|---|---|---|---|---|
| 1. Demerol | 2 mg/kg | IM | 1.2 mg/kg | 0.6 mg/kg |
| Phenergan | 1 mg/kg | | 0.3 mg/kg | 0.15 mg/kg |
| Thorazine | 1 mg/kg | | 0.3 mg/kg | 0.15 mg/kg |

Comments:
- max. dose = 50 mg Demerol
- give deep IM in single syringe
- adequate sedation and analgesia
- partially reversible with naloxone

| | | | | |
|---|---|---|---|---|
| 2. Chloral Hydrate | 25-100 mg/kg | PO | | |

Comments:
- less respiratory depression
- avoid large doses in severe cardiac disease
- no analgesic or amnestic properties

| | | | | |
|---|---|---|---|---|
| 3. Fentanyl | 1-2 mcg/kg | IM | | |
| Hydroxyzine | 1 mg/kg | IM | | |

Comments:
- respiratory depressant effects may outlast analgesia
- no amnestic effect
- partially reversible with Narcan

| | | | | |
|---|---|---|---|---|
| 4. Fentanyl | 1-2 mcg/kg | IM or slow IV | | |
| Diazepam | 0.1-0.2 mg/kg | IM or slow IV | | |

(Midazolam IM or IV may be substituted for diazepam.)

Comments:
- respiratory depressant effects may outlast analgesia
- has sedative, analgesic, and amnestic properties
- partially reversible with naloxone

Ref: Taylor, M, Anesthesia 1986; 41:21.

## DRUGS FOR SEXUALLY TRANSMITTED DISEASES

The recommendations below are based on the 1985 STD Treatment Guidelines issued by the Centers for Disease Control. For more extensive discussion as well as for recommendations for other diseases refer to Morbidity and Mortality Weekly Report 1985; 34:1-35.

I.  Pelvic Inflammatory Disease (PID) in Children > 45 kg:

A.  Intravenous therapy (Use one of the 2 regimens below.)

1.  Doxycycline 100 mg/dose IV Q12h and cefoxitin 2.0 gm/dose IV Q6h.
2.  Clindamycin 600 mg/dose IV Q6h and gentamicin 2 mg/kg IV x 1, then 1.5 mg/kg/dose Q8h.

Continue intravenous therapy at least 4 days and at least 48 hours after the patient improves. Then continue doxycycline 100 mg/dose PO BID or clindamycin 450 mg/dose PO QID to complete 10-14 days of therapy.

B.  Outpatient therapy

Use any one of the 5 regimens below followed by doxycycline 100 mg/dose PO BID x 10-14 days (tetracycline 500 mg/dose PO QID is an alternative.)

1.  Cefoxitin: 2.0 gm IM, probenecid 1.0 gm PO.
2.  Amoxicillin: 3.0 gm IM, probenecid 1.0 gm PO.
3.  Ampicillin: 3.5 gm IM, probenecid 1.0 gm PO.
4.  Procaine pen G: 4.8 million U IM at 2 sites, probenecid 1.0 gm PO.
5.  Ceftriaxone: 250 mg IM.

Alternative regimens active against chlamydia for patients in whom tetracyclines are contraindicated or not tolerated:

1.  Erythromycin base or stearate: 500 mg PO QID x 7-10 days.
2.  Erythromycin ethylsuccinate: 800 mg PO QID x 7-10 days.

II.  Gonorrhea in Children < 45 kg

A.  Amoxicillin 50 mg/kg PO with probenecid 25 mg/kg (max. 1 gm) or ceftriaxone 125 mg IM. (Ceftriaxone is preferable when proctitis or pharyngitis are present.) In patients allergic to penicillins or cephalosporins: spectinomycin 40 mg/kg IM.

## DRUGS AND CHEMICALS TO BE AVOIDED BY PERSONS WITH "REACTING" (PRIMAQUINE SENSITIVE) RED CELLS (G6PD DEFICIENCY)

### Antimalarials

Primaquine

### Sulfonamides

1. Sulfanilamide
2. Sulfisoxazole (Gantrisin)*
3. Salicylazosulfapyridine (Azulfidine)
4. Sulfacetamide (Sulamyd)
5. Trisulfapyrimidine (Sultrin)

### Nitrofurans

1. Nitrofurantoin (Furadantin)
2. Furazolidone (Furoxone)

### Antipyretics and Analgesics

1. Acetylsalicylic Acid*
2. Acetophenetidin (Phenacetin)*
3. Antipyrine
4. p-Aminosalicylic Acid

### Others

1. Sulfoxone*
2. Naphthalene
3. Methylene Blue*
4. Probenecid
5. Fava Bean
6. Vitamin K - water soluble analogs only
7. Aniline dyes
8. Ascorbic acid§
9. Chloramphenicol†

\* Only slightly hemolytic to G6PD A⁻ patients in very large doses.
† Hemolytic in G6PD Mediterranean but not in G6PD A⁻ or Canton.
§ In massive doses

NOTE: Many other compounds have been tested, but are free of hemolytic activity. Penicillin, the tetracyclines, and erythromycin, for example, will not cause hemolysis. Also, the incidence of allergic reaction in these individuals is not any greater than that observed in normals. Any drug, therefore, which is not included in the list known to cause hemolysis, may be given.

## MATERNAL MEDICATIONS AND BREAST FEEDING

I. <u>Drugs</u> <u>that</u> <u>are</u> <u>contraindicated</u> <u>during</u> <u>breast</u> <u>feeding</u>

Antimetabolites
  Cyclophosphamide, methotrexate
Bromocriptine
Cimetidine
Clemastine (an antihistamine)
Ergotamine
Gold Salts
Methimazole
Phenindione
Thiouracil

II. <u>Drugs</u> <u>that</u> <u>require</u> <u>temporary</u> <u>cessation</u> <u>of</u> <u>breast</u> <u>feeding</u>

Metronidazole
Radioactive diagnostic and therapeutic agents

<u>Ref</u>:  Committee on Drugs, AAP.  Pediatrics 1983; 72:375-83.

## USE OF DRUGS IN RENAL FAILURE

To adjust maintenance dosage in patients with renal insufficiency, one may lengthen the intervals between individual doses, keeping the dosage size normal. This method is known as the "interval extension" method. Alternatively, one may reduce the amount of individual doses, keeping the interval between doses normal. This "dose reduction" method is recommended especially for drugs in which a relatively constant blood level is desired. In the following tables after identification of the method used (D for dose reduction or I for interval extension) recommendations are given for various levels of renal function as estimated by glomerular filtration rate. In the dose reduction method, the percentage of the usual dose that should be given at the normal dose interval is shown, whereas for the interval extension method the number of hours between doses of normal amount is given.

These dosage modifications are approximations only. The individual patient must be followed closely for signs of drug toxicity, serum levels of the drugs must be measured when available, and the dosage and interval modified accordingly.

In the following tables, the quantitative effects of hemodialysis (He) and peritoneal dialysis (P) on drug removal are shown. "Yes" refers to removal of enough drug to warrant a supplemental dosage for maintenance of adequate therapeutic blood levels. "No" indicates no need for dosage adjustment with dialysis. The designation "no" does not preclude the use of dialysis or hemoperfusion for drug overdose.

The data in these tables are adapted from Bennett, WM, et al, Ann Int Med 1980; 93:62; Bennett, WM, et al. Amer J Kidney Dis 1983; 3:155-193.

USE OF DRUGS IN RENAL FAILURE:
DRUGS REQUIRING ADJUSTMENT
(Antimicrobials)

| Drug | Route of Excretion | Normal Half-Life (hours) | Normal Dose Interval | Method | Creatinine Clearance (ml/min) | | | Supplemental Dose for Dialysis |
|---|---|---|---|---|---|---|---|---|
| | | | | | >50 | 10-50 | <10 | |
| Acyclovir | Ren | 2.1-3.8 | Q8h | I | Q8h | Q24h | Q48h | Yes (He) |
| Amikacin | Ren | 2-2.5 | Q8-12h | I / D | Q12-18h / 60-90% | 24 / 30-70% | 24 / 20-30% | Yes (He, P) |
| Amphotericin B | NonRen | 24 | Q24h | I | Q24h | Q24h | Q24h-36h | No (He, P) |
| Ampicillin | Ren (Hep) | 0.8 | Q6h | I | Q6h | Q6-12h | Q12-16h | Yes (He) / No (P) |
| Cefotaxime | Ren (Hep) | 1 | Q6-8h | I | Q6-8h | Q8-12h | Q12-24h | Yes (He) |
| Cefuroxime | Ren | 1.6-2.2 | Q6-8h | I | Q6h | Q6-8h | Q8h | Yes (He, P) |
| Cephalexin | Ren | 0.9 | Q6h | I | Q6h | Q6-8h | Q9-12h | Yes (H) |
| Cephalothin | Ren (Hep) | 0.5-0.9 | Q6h | I | Q6h | Q6h | Q8-12h | Yes (He, P) |
| Ethambutol | Ren | 4 | Q24h | I | Q24h | Q24-36h | Q48h | Yes (He, P) |
| Flucytosine | Ren | 3-6 | Q6h | I | Q6h | Q12-24h | Q24-48h | Yes (He, P) |
| Gentamicin | Ren | 2 | Q8h | D / I | 60-90% / Q8-12h | 30-70% / Q12h | 20-30% / Q24h | Yes (He, P) |
| Isoniazid | Hep (Ren) | 2-4 (slow) 0.5-1.5 (fast) | Q24h | D | 100% | 100% | 65-75% | Yes (He, P) |

PHARMACOKINETICS

ADJUSTMENTS IN RENAL FAILURE
(see previous page for explanation)

USE OF DRUGS IN RENAL FAILURE (continued)
DRUGS REQUIRING ADJUSTMENT
(Antimicrobials)

| | PHARMACOKINETICS | | | | ADJUSTMENTS IN RENAL FAILURE | | | | |
|---|---|---|---|---|---|---|---|---|---|
| Drug | Route of Excretion | Normal Half-Life (hours) | Normal Dose Interval | Me-thod | Creatinine Clearance (ml/min) | | | Supplemental Dose for Dialysis |
| | | | | | >50 | 10-50 | <10 | |
| Kanamycin | Ren | 2-3 | Q8h | I D | Q24h 75% | Q24-72h 50% | Q72-96h 25% | Yes (He, P) |
| Methicillin | Ren (Hep) | 0.5 | Q4h | I | Q4h | Q4h | Q8-12h | No (He, P) |
| Metronidazole | Ren (Hep) | 6-14 | Q8h | I | Q8h | Q12h | Q24h | |
| Penicillin G | Ren (Hep) | 0.5 | Q4-6h | I | Q6-8h | Q8-12h | Q12-16h | Yes (He) No (P) |
| † Ticarcillin | Ren | 1-1.5 | Q8h | I | Q8-12h | Q12-24h | Q24-48h | Yes (He, P) |
| § Tobramycin | Ren | 2.5 | Q8h | D I | 60-90% Q8-12h | 30-70% Q12h | 20-30% Q24h | Yes (He, P) |
| Trimethoprim | Ren (Hep) | 8-15 | Q12h | I | Q12h | Q18h | Q24h | Yes (H) |
| Sulfamethoxazole | Hep (Ren) | 9-11 | | | | | | No (P) |
| Vancomycin | Ren | 6-8 | Q24h | I | Q24-72h | Q72-240h | Q240h | No (He, P) |

† May inactivate aminoglycosides in patients with renal impairment
§ May add 4-5 mg/L to peritoneal dialysate to obtain adequate serum levels

USE OF DRUGS IN RENAL FAILURE:
DRUGS REQUIRING ADJUSTMENT
(Non-Antimicrobials)

| Drug | PHARMACOKINETICS | | | ADJUSTMENTS IN RENAL FAILURE | | | | |
|---|---|---|---|---|---|---|---|---|
| | Route of Excretion | Normal Half-Life (hours) | Normal Dose Interval | Method | Creatinine Clearance (ml/min) | | | Supplemental Dose for Dialysis |
| | | | | | >50 | 10-50 | <10 | |
| Acetaminophen | Hep | 2 | Q4h | I | Q4h | Q6h | Q8h | Yes (He) No (P) |
| †Acetylsalicylic acid | Hep (Ren) | 2-4.5 | Q4h | I | Q4h | Q4-6h | Avoid | Yes (He, P) |
| Allopurinol | Ren | 0.7 | Q12-24h | D I | none Q8h | none Q8-12h | 50% Q12-24h | ? |
| Captopril | Ren (Hep) | 1.9 | Q8h | D | none | none | 50% | Yes (He) |
| Carbamazepine | Hep (Ren) | 35 | Q8h | D | none | none | 75% | No (He) |
| Cimetidine | Ren | 1.5-2 | Q6h | D I | 100% Q6h | 75% Q8h | 50% Q12h | No (He, P) |
| §Digoxin | Ren (NonRen 15-40%) | 36-44 | Q24h | D I | 100% Q24h | 25-75% Q36h | 10-25% Q48h | No (He, P) |
| Diphenhydramine | Hep | 4-7 | Q6h | I | Q6h | Q6-9h | Q9-12h | ? |
| ††Hydralazine | Hep (GI, Ren) | 2-4.5 | Q8h (fast) Q12h (slow) | I | none | none | Q8-16h (fast) Q12-24h (slow) | No (He, P) |

† T1/2 given for <500 mg dose. With large doses T1/2 prolonged up to 30 hrs.
§ Decrease loading dose 50% in end stage renal disease because of decreased volume of distribution.
†† Dose interval varies for rapid and slow acetylators with normal and impaired renal function.

USE OF DRUGS IN RENAL FAILURE (continued):
DRUGS REQUIRING ADJUSTMENT
(Non-Antimicrobials)

| Drug | PHARMACOKINETICS | | | ADJUSTMENTS IN RENAL FAILURE | | | | |
|------|------|------|------|------|------|------|------|------|
| | Route of Excretion | Normal Half-Life (hours) | Normal Dose Interval | Me-thod | Creatinine Clearance (ml/min) | | | Supplemental Dose for Dialysis |
| | | | | | >50 | 10-50 | <10 | |
| Insulin (Reg) | Hep (Ren) | 9 min. | Variable | D | 100% | 75% | 50% | ? |
| Methotrexate | Ren | Triphasic 0.1, 2.3, 27 | Single treatment | D | Un-changed | 50% | avoid | Yes (He) No (P) |
| Phenobarbital | Hep (Ren 30%) | 65-150 | Q8h | I | none | none | Q12-16h | Yes (He, P) |
| Primidone | Hep (Ren < 20%) | 3-12 | Q8h | I | Q8h | Q8-12h | Q12-24h | Yes (He) |
| Spironolactone | Ren | 10-35 | Q6h | I | Q6-12h | Q12-24h* | Avoid | ? |
| Thiazides | Ren | 1-2 | Q12h | D | none | none | Avoid | ? |

* Hyperkalemia common with GFR<30 ml/min.

## USE OF DRUGS IN RENAL FAILURE:
## DRUGS REQUIRING <u>NO</u> ADJUSTMENT

### Antibiotics

| Drug | Supplemental Dose for Dialysis | Drug | Supplemental Dose for Dialysis |
|---|---|---|---|
| Chloramphenicol | X | Isoniazid | X |
| Clindamycin | | Nafcillin | |
| Cloxacillin | | Pyrimethamine | |
| Erythromycin | | Rifampin | |

### Non-Antibiotics

| Drug | Supplemental Dose for Dialysis | Drug | Supplemental Dose for Dialysis |
|---|---|---|---|
| Adriamycin | | Indomethacin | |
| Amitriptyline | | Lidocaine | |
| Busulfan | | Meperidine | |
| Chlorpheniramine | | Metolazone | |
| Chlorpromazine | | Morphine | |
| Clonidine | | Naloxone | |
| Codeine | | Nifedipine | |
| Corticosteroids (any) | | Nitroprusside | X |
|   cortisone | | Pentazocine | X |
|   methylprednisolone | | Pentobarbital | |
|   prednisone | X | Phenytoin | |
| Cytosine Arabinoside | | Prazosin | |
| Diazepam | | Propoxyphene | |
| Diazoxide | X | Propranolol | |
| Diltiazem | | Quinidine | X |
| 5-Fluorouracil | X | Secobarbital | |
| Flurazepam | | Succinylcholine | |
| Furosemide | | Theophylline | X |
| Haloperidol | | Valproic Acid | |
| Heparin | | Verapamil | |
| Ibuprofen | | Vincristine | |
| Imipramine | | Warfarin | |

PART III

THERAPEUTIC DATA

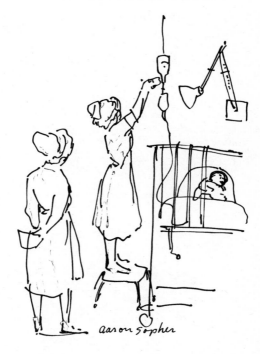

aaron sopher

# FLUID AND
# ELECTROLYTE THERAPY

1. ## General Considerations

    A. ### Atomic Weights

    | | | | |
    |---|---|---|---|
    | Aluminum (Al) | 26.97 | Lead (Pb) | 207.21 |
    | Calcium (Ca) | 40.08 | Magnesium (Mg) | 24.32 |
    | Carbon (C) | 12.01 | Manganese (Mn) | 54.93 |
    | Chlorine (Cl) | 35.46 | Nitrogen (N) | 14.01 |
    | Copper (Cu) | 63.57 | Oxygen (O) | 16.00 |
    | Fluorine (F) | 19.00 | Phosphorus (P) | 30.98 |
    | Gold (Au) | 197.20 | Potassium (K) | 39.10 |
    | Hydrogen (H) | 1.01 | Sodium (Na) | 23.00 |
    | Iodine (I) | 126.92 | Sulfur (S) | 32.06 |
    | Iron (Fe) | 55.85 | | |

    B. ### Ion Calculations
    1) Moles:

    | Mole | = molecular weight in grams |
    |---|---|
    | Millimole | = molecular weight in milligrams |

    Na 23
    Cl 35.5
    NaCl 58.5 gm = 1 mole
    58.5 mg = 1 mM

    2) Equivalents (number of electric charges per liter):
    Equivalent = atomic weight divided by valence

    | mEq | = equivalent weight in mg |
    |---|---|
    | $\mu$Eq | = equivalent weight in $\mu$g |

    For single valence ions 1 mM = mEq.
    For divalent ions 1mM = 2 mEq.

    3) Osmolality (number of particles per liter):
    Osmole = molecular weight divided by number of
    particles exerting osmotic pressure

    $$1 \text{ mM } Na^+ = 1 \text{ mOsm}$$
    $$1 \text{ mM NaCl} = 2 \text{ mOsm } (Na^+ + Cl^-)$$
    $$1 \text{ mM } Na_2SO_4 = 3 \text{ mOsm } (2Na^+ + SO_4^{--})$$

    Osmolality is the preferred term rather than
    osmolarity and represents solute concentration per
    unit solvent (water) rather than solution (serum).

    4) Approximate serum osmolality =
    $$2 \text{ (Na)} + \frac{glucose \text{ (mg/dl)}}{18} + \frac{BUN \text{ (mg/dl)}}{2.8}$$

    Usual range 285-295 mOsm/L.

2.   Calculation of Maintenance Requirements

   A.   Caloric Expenditure Method: based on the understanding
        that water and electrolyte requirements parallel caloric
        expenditure but not body weight.   This method is
        effective for all ages, shapes, and clinical states.
        1)   Start by determining the child's standard basal
             caloric expenditure:

STANDARD BASAL CALORIES

| AGE | WEIGHT (KG) | CALORIC EXPENDITURE (CAL/KG/24 HOURS) |
|---|---|---|
| Newborn | 2.5-4 | 50 |
| 1 week-6 months | 3-8 | 65-70 |
| 6-12 months | 8-12 | 50-60 |
| 1-2 years | 10-15 | 45-50 |
| 2-5 years | 15-20 | 45 |
| 5-10 years | 20-35 | 40-45 |
| 10-16 years | 35-60 | 25-40 |
| Adult | 70 | 15-20 |

        2)   Add 12% of the standard basal calories for each
             degree Centigrade above the basal rectal tempera-
             ture of 37.8°C.
        3)   Add 0-30% of the standard basal calories for bed
             activity; e.g., coma or thrashing about.
        4)   For each 100 calories metabolized per 24 hours, the
             average patient will need 100-120 cc $H_2O$, 2-4 mEq
             Na+, and 2-3 mEq $K^+$.  These estimates are derived
             from the following table.

Average Water and Electrolyte Expenditures Per 100
Calories Metabolized Per 24 Hours

| ROUTE | USUAL | | | RANGE ¶ | | |
|---|---|---|---|---|---|---|
| | $H_2O$* | Na** | K** | $H_2O$* | Na** | K** |
| Lungs | 15 | 0 | 0 | 10- 60 | 0 | 0 |
| Skin | 40 | 0.1 | 0.2 | 20-100 | 0.1- 3.0 | 0.2- 1.5 |
| Stool | 5 | 0.1 | 0.2 | 0- 50 | 0.1- 4.0 | 0.2- 3.0 |
| Urine | 65 | 3.0 | 2.0 | 0-400 | 0.2-30 | 0.4-30 |
| TOTAL | 125 | 3.2 | 2.4 | 30-610 | 0.4-37 | 0.8-34.5 |

*cc/100 calories metabolized
**mEq/100 calories metabolized
¶abnormally high values represent abnormal losses due to environ-
mental variation or pathological states.

Note:   Despite 125 ml $H_2O$ being lost for every 100
        cal/24 hr, the usual $H_2O$ requirement is 5-15 ml less
        (i.e., 110-120 ml) because of the production of
        endogenous $H_2O$ through oxidation of carbohydrate,
        fat and protein.

5)  Average Water and Electrolyte Requirements for
    Different Clinical States per 100 Calories per 24
    Hours
    Based on data in preceding table.

|  | ml $H_2O$ | mEq Na | mEq K |
|---|---|---|---|
| *Average patient receiving parenteral fluids | 110-120 | 2-4 | 2-3 |
| Anuria | 45 | 0 | 0 |
| Acute CNS infections and inflammation | 80-90 | 2-4 | 2-3 |
| Chronic renal disease with fixed specific gravity | 140 | variable | variable |
| Diabetes insipidus | Up to 400 | variable | variable |
| Hyperventilation | 120-210 | 2-4 | 2-3 |
| Heat stress | 120-240 | variable | variable |
| High humidity environment | 80-100 | 2-4 | 2-3 |

*Adequate maintenance solution
Na and Cl: 30 mEq/L
K: 20 mEq/L
Glucose: 5% or 10% as needed
i.e., Dextrose 5% in 0.2% NaCl + 20 mEq/L KCl.

B.  Holliday - Segar Method:
    A quick, simple formula which estimates caloric
    expenditure from weight alone. Assumes that for each
    100 calories metabolized, 100 cc $H_2O$ will be required.

| Water | | Electrolytes | |
|---|---|---|---|
| 100cc/kg-for 1st 10 kg of body weight | | Na+ | 3mEq/100cc $H_2O$ |
| 50cc/kg -for 2nd 10 kg of body weight | | Cl⁻ | 2mEq/100cc $H_2O$ |
| 20cc/kg -for each additional kg | | K+ | 2mEq/100cc $H_2O$ |

    This method is not ideal for infants during the first
    10-14 days, nor is it well suited to conditions in which
    there are increased or decreased losses (e.g.,
    hypermetabolic states, anuria).

C.  Body Surface Area Method:
    Based on the assumption that caloric expenditure is
    proportional to surface area.

$$H_2O \qquad 1500 \ cc/M^2/24 \ hrs.$$
$$Na^+ \qquad 30\text{-}50 \ mEq/M^2/24 \ hrs.$$
$$K^+ \qquad 20\text{-}40 \ mEq/M^2/24 \ hrs.$$

The body surface area method should not be used for children $\leq$10kg. It provides no convenient method of taking into account changes in metabolic rate.

Ref: Finberg L, et al. Water and Electrolytes in Pediatrics. Philadelphia: WB Saunders, 1982. Behrman R, et al. Nelson Textbook of Pediatrics. 12th ed. Philadelphia: WB Saunders, 1983.

3. Deficit Therapy

A. Clinical Estimate of Fluid Deficit in Isotonic Dehydration *

| % Dehydration | Clinical Observation |
|---|---|
| 5% | ↑HR (10-15% above baseline)<br>Dry mucous membranes<br>Concentration of the urine<br>Poor tear production |
| 10% | Decreased skin turgor<br>Increased severity of above signs<br>Oliguria<br>Sunken eyeballs<br>Sunken anterior fontanelle |
| 15% | Markedly increased severity of above<br>Decreased blood pressure<br>Poor tissue perfusion (delayed capillary refill and acidosis) |

* In hypotonic dehydration ($Na^+$ <130) all manifestations appear at lesser degrees of deficit, while in hypertonic dehydration (Na >150) the circulating volume is relatively preserved at the expense of cellular water, and less circulatory disturbance is seen for a given amount of fluid deficit.

B.  Calculation of Deficits

PROBABLE DEFICITS OF WATER AND ELECTROLYTES IN
INFANTS WITH SEVERE DEHYDRATION (10-12 PERCENT)

| Condition | H$_2$O ml | Na mEq | K* mEq | Cl mEq |
|---|---|---|---|---|
| | | Per Kg of Body Weight | | |
| Fasting and thirsting | 100-120 | 5- 7 | 1- 2 | 4- 6 |
| Diarrhea | | | | |
|   Isotonic | 100-120 | 8-10 | 8-10 | 8-10 |
|   Hypertonic | 100-120 | 2-4 | 0-4 | -2-6** |
|   Hypotonic | 100-120 | 10-12 | 8-10 | 10-12 |
| Pyloric stenosis | 100-120 | 8-10 | 10-12 | 10-12 |
| Diabetic acidosis | 100-120 | 8-10 | 5-7 | 6-8 |

*Converted for breakdown of tissue cells:
 3 mEq K for each gram of nitrogen lost by catabolism
**Negative balance of chloride indicates excess at beginning of
therapy.

C.  Fluid Administration
    1)  Initial step:  For significant dehydration, rapidly
        expand the extracellular volume in order to improve
        the circulation and renal function.  Blood is used
        only for shock not responding to Ringer's lactate,
        or in the event of acute blood loss.
        a)  Ringer's lactate 20 ml/kg/1st hr.
        b)  Blood or plasma 10 ml/kg, if indicated.
        For shock give isotonic fluids at a maximal rate
        until a clinical response is seen.
    2)  Replace intracellular deficits slowly over 24-48 hrs.
        See table above for approx. magnitude of deficits.
    3)  Maintenance therapy for usual losses.
    4)  Replace continued abnormal losses.

D.  Correction of Persistent Symptomatic Disturbances of
    Electrolyte Concentration
    Formula:  (CD - CA) x fD x Wt* in kg = mEq required

        CD= concentration desired (mEq/L)
        CA= concentration present (mEq/L)
        fD = apparent distribution factor as fraction of body
            weight
    *Baseline weight prior to illness.

| Electrolyte | Apparent Distribution Factor (fD) |
|---|---|
| Bicarbonate | 0.4-0.5 |
| Chloride | 0.2-0.3 |
| Sodium | 0.6-0.7 |

Note:  With hyperglycemia, serum Na+ decreases 1.6 mEq/L for
      each 100 mg/dl rise in glucose.

4.  Replacement of Concurrent Losses in Addition to Maintenance Requirements

COMPOSITION OF EXTERNAL ABNORMAL LOSSES*

| Fluid | Na | K (mEq/L) | Cl | Protein Gm% |
|---|---|---|---|---|
| Gastric | 20- 80 | 5-20 | 100-150 | --- |
| Pancreatic | 120-140 | 5-15 | 40- 80 | --- |
| Small intestine | 100-140 | 5-15 | 90-130 | --- |
| Bile | 120-140 | 5-15 | 80-120 | --- |
| Ileostomy | 45-135 | 3-15 | 20-115 | --- |
| Diarrheal | 10- 90 | 10-80 | 10-110 | --- |
| Burns | 140 | 5 | 110 | 3-5 |

*These losses should be determined Q6h-Q8h. Because of the wide range of normal values, specific analyses are suggested in individual cases.

5.  Mean Insensible Water Loss From the Skin in Newborn Infants (ml/kg body weight/24 hrs) - at ambient humidity of 50%

| | Gestational age (weeks) | Mean birth weight | Post-natal age (days) | | | | | | | |
|---|---|---|---|---|---|---|---|---|---|---|
| | | | <1 | 1 | 3 | 5 | 7 | 14 | 21 | 28 |
| AGA | 25-27 | 0.86 | 129 | 110 | 71 | 51 | 43 | 32 | 28 | 24 |
| | 28-30 | 1.34 | 42 | 39 | 32 | 27 | 24 | 18 | 15 | 15 |
| | 31-36 | 2.11 | 12 | 11 | 12 | 12 | 12 | 9 | 8 | 7 |
| | 37-41 | 3.60 | 7 | 6 | 6 | 6 | 6 | 6 | 6 | 7 |
| SGA | 28-30 | 0.78 | 39 | 34 | 34 | 28 | 26 | 23 | 23 | 23 |
| | 31-36 | 1.38 | 13 | 13 | 13 | 13 | 12 | 11 | 11 | 10 |
| | 37-39 | 2.14 | 6 | 6 | 7 | 7 | 7 | 7 | 9 | - |

Ref: Hammarlund K, et al. Acta Pediatr Scand 1983; 72:725.

6.  Anion Gap

    A.  The anion gap represents the difference between unmeasured cations (UC) and unmeasured anions (UA). Clinically it is measured by:

    $$AG = UC - UA = Na - (Cl + HCO_3)$$
    Normal: 12 mEq/L $\pm$ 2 mEq/L

B. Causes of Increased Anion Gap
    1) Decreased unmeasured cation: hypokalemia, hypo-calcemia, hypomagnesemia.
    2) Increased unmeasured anion:
       a) Organic anions: lactate, ketones.
       b) Inorganic anions: phosphate, sulfate.
       c) Proteins: hyperalbuminemia (transient).
       d) Exogenous anions: salicylate, formate, nitrate, penicillin, carbenicillin, etc.
       e) Incompletely identified: anion accumulating in paraldehyde, ethylene glycol, methanol and salicylate poisoning, uremia, hyperosmolar hyperglycemic nonketotic coma.
    3) Laboratory error:
       a) Falsely increased serum sodium.
       b) Falsely decreased serum chloride or bicarbonate.

C. Causes of Decreased Anion Gap
    1) Increased unmeasured cation:
       a) Increased concentration of normally present cation: hyperkalemia, hypercalcemia, hyper-magnesemia.
       b) Retention of abnormal cation: IgG globulin, tromethamine (TRIS buffer), lithium.
    2) Decreased unmeasured anion: hypoalbuminemia.
    3) Laboratory error:
       a) Systematic error: hyponatremia due to viscous serum, hyperchloremia in bromide intoxication.
       b) Random error: falsely decreased serum sodium, falsely increased serum chloride or bicar-bonate.

Ref: Emmett M, Narins R. Medicine 1977; 56:38. Oh MS, Carroll HJ. New Eng J Med 1977; 297:814.

7. Lab studies to differentiate prerenal azotemia from intrinsic renal failure

|  | Adult/Child | | Newborn Infant | |
|---|---|---|---|---|
|  | Prerenal | Intrinsic | Prerenal | Intrinsic |
| U/P osmolatity | >1.3 | <1.1 | >1.3 | <1.0 |
| U/P creatinine | >40 | <20 | >30 | <10 |
| FE Na (%) | <1 | >2 | <2.5 | >2.5 |

U/P = urine/plasma ratio
FE Na = fractional excretion of sodium. Defined as: U/P Na ÷ U/P creatinine x 100%

Ref: Feld LG, et al. J Pediatr 1986; 109:404.

COMPOSITION OF FREQUENTLY USED ORAL SOLUTIONS

| Liquid | CHO gm/100 ml | Prot.* gm/100 ml | Cal/L | Na | K mEq/L†† | Cl | HCO** | Ca | P+ mg/dl |
|---|---|---|---|---|---|---|---|---|---|
| Infalyte | 2.0 | -- | 80 | 50 | 20 | 40 | 30 | | |
| Lytren | 2.0 | -- | 80 | 50 | 25 | 45 | 30 | | |
| Pedialyte | 2.5 | -- | 100 | 45 | 20 | 35 | 30 | | |
| Pedialyte - RS | 2.5 | -- | 100 | 75 | 20 | 65 | 30 | | |
| Resol | 2.0 | -- | 80 | 50 | 20 | 50 | 34 | | |
| WHO solution | 2.0 | -- | 80 | 90 | 20 | 80 | 30 | | |
| | | | | | | | | | |
| Apple juice | 11.9 | -- | 483 | 0.43 | 25 | -- | -- | 6 | 16 |
| Coca Cola | 10.0 | -- | 400 | 3.6 | -- | -- | 13.4 | 3.0 | 16 |
| Gatorade | 4 | -- | 170 | 23.5 | 2.5 | 17 | -- | 23 | -- |
| Ginger ale | 7.5 | -- | 300 | 4.5 | 0.1 | -- | 3.6 | 2.7 | -- |
| Grape juice | 18.0 | -- | 660 | 0.8 | 29.6 | -- | 32 | 10.9 | 12 |
| Jell-O (1/2 strength) | 9.7 | 0.8 | 404 | 5.5-16.5§ | 0.1-0.2§ | -- | 1 | 2.5 | -- |
| Kool-Aid# (sweetened) | 10.0 | -- | 416 | 0.2 | 0.1 | -- | -- | 1 | 18 |
| Milk (skim) | 4.8 | 3.6 | 425 | 22 | 38 | 29 | -- | 110 | 90 |
| Milk (whole) | 4.8 | 3.37 | 670 | 22 | 37.5 | 28 | 30 | 110 | 90 |
| Orange juice (unsweetened) | 11.0 | -- | 451 | 0.35 | 51.2 | -- | 50 | 10 | 18 |
| Pepsi-Cola | 10.8 | -- | 480 | 1.1 | 1.0 | -- | 7.3 | -- | -- |
| 7-UP | 10.0 | -- | 411 | 0.5 | -- | -- | -- | -- | -- |
| Sprite | 10.0 | -- | 400 | 7.6 | -- | 4 | -- | 3 | 0 |
| Water (Balto City) | -- | -- | -- | 3 | 0.5 | 4 | -- | -- | 6.8 |

* Protein or amino acid equivalent
** Actual or potential bicarbonate, such as lactate, citrate, or acetate
† Calculated according to valence of 1.8
†† Approximate values: actual values may vary somewhat in various localities depending on electrolyte composition of water supply used to reconstitute solution.
§ Depends on flavor (concord grape, black raspberry-lowest Na; wild cherry-highest Na)
# Does not include electrolyte contribution from local water.
Adapted from: USDA Handbook #456, JHH Diet Manual, and Facts and Comparisons, 1986.

## COMPOSITION OF FREQUENTLY USED PARENTERAL FLUIDS

| Liquid | CHO gm/100 ml | Prot.* gm/100 ml | Cal/L | Na | K (mEq/L++) | Cl | HCO** | Ca (mg/dl) | P+ |
|---|---|---|---|---|---|---|---|---|---|
| D$_5$W | 5 | -- | 170 | -- | -- | -- | -- | -- | -- |
| D$_{10}$W | 10 | -- | 340 | -- | -- | -- | -- | -- | -- |
| Normal saline (0.9% NaCl) | -- | -- | -- | 154 | -- | 154 | -- | -- | -- |
| 1/2 Normal saline (0.45% NaCl) | -- | -- | -- | 77 | -- | 77 | -- | -- | -- |
| D5 (0.2% NaCl) | 5 | -- | 170 | 34 | -- | 34 | -- | -- | -- |
| 3% Saline | -- | -- | -- | 513 | -- | 513 | -- | -- | -- |
| 8.4% Sodium Bicarbonate (1 mEq/ml) | -- | -- | -- | 1000 | -- | -- | 1000 | -- | -- |
| Ringer's | 0-10 | -- | 0-340 | 147 | 4 | 155.5 | -- | 4.5 | -- |
| Ringer's Lactate | 0-10 | -- | 0-340 | 130 | 4 | 109 | 28 | 3 | -- |
| Amino Acid 8.5% (Travasol) | -- | 8.5 | 340 | 3 | -- | 34 | 52 | -- | -- |
| Plasmanate | -- | 5 | 200 | 110 | 2 | 50 | 29 | -- | -- |
| Albumin 25% (Salt Poor) | -- | 25 | 1000 | 100-160 | <1 | <120 | -- | -- | -- |
| Intralipid (Cutter)§ | 2.25 | -- | 1100 | 2.5 | 0.5 | 4.0 | -- | -- | 0.8 |

\* Protein or amino acid equivalent

\*\* Bicarbonate or equivalent (citrate, acetate, lactate)

+ Approximate values: actual values may vary somewhat in various localities depending on electrolyte composition of water supply used to reconstitute solution

§ Values are approximate – may vary from lot to lot

POISONING

1.   The Unknown Poison (Partial Listing)

| Sign or Symptom | Poison |
|---|---|
| | EYES |
| Pupillary dilatation | Belladonna alkaloids, atropine, meperidine, sympathomimetics, parasympatholytics, antihista-mines, cocaine, camphor, benzene, botulinus toxin, cyanide, carbon monoxide, LSD, mesca-line, thallium, alcohols, tricyclics. |
| Pupillary constriction | Opiates, sympatholytics, parasympathomimetics, barbiturates, cholinesterase inhibitors, chloral hydrate, phenothiazines, ethanol, organophos-phate insecticides, phencyclidine. |
| Nystagmus | Phenytoin, PCP, barbiturates, sedatives, tricyclic antidepressants. |
| Ptosis | Botulinus toxin, phenytoin. |
| Strabismus | Botulinus toxin, thallium. |

FACE AND SCALP

| Alopecia | Arsenic, radioactive agents, cancer chemothera-peutic agents, vitamin A, lead, boric acid, thallium |
|---|---|
| Facial twitchings | Lead, mercury |

SKIN AND MUCOUS MEMBRANES

| Sweating | Cholinergics, organophosphate insecticides, nicotine, phencyclidine |
|---|---|
| Hot, dry skin | Atropine, belladonna alkaloids, botulinus toxin, sympathomimetics |
| Flushing | Sympathomimetics, anticholinergics, boric acid, carbon monoxide, alcohol, snake bites, atro-pine, antihistamines, phenothiazines |
| Salivation | Caustics, arsenic, mercury, bismuth, choliner-gics, organophosphate insecticides, muscarine-containing mushrooms, salicylates, nicotine, fluoride, phencyclidine |
| Dry mouth | Atropine, belladonna alkaloids, botulinus toxin, antihistamines, sympathomimetics, narcotics, anticholinergics |
| Burns | Corrosives, thallium, boric acid |
| Stomatitis | Cancer chemotherapeutic agents |
| Pink | Carbon monoxide, cyanides, boric acid |

| Yellow | Jaundice from hepatic injury (chlorinated compounds, heavy metals, mushrooms and many drugs), jaundice from hemolytic anemias (aniline, fava beans, many drugs); quinacrine, vitamin A |
|---|---|
| Cyanotic, brown bluish (in absence of respiratory depression or shock) | Nitrobenzene, chlorates, carbon dioxide, ethylene glycol, iron, nitrites, nitrates, ergot, and well over 100 other drugs and chemicals, methemoglobinemias. |
| Red orange | Rifampin. |

NERVOUS SYSTEM

| Obtundation, coma | Opiates, all hypnotics, sedatives and general anesthetics, barbiturates, chloral hydrate, paraldehyde, chloroform, ethers, bromides, alcohols, lead, cyanide, carbon monoxide, carbon dioxide, nicotine, benzene, atropine, scopolamine, irreversible cholinesterase inhibitors, insulin, aniline derivatives, mushrooms, salicylates, anticonvulsants, phencyclidine. |
|---|---|
| Delirium, agitation | Atropine, belladonna alkaloids, cocaine, alcohol, caffeine, lead, marijuana, arsenic, amphetamines, antihistamines, camphor, LSD, PCP, benzene, barbiturates, DDT, aniline dyes, theophylline, digitalis, tricyclics. |
| Convulsions | Strychnine, camphor, cocaine, atropine, belladonna alkaloids, organophosphate insecticides, amphetamines, nicotine, lead, mushrooms, caffeine, theophylline, cyanides, tricyclic antidepressants, salicylates, narcotics, barbiturate withdrawal, boric acid, mercury, phenothiazines, antihistamines, arsenic, DDT, hydrocarbons, fluoride, digitalis, thallium, alcohols, PCP, propoxyphene, phenytoin |
| Headache | Organophosphate insecticides, carbon monoxide, benzene, anilines, lead, caffeine |
| Muscle spasms | Atropine, strychnine, lead, spider and scorpion bites, phenothiazines, camphor, fluorides, phencyclidine. |
| Paresthesias, weakness, paralysis | Carbon monoxide, botulinus toxin, alcohols, curare, DDT, nicotine, cyanide, mercury, lead, arsenics, thallium, organophosphates, fluorides |

## GI TRACT

| | |
|---|---|
| Nausea, vomiting, diarrhea, abdominal pain | Arsenic, iron, corrosives, lead, spider bites, boric acid, organophosphates, phosphorus, nicotine, fluorides, thallium, methanol, mushrooms, digitalis, opiates, DDT, botulinus toxin, cocaine, salicylates, theophylline, snake bites, food poisoning, mercury, naphthalene |
| Dysphagia | Caustics, botulinus toxin, camphor, iodine, arsenics |
| Hematemesis | Caustics, fluoride, iron, arsenic, salicylates, theophylline, warfarin, phosphorus |

## EAR

| | |
|---|---|
| Tinnitus | Salicylates, quinine, quinidine, aminoglycosides, camphor, nicotine, methanol, diuretics |

## RENAL

| | |
|---|---|
| Proteinuria | Arsenic, mercury, phosphorus |
| Hematuria and/or hemoglobinuria | Arsenic, mercury, naphthalene, and other potential hemolytic oxidizers, cyclophosphamide. |

## HEMATOLOGIC

| | |
|---|---|
| Anemia | Lead, naphthalene and other potentially hemolytic agents, snake venom |
| Hemorrhage | Warfarin, thallium |
| Methemoglobinemia | Nitrates, nitrites, anilines |

## RESPIRATORY

| | |
|---|---|
| Respiratory depression and failure | Opiates, fluorides, cyanides, barbiturates, alcohols, snake venom, carbon monoxide, benzodiazepines, phenothiazines, organophosphates |
| Tachypnea and hyperpnea | Atropine, belladonna alkaloids, cocaine, amphetamines, strychnine, salicylates, camphor, hydrocarbons, snake venoms, cyanides, carbon monoxide, talc, caustics |
| Dyspnea | Cyanides, carbon monoxide, carbon dioxide, snake venoms, volatile organic solvents (benzene) |

## CARDIOVASCULAR

| | |
|---|---|
| Bradycardia | Digitalis, mushrooms, quinine, quinidine, lead, barbiturates, opiates, organophosphates, beta blockers |

| Tachycardia | Amphetamines, atropine, cocaine, sympathomimetics, caffeine, theophylline |
|---|---|
| Hypertension | Amphetamines, sympathomimetics, lead, nicotine, cortisone |
| Hypotension | Chloral hydrate, phenothiazines, iron, sympatholytics, tricyclic antidepressants. |
| Cardiovascular collapse (shock) | Leads, acids, alkalis, opiates, endotoxins, food poisoning, iron |
| Dysrhythmias | Digitalis, tricyclic antidepressants, theophylline, narcotics, amphetamines, phenothiazines, solvents |

BREATH ODOR

| Alcoholic | Phenols, chloral hydrate, alcohol |
|---|---|
| Sweet | Chloroform, acetone, ether |
| Bitter almond | Cyanides |
| Pears | Chloral hydrate |
| Garlic | Phosphorus, arsenic, organophosphate insecticides |
| Wintergreen | Methyl salicylate |
| Violets | Turpentine |
| Pine | Pine oil |

GENERAL

| Fever | Atropine, salicylates, food poisoning, antihistamines, phenothiazines, camphor, alcohols, theophylline, quinine, belladonna alkaloids |
|---|---|

Adapted from: Arena JM. Poisoning. Springfield: Charles C Thomas, 1985:15-19.

Other General References: Skoutakis VA. Clinical Toxicology of Drugs: Principles and Practice. Philadelphia: Lea and Febiger, 1982; Haddad LM and Winchester JF. Clinical Management of Poisoning and Drug Overdose. Philadelphia: W B Saunders, 1983.

2.   Prevention of Systemic Absorption

   A.   Emesis
        1)   Recommended for most ingestions

| Contraindication | Relative Contraindication |
|---|---|
| a. Decreased level of consciousness | a. Under 6 months of age |
| b. Caustic ingestions | b. Severe cardiac/respiratory disease |
| c. Hematemesis | c. Late stage pregnancy |
| d. Seizures | d. Uncontrolled hypertension |
| | e. Most hydrocarbons |

2) Syrup of Ipecac dosages:
   a) 6-12 months of age    – 10 ml
   b) 1-12 years of age     – 15-30 ml
   c) >12 years of age      – 30-60 ml
3) Follow ipecac with 100-500 ml of clear fluids, according to age.
4) If no emesis occurs in 20 min, repeat the dose only once and give more fluids.

B. Gastric lavage
   1) Indications:
      a) Ipecac failure
      b) Infants <6 months of age
      c) Stuporous and comatose patients
      d) Post-ictal patients (emesis during a second seizure could be dangerous)
   2) Contraindications:
      a) Caustic ingestions
      b) Hydrocarbon ingestions (see Section H)
   3) Insertion and inflation of a cuffed endotracheal tube prior to gastric lavage protects against aspiration of gastric contents, especially in the patient with altered mental status or a depressed gag reflex.
   4) Method:
      a) Position patient on left side, with the head slightly lower than the body.
      b) Insert large-bore orogastric tube.
      c) Lavage with 0.9% normal saline 15 ml/kg/cycle to maximum to 200-400 cc/cycle in adults, until gastric contents are clear. This may require several liters. Save initial pass for toxicologic examination. Add activated charcoal to the lavage solution to increase the amount of poison removed.

C. Activated charcoal
   1) Indicated after emesis or lavage in all ingestions except caustics, hydrocarbons, alcohols, iron, boric acid, or cyanide. (Do not give before emesis, as charcoal will inactivate ipecac.)

2)   Effectively adsorbs and prevents systemic absorption of toxins.

3)   <u>Initial Dose</u>:   Small children:   15-30 gm activated charcoal PO or NG in 70% sorbitol solution. Children >12 years of age 50-60 gm PO or NG.

Note:   Consider multiple dose charcoal regimen for severe intoxication with theophylline, phenobarbital, tricyclic antidepressants, digoxin, or tegretol.
Regimen:  a) Give 1/2 the initial dose every 4 hours
          b) Endpoint is nontoxic blood levels or lack of signs/symptoms of clinical toxicity after 12-24 hours. Watch for hypernatremia.

D.   Cathartics
1)   Recommended in conjunction with activated charcoal therapy.
     <u>Dose</u>:   (a) Sorbitol administered in 70% solution with appropriate dose of charcoal (preferred) or (b) magnesium citrate 4 ml/kg - max dose of 200 ml in adult.

2)   <u>Contraindications</u>:   Caustic ingestions, absent bowel sounds or recent bowel surgery. Avoid Mg containing cathartics in patients with compromised renal function.

Ref:   Rogers GC, et al. Pediatr Clin North Am 1986; 33:261.  Curr Probl Pediatr 1986; 16:85-233.

E.   Dialysis
1)   Indicated in severe ingestions of dialyzable substances (i.e. low volume of distribution, low molecular weight, decreased binding to plasma proteins) which are unresponsive to standard care.
2)   Hemoperfusion is useful for specific toxins.
3)   Dialyzable poisons (partial list)

| | |
|---|---|
| Ammonia | Iodides |
| Amphetamines | Isoniazid |
| Anilines | Meprobamate |
| Antibiotics | Paraldehyde |
| Barbiturates (long acting) | Potassium |
| Boric Acid | Quinidine |
| Bromides | Quinine |
| Calcium | Salicylates |
| Chloral Hydrate | Strychnine |
| Fluorides | Thiocyanates |

Ref:   Arena JM, Poisoning. Springfield:   Charles C Thomas, 1985.  Gellis SS, Kagan BM, Current Pediatric Therapy. Philadelphia:  WB Saunders, 1986.

3.   Specific Poisonings

   A.   Salicylate Poisoning
        1)   Symptoms:  hyperpnea, hyperthermia, lethargy,
             nausea, vomiting, tinnitus, dehydration, metabolic
             acidosis, coma
        2)   Establish the severity of ingestion
             a)   The acute toxic dose (single-dose ingestion):
                  150 mg/kg
             b)   Chronic overdosage can produce toxicity at
                  much lower doses
             c)   Preparations:
                  (1)   Children's aspirin:  1¼ grain  (81 mg)
                        tablets (36 tabs per bottle)
                  (2)   Adult aspirin:  5 grain (325 mg) tablets
                  (3)   Methyl salicylate (oil of wintergreen):
                        1.4 gm/ml
        3)   Test of salicylates

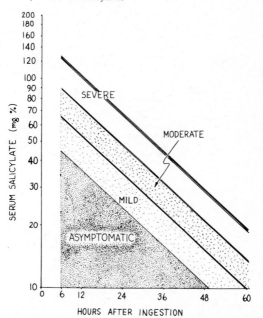

   <u>Done Nomogram</u>: the nomogram relates serum
   salicylate and expected severity of intoxication
   at varying intervals following ingestion of a
   <u>single</u> dose of salicylate, starting six hours
   after the ingestion.

a) Urine ferric chloride: Mix one ml of urine with one ml 10% $FeCl_3$ solution. Purple color change indicates a positive test. However, even an insignificant amount of salicylate will produce a positive test. Urinary ketones also will produce a false positive test; these can be removed by first boiling the urine.

b) Serum salicylate level: therapy must be based upon quantitative serum level and not upon the above presumptive tests. At least two levels obtained several hours apart are necessary to determine the severity of ingestion, as continued slow absorption may increase the serum level for up to 24 hours.

4) Treatment

a) Institute therapy immediately. Do not wait for the salicylate level to return.

b) Empty the stomach by emesis (preferably), or lavage using 0.9% normal saline. Administer activated charcoal and cathartic.

c) Monitor serum electrolytes, calcium, arterial blood gases, glucose, urine pH and SG, and coagulation studies as needed.

d) Treat fluid and solute deficits

(1) replenish intravascular volume with D5 Ringer's Lactate at 20 ml/kg/hr for 1-2 hrs until adequate urine output is established.

(2) then begin infusing D5 with 50 mEq Na $HCO_3$/L and 20-40 mEq K/L at rates of 3-6 L/ $M^2$/day (i.e., 2-4 times maintenance fluids). Aim for a urine output of 2 ml/kg/hr, as this will enhance salicylate excretion. Adjust concentrations of the electrolytes as needed to correct serum electrolyte abnormalities (esp. hypokalemia, which inhibits salicylate excretion), and to maintain a urinary pH >7.0.

e) Administer parenteral vitamin K as indicated by coagulation studies (especially in chronic intoxications).

f) Continue fluid therapy until the patient is asymptomatic for several hours, regardless of the serum salicylate level.

g) Proceed to hemodialysis in the presence of unresponsive acidosis (pH <7.10), renal failure, seizures unresponsive to calcium gluconate and anticonvulsants, or progressive deterioration when all other methods have been carried out appropriately.

Ref: Snodgrass WR, Pediatr Clin North Am 1986; 33:381-91. Temple AR, Arch Intern Med, 1981; 141:364-9.

247

B. Acetaminophen Poisoning
   1) Symptoms: nausea, vomiting, and malaise for 24
      hrs, improvement over the next 48 hrs, followed by
      clinical or laboratory evidence of hepatic dysfunc-
      tion. Death can occur due to fulminant hepatic
      failure.
   2) Likelihood of hepatic toxicity related to:
      a) Dose: 140 mg/kg is considered toxic.
      b) Plasma level: Draw level at 4 hrs post
         ingestion and plot on nomogram.
      c) Delay in treatment: N-acetylcysteine (NAC) is
         most effective if administered within 10 hrs of
         the ingestion. Efficacy is lower between 10-16
         hrs post-ingestion. Few deaths have been
         reported when NAC is used within 24 hours.

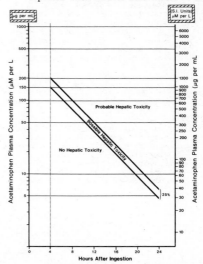

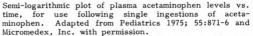

Semi-logarithmic plot of plasma acetaminophen levels vs.
time, for use following single ingestions of acetaminophen. Adapted from Pediatrics 1975; 55:871-6 and
Micromedex, Inc. with permission.

3) Therapy: If time since ingestion is < 1 hr, give ipecac; after emesis give charcoal; draw plasma level at 4 hrs. If ingestion was 1-4 hrs ago, give charcoal and draw acetaminophen level at 4 hrs. After 4 hrs, draw level and treat with NAC orally or IV if level is in toxic range. <u>NB</u>: Charcoal adsorbs oral NAC; avoid simultaneous administration.

Oral NAC Regimen (PO or NG): Give 20% NAC diluted 1:4 in a carbonated beverage as a loading dose of 140 mg/kg, then 70 mg/kg q4h for 17 doses.

IV NAC Regimen: (Approved in Canada and UK, but not by USFDA. To use IV NAC in U.S., contact local Poison Center.) Use 20% NAC solution: Give 150 mg/kg in 200 mL of D5W over 15 minutes. Then 50 mg/kg in 500 mL of D5W over 4 hours. Then 100 mg/kg in 1000 mL of D5W over next 16 hours. Check plasma level at 24 hours. Small risk of anaphylaxis with IV NAC.

Ref: Rumack, BH. Pediatr Clin North Am 1986; 33:691-701; Tenenbein M, Curr Probl Pediatr 1986; 16:185-233; Prescott LF, Drugs 1983; 25:290-314; Peterson RG, Personal Communication, 1988.

C. Hyperkalemia
   1) Diagnosis based on serum level and EKG abnormalities (see Cardiology section, page 74). Serum levels often do not correlate directly with EKG abnormalities.
   2) Treatment
      a) Serum level >6.0 mEq/L: discontinue all exogenous potassium sources and K-sparing diuretics.
      b) Significant EKG abnormalities: Begin continuous EKG monitoring and institute one or more of the following therapies either sequentially or concurrently and repeat them as necessary.
         (1) Administer 0.5 ml/kg of calcium gluconate 10% solution IV over 5-10 min, while monitoring for bradycardia and hypotension. Adult maximum dose is 10-20 ml.
         (2) Administer 1-2 mEq/kg sodium bicarbonate IV over 5-10 min.

NOTE: Sodium bicarbonate and calcium gluconate are incompatible solutions and will precipitate if given through the same IV line without flushing between doses.

(3) Administer IV over 2 hrs: 0.5 gm/kg of glucose with 0.3 units regular insulin added per gram of glucose.

c) Administer Kayexalate (sodium polystyrene sulfonate resin) 1-2 gm/kg/day orally divided Q6h in 70% sorbitol solution (3 ml/gm resin) or as a retention enema in 20% sorbitol solution (5 ml/gm resin). One gram of Kayexalate per kg body weight should lower serum potassium approximately 1 mEq/L.

d) Proceed rapidly to dialysis if hyperkalemia appears imminently life-threatening. Arrhythmias which significantly compromise cardiac output may require temporary artificial pacing.

D. Digoxin Intoxication

1) Symptoms: major manifestations are GI (anorexia, nausea, vomiting), CNS (headache, disorientation, somnolence, seizures), and CARDIAC (any new rhythm, esp. those combining increased automaticity of ectopic pacemakers and impaired conduction). Most cases result in GI symptoms with mild CNS and cardiac disturbances.

2) Evaluation

a) Determine serum digoxin level and electrolytes (including Mg and Ca) stat

b) Doses of >0.07 mg/kg (or 2-3 mg in adolescent) are associated with toxicity

c) Signs and symptoms predict digoxin level >2 ng/ml however absence of symptoms when level >2 ng/ml cannot predict potential for toxicity.

d) Quinidine, amiodarone, or poor renal function will increase the digoxin level. Low K, Mg or $T_4$ will increase digoxin toxicity at a given level, as will high Ca.

e) Hyperkalemia correlates with a high digoxin level.

3) Treatment

a) Ipecac, charcoal (even several hours after ingestion), and cathartic.

b) Start continuous ECG monitoring.

c) In cardiac rhythm disturbances:

(1) AV block: atropine alone 0.01 mg/kg IV may reverse sinus bradycardia or AV block. Repeated doses may be necessary. Avoid propranolol, quinidine, procainamide, or disopyramide if AV block is present.

(a) Phenytoin improves AV conduction. Dose is 1-2 mg/kg, no faster than 50 mg/min. Repeat Q5 min until arrhythmia is controlled or maximum dose is reached.

          (b)  Transvenous ventricular pacing is usually effective if atropine and phenytoin fail.

      (2)  Ventricular tachycardia, PVCs: phenytoin and lidocaine are effective.

   d)  In severe poisonings with uncontrollable dysrhythmia and/or hyperkalemia, administer purified digoxin specific Fab fragments. Since this therapy can be life saving, continue CPR for prolonged periods if Fab fragments are available.

Dose: Digoxin Immune FAB (Digibind) available in 40 mg vial. Each vial will bind approximately 0.6 mg of digoxin.
Estimate of body load in mg based on:

      (1)  Known acutely ingested dose (x 0.8 to correct for incomplete absorption of tablets) or

      (2)  Serum drug concentration x 5.6 x wt. in kg ÷ 1000 (volume of distribution of digoxin 5.6 L/kg)

Dose in # of vials = $\dfrac{\text{Body load (mg)}}{0.6 \text{ mg/vial}}$

Administer IV over 30 minutes. Give as bolus injection if cardiac arrest is imminent.

Ref: Smith TW, et al. New Engl J Med 1982; 307:1357; Tenenbein M. Curr Probl Pediatr 1986; 16:185, 1986; Lewander WJ, et al. Am J Dis Child 1986; 140:770; Murphy DJ, et al. Pediatr 1982; 70:472.

E.  Iron Poisoning
   1)  Diagnosis
      a)  Symptoms
          (1)  First phase: GI toxicity (30 min - 12 hrs after ingestion) - nausea, vomiting, diarrhea, abdominal pain, hematemesis, melena. Rarely - shock, seizures, coma.

          (2)  Second phase: latent period (8-36 hrs after ingestion) - improvement in clinical symptoms.

          (3)  Third phase: systemic toxicity (12-48 hrs after ingestion) - hepatic injury or failure, hypoglycemia, metabolic acidosis, bleeding, shock, coma, convulsions, death.

          (4)  Fourth phase: late complications (4-8 wks after ingestion) - pyloric or antral stenosis, CNS sequelae. Post intoxication liver cirrhosis not seen in children.

      b)  Determination of estimated dose (for children

less than 5 years old):

| Elemental Fe | Therapy |
|---|---|
| <20 mg/kg | No Therapy |
| 20-60 mg/kg | Syrup of Ipecac, home mgmt |
| >60 mg/kg | Physician evaluation |

c)  Deferoxamine challenge test: give 1 gm IM. Presence of "vin rose" color to urine indicates significant ingestion of iron.

d)  Determine serum iron concentration 4-6 hours post ingestion.

| Level | Therapy |
|---|---|
| 300-500 mcg/dl | Begin chelation if iron concentration exceeds TIBC or if patient showing signs/symptoms of toxicity. |
| >500 mcg/dl | 20% risk of shock. Institute chelation therapy immediately. |

Note: Serum iron levels obtained beyond 6 hours after ingestion may not be elevated, even in the presence of severe poisoning.

2)  Treatment

a)  Induce emesis if patient awake, alert.

b)  Lavage all patients after emesis with 5% NaHCO$_3$ solution.

c)  Obtain abdominal X-ray after lavage.

d)  Deferoxamine should be given IV at 15 mg/kg/hr in all cases of serious poisoning. If serum iron concentration >500 mcg/dl continue chelation until serum iron <300 mcg/dl. When traditional "vin rose" urine does occur, continue chelation until 24 hours after the child is producing an adequate volume of normally colored urine.

e)  Above all, supportive care is the most important therapy. Large IV fluid volumes may be needed in first 24 hours to avoid hypovolemic shock and acidemia. Hydrating solution should contain 1-2 meq/kg/L of NaHCO$_3$ and urine output should be maintained at >2 ml/kg/hr.

Ref: Banner W Jr, Tong TG. Pediatr Clin North Am, 1986; 33:393-409. Gellis SS, Kogan BM. Current Pediatric Therapy. WB Saunders, 1986.

F.  Lead Poisoning

1)  Diagnosis

a)  Establish presumptive diagnosis with peripheral blood count and smear for basophilic stippling, long bone x-rays for "lead lines," and abdominal x-ray for radiopaque foreign matter.

b) Definitive diagnosis is based on blood lead (Pb) and erythrocyte protoporphyrin levels by the extraction method (EP) or zinc protoporphyrin (Zn PP) by hematofluorometer (see table below). Note that EP levels may be elevated (but less than 300 mcg/dl) in iron deficiency.

### Risk Classification of Asymptomatic Children

| Pb (mcg/dl) | EP values in mcg/dl | | | |
|---|---|---|---|---|
| | <35(<35)* | 35-109(35-74)* | 110-249(75-174)* | >250(>175)* |
| <24 | I | Ia | Ia | EPP |
| 25-49 | Ib | II | III | III |
| 50-69 | N | III | III | IV |
| >70 | N | N | IV | IV |

* Zn PP values in parentheses.

| | | |
|---|---|---|
| I, Ib = Low risk | II = moderate risk | N = not observed |
| Ia = Low risk seen in iron deficiency | III = high risk IV = urgent risk | EPP = erythropoietic protoporphyria |

Note: Diagnostic classification is more urgent than the classification indicated for children with symptoms compatible with lead toxicity, children <3 years of age, children in the upper part of a particular class, or children with siblings in a higher class.

Ref: Centers for Disease Control   Preventing Lead Poisoning in Young Children, 1985.

2) Treatment of Asymptomatic Cases
   a) Class I - none required
   b) Class II
      (1) remove patient from lead sources
      (2) stringent dust control
      (3) treat iron deficiency
      (4) Low fat, lead free diet with adequate calcium, magnesium, zinc, copper, and iron.
      (5) Monitor Pb and FEP every 3 months for at least 18 months to determine status.
   c) Class III
      (1) Remove patient from lead source and institute above diet.
      (2) Limit chelation therapy to children with one or more of following:
          (a) Pb >45-50 mcg;
          (b) 24 hr CaEDTA mobilization test >0.75 mcg Pb excreted/mg CaEDTA;
          (c) behavioral changes and mild non-specific Sx suggestive of early clinical plumbism.

NOTE: The FEP is of no value in making the decision regarding chelation therapy.

Therapy for class III toxicity consists of:
CaEDTA 500 mg/M²q12° IM x 5 days (if given IV infuse over 6° and use cardiac monitor). Follow with either (a) 1-3 additional 5 day courses of CaEDTA (allowing 1 week between each 5 day course of therapy) or (b) oral D-penicillamine 500 mg/M²/day. Give on empty stomach 2 hrs before breakfast. Contents may be mixed with chilled fruit or fruit juice. Give 25mg of pyridoxine QD concomitantly.

NOTE: CaEDTA is excreted unchanged exclusively by glomerular filtration. Therefore with significantly impaired renal function withhold CaEDTA therapy. Untoward reactions to CaEDTA include ↑Ca, ↑BUN proteinuria, microscopic hematuria, and fever.

D-penicillamine is contraindicated with renal disease and a history of sensitivity to penicillin. Neutropenia, proteinuria, hypersensitivity reactions, and erythematous rashes are contraindications to further use.

d)  Class IV
    CaEDTA 500 mg/M² q12hr IM x 5 days. Urine output in first 24 hours used to determine chelatable lead (mcg Pb excreted/mg CaEDTA administered/day).
    BAL not given unless symptomatic or Pb >100 mcg/dl.

3)  Treatment of Symptomatic Cases
    Children with one or more of following: persistent vomiting, ataxic gait, gross irritability, severe anemia, seizures, or alteration in state of consciousness are treated as potential cases of acute encephalopathy.

    Therapy:
    a)  Establish urine output with 10-20 ml/kg IV if necessary. Then adjust fluid therapy to maintain urine output of 350-500 ml/M²/day.
    b)  Control seizures initially with diazepam and thereafter with paraldehyde. Phenobarbital and/or phenytoin may be necessary for long term seizure control.
    c)  Chelate with BAL-CaEDTA in combination.
        Dosage:  BAL 83 mg/M²/dose IM Q4H
                 CaEDTA 250 mg/M²/dose IM Q4H
        Administration:  For first dose inject BAL (IM)

only. Beginning 4 hours later and every 4 hours thereafter for 5 days inject BAL and CaEDTA simultaneously at separate and deep IM sites; rotate injection sites.

NOTE: Usual 5 day course may be extended to 7 days cautiously if clinical evidence of encephalopathy persists beyond 4 days.

Serial Pb measurements should be made after the last doses of BAL and CaEDTA and at day 7, 14, and 21 thereafter.

If Pb rebounds to 40 mcg/dl or more, additional 5 day courses of CaEDTA are indicated. Rebound is minimized if the initial course of BAL/CaEDTA is followed by oral D-penicillamine.

NOTE: BAL contraindicated in acute hepatocellular injury and G6PD deficiency. BAL should not be given concomitantly with medicinal iron.

Most dosage recommendations are from: Chisholm JJ. In: Gellis SS, Kagen BM. Current Pediatric Therapy. 12th Edition. Philadelphia: WB Saunders, 1986. See also Piomelli S, et al. J Pediatr 1984;105: 523-32.

G. Caustic Ingestions (Strong Acids and Alkalis)
   1) All patients with a history of caustic ingestion should be hospitalized for endoscopy. Absence of oropharyngeal damage does not exclude esophageal burns.
   2) Maintain patient NPO. Attempts to "neutralize" the burn are ineffective and obscure and delay endoscopy. Ipecac or lavage is contraindicated.
   3) Begin intravenous fluid therapy.
   4) Begin intravenous ampicillin 100-200 mg/kg/day.
   5) Begin intravenous hydrocortisone sodium succinate 10-20 mg/kg/day.
   6) Provide tetanus prophylaxis as indicated.
   7) Obtain blood count, chest x-ray, blood type and crossmatch. Chest x-ray may demonstrate esophageal perforation.
   8) Proceed to endoscopy. Do not pass NG tube. Discontinue endoscopy immediately if esophageal burn identified.
   9) In the absence of esophageal burn, antibiotics and steroids may be discontinued. Provide care for local burns.
   10) In the presence of esophageal burns, continue antibiotics for at least 5-7 days and steroids for 3 wks. Advance diet slowly after patient is able to handle

own secretions well. Steroids may be changed to oral prednisone 2 mg/kg/day if tolerated. Taper prednisone slowly after full 3 wk course.

11) Provide close follow-up and further surgical therapy for esophageal or antral/pyloric strictures, as required. Risk of developing esophageal carcinoma after caustic ingestion is markedly increased.

NOTE: Ingestion of alkaline button batteries can lead to esophageal and gastric burns. If initial X-ray shows battery to be lodged in esophagus, immediate endoscopic retrieval is indicated. If the disc is beyond the esophagus, patient is discharged and follow up X-rays performed only if battery not passed in 4-7 days.
For batteries >23 mm diameter a 48 hour X-ray should be performed to exclude persistent gastric position and need for endoscopic retrieval.

Ref: Rothstein FC. Pediatr Clin North Am 1986; 33:665-74. Moore WR. Clin Pediatr 1986; 25:192-6. Wason S. Emerg Med, 1985; 2:175-182.

H. Hydrocarbon Ingestions
1) Symptoms: Pulmonary: tachypnea, dyspnea, tachycardia, cyanosis, grunting, cough; CNS: lethargy, seizures, coma.
2) Evaluation:
   a) Aliphatic hydrocarbons have the greatest aspiration hazard and pulmonary toxicity. They include: gasoline, kerosene, mineral seal oil, lighter fluid, tar, mineral oil, lubricating oils, turpentine.
   b) Aromatic hydrocarbons (benzene, toluene, xylene) and halogenated hydrocarbons (carbon tetrachloride) have mainly CNS and hepato-toxicity.
3) Therapy
   a) Removal of toxin
      (1) Avoid emesis or lavage if possible as these increase the risk of aspiration.
      (2) If the hydrocarbon contains a potentially toxic substance (insecticide, heavy metal, camphor) and a toxic amount has been ingested, induce emesis with ipecac in the fully conscious patient. In lethargic patients, intubate with a cuffed ETT then lavage.
      (3) Avoid charcoal. It does not bind aliphatics and will increase the risk of aspiration.
   b) Obtain CXR and arterial blood gases on patients with pulmonary symptoms.
   c) Observe patient for 6 hours.

       (1)   If child asymptomatic for 6 hours and CXR normal discharge home.

       (2)   If child becomes symptomatic in 6 hour period-admit.

       (3)   If asymptomatic but CXR abnormal consider admission for further observation. Discharge only if close follow up can be ensured.

    d)   Treat pneumonitis with oxygen, PEEP. Antibiotics and steroids are not routinely warranted.

Ref: Tenenbein M. Curr Probl Pediatr 1986; 16:185-233. Klein BL. Pediatr Clin North Am 1986; 33:411-9.

I.   **Theophylline Toxicity**

   1)   Symptoms: GI: vomiting, hematemesis, abdominal pain, bloody diarrhea; CV: tachycardia, arrhythmia, cardiac arrest; CNS: seizures, agitation, coma, hallucinations.

   2)   Evaluation:

      a)   Obtain a theophylline level stat and again in 1-4 hours to see the pattern of absorption. Peak absorption has been reported to be delayed as long as 13-17 hrs after ingestion.

      b)   Levels >20 mcg/ml associated with increasing toxicity; especially >40 mcg/ml.

      c)   Levels >40 mcg/ml or patients with neurotoxicity require admission and careful monitoring.

      d)   Hypokalemia may occur.

   3)   Therapy:

      a)   Ipecac (preferably) or lavage.

      b)   Charcoal followed by cathartic, regardless of the length of time after ingestion. For severe intoxication begin multiple dose charcoal regimen as outlined earlier.

      c)   Establish IV access and treat dehydration.

      d)   Charcoal hemoperfusion: an effective and safe method of rapidly lowering theophylline levels. Start hemoperfusion whenever signs of neurotoxicity (seizures, coma) are present. Whether a high theophylline level alone is an indication for hemoperfusion is controversial.

Ref: Gaudreault P, et al. J Pediatr 1983; 102:474; Sahney S, et al. Pediatrics 1983; 71:615.

J.   **Anticholinergic Toxicity**

   1)   Agents: tricyclics, antihistamines, antiparkinsonians, scopolamine, belladonna, jimson weed, ophthalmic mydriatics, atropine.

   2)   Symptoms: "mad as a hatter, red as a beet, blind

as a bat, hot as a hare, dry as a bone", oral
dryness and burning, speech and swallowing diffi-
culties, thirst, blurred vision, photophobia,
mydriasis, skin flushing, tachycardia, fever, urinary
urgency, delirium, hallucinations, cardiovascular
collapse.

3) Treatment:
   a) Emesis or lavage, activated charcoal, and
      cathartic as above.
   b) Observation is all that is necessary in mild
      cases.
   c) In life-threatening emergencies (arrhythmias,
      hypertension, myoclonic seizures, severe hallu-
      cinations), physostigmine will reverse symp-
      toms.

   NOTE: Neostigmine and pyridostigmine will not
   affect the CNS symptoms. Do not use physostigmine
   simply to maintain an alert state in an otherwise
   stable patient in coma.

      (1) dose: in children <5 yrs, give physo-
          stigmine 0.5 mg IV every 5 min until a
          therapeutic effect is seen or a total dose
          of 2.0 mg is achieved. In those >5 yrs,
          give 1-2 mg IV. Repeat in 10 min if
          ineffective. Max. dose = 4 mg in 30 min.
      (2) rate: infuse at 1 mg/min. Faster rates
          can cause seizures or precipitate a cholin-
          ergic crisis. Effective within 3-5 min.
      (3) reversal: atropine should be available to
          reverse excess cholinergic side effects, in
          a dose of 0.5 mg for each 1 mg of physo-
          stigmine just given.

      Ref: Rumack BH. Pediatrics 1973; 52:449.

K. Tricyclic Antidepressant Overdose
   1) Symptoms: choreoathetosis, myoclonus, hypo- or
      hypertension, arrhythmias, in addition to the symp-
      toms of anticholinergic toxicity.
   2) Evaluation:
      a) Toxicity associated with doses >10 mg/kg. A
         dose of >30 mg/kg can be lethal.
      b) EKG: QRS duration >0.10 sec predicts risk of
         seizures and ventricular dysrhythmia in acute
         oversdose.
      c) Serum drug levels are not of predictive value.
   3) Therapy:
      a) Treat life-threatening symptoms (as in anti-
         cholinergic toxicity). Treat seizures with
         diazepam then phenytoin. For arrhythmias
         refractory to physostigmine, give NaHCO$_3$ 1-2

mEq/kg to keep pH >7.4 (lessens risk of arrhythmia), and phenytoin 1 mg/kg (increases AV conduction). Phenytoin may be repeated up to a maximum loading dose of 15-18 mg/kg.
b) Give charcoal and cathartic. For severe intoxication begin multiple dose charcoal regimen as outlined earlier.
c) Cardiac monitoring: once the level of consciousness and QRS duration return to normal, the risk of arrhythmia or sudden death is minimal.
d) Symptomatic and supportive care.

Ref: Boehnert MT, Lovejoy FH: New Eng J Med 1985; 313:474-9. Braden NJ. Pediatr Clin North Am 1986; 33:287-97.

L. Narcotics, Opiates, and Morphine Analogs
1) Suspect in any patient with depressed mental status of unknown etiology.
2) Pupillary signs may be variable.
3) Administer IV nalaxone (Narcan) 0.01 mg/kg. If this is ineffective, administer 0.1 mg/kg. Improvement in mental status indicates a clinical response.
4) Careful inpatient monitoring is required due to the short half life of naloxone compared to most opiates.
5) Indications for continuous naloxone infusion include:
a) requirement for repeat bolus therapy
b) requirement of large initial bolus
c) ingestion of large amount of opiate or long acting opiate
d) decreased opiate metabolism.
Suggested regimen is as follows:
a) Administer as loading dose the previously successful bolus.
b) Administer as an hourly infusion dose the above loading dose.
c) Attempt to discontinue infusion every 12 hours.

Ref: Moore R, et al. Am J Dis Child 1980; 134:156. Tenebein M, J Pediatr 1984; 105:645.

M. Carbon Monoxide Poisoning
1) Diagnosis
a) Symptoms: headache, confusion, dizziness, nausea, weakness, syncope, seizures, or coma.
b) Sources: fire, automobile exhaust, gasoline or propane engines operating in enclosed spaces, faulty furnaces or gas stoves, charcoal burners, paint removes with methylene chloride.
c) Obtain carboxyhemoglobin (COHb) level in blood.
2) Treatment

a) Administer 100% $O_2$
b) Ensure adequate airway; prevent ↑ $PCO_2$
c) Proceed to hyperbaric $O_2$ therapy if COHb level >25%, patient has impaired mentation, or patient is pregnant.
   If hyperbaric $O_2$ unavailable administer 100% $O_2$ until COHb level decreases below 10%.
d) Complications of severe CO poisoning include cardiac dysrhythmias, pulmonary edema, myoglobinuria with acute renal failure, temporary blindness, encephalopathy and cerebral edema.

Ref: Zimmerman SS, Truxal B. Pediatrics 1981; 68:215-24; Gozal D, et al. Clin Pediatr 1985; 24:132-6. Ann Emerg Med 1985; 14:1168-71.

N. Phenothiazine and Butyrophenone Intoxication
1) Diagnosis
   a) Symptoms: (may be delayed 6-24 hours post ingestion). Depressed neurologic status, meiosis, hypotension, dysrhythmias, extrapyramidal signs or neuroleptic malignant syndrome (fever, diaphoresis, rigidity, tachycardia, coma).
2) Treatment
   a) Support and monitoring of respiratory and cardiovascular status.
   b) Ipecac followed by activated charcoal if patient awake and cooperative. Otherwise gastric lavage recommended. Dialysis contraindicated.
   c) Extrapyramidal Signs: IV diphenhydramine 2 mg/kg slowly over 2-5 minutes, OR IV benztropine mesylate 0.5 mg/kg.
   d) Dysrhythmias:
      (1) Ventricular: Phenytoin 10-15 mg/kg IV slowly or Lidocaine 1 mg/kg IV push.
      (2) Supraventricular: supportive, however if hemodynamically unstable proceed to cardioversion.
      (3) AV dissociation: Pacemaker.
   e) Neuroleptic Malignant Syndrome:
      (1) Reduce hyperthermia with lavage and cooling blankets.
      (2) Support respiratory and cardiovascular status - monitor neurologic and fluid status.
      (3) Use of dantrolene (0.5 mg/kg PO Q12hr) to reduce muscle rigidity and oxygen consumption is experimental.

Ref: Knight ME, et al. Pediatr Clin North Am, 1986; 33:299-309.

# BURNS

I. Initial Assessment

   A. Vital Signs
      Assess and establish adequate airway, breathing, circulation. Intubation should be considered if evidence of inhalation injury is present--singed nares, cough, wheezes, hoarseness, facial burns, charring of lips, carbonaceous secretions, or history of fire in enclosed space--or if necessary for pulmonary toilet. (Inhalation injury is present in approximately 30% of victims of major burns. Mortality of patients with inhalation injury is increased.)

   B. Monitor pulmonary status with serial ABG's. Clinical monitoring of resp. rate hourly, noting increasing tachypnea, is critical in early dx. of pulmonary insufficiency caused by acute asphyxia and CO toxicity, upper airway obstruction secondary to edema, or overwhelming parenchymal damage. Delivery of high concentrations of $O_2$ counteracts the effects of CO and speeds its clearance. (CXR may not show changes for 24-72 hours)

   C. Assess and begin treatment for any other injuries. Include EKG. (Electrical injuries may produce extensive deep tissue damage, intravascular thrombosis, cardiac and respiratory arrest, fractures due to muscle contractions, and cardiac arrhythmias).

   D. Establish IV access and begin fluid resuscitation immediately on infants with burns greater than 10% of body surface area (BSA) or children with >15% BSA burned. Begin with Ringer's lactate at approximately 500 cc/m$^2$BSA per hour (enough to maintain a urine output of (0.5-1.5 cc/kg/hr).

   E. Insert NG tube (ileus common in major burns) and Foley catheter. Maintain NPO for 24 hrs. except for Maalox 15-30 cc/m$^2$/hr. per NG to decrease the incidence of stress ulcers.

   F. Tetanus toxoid 0.5 cc IM as needed. If it is to be used, begin penicillin prophylaxis (see section III. D. 2. c. below).

   G. IV analgesia is often necessary to treat pain.

II. Burn Assessment
    Obtain weight and height to calculate surface area. See pg. 330 for BSA nomogram.

261

A. Using the burn assessment chart map the areas of 2nd and 3rd degree burn and calculate the total BSA burned. Extent of tissue damage with electrical burns may not be initially apparent.

B. Depth of burns
   1) 1st degree - only epidermis involved - painful and erythematous.
   2) 2nd degree - epidermis and dermis involved but dermal appendages are spared. Superficial 2nd degree burns are blistered and painful. Deep 2nd degree burns may be white and painless, may require grafting, and can be converted to full thickness burns with wound sepsis.
   3) 3rd degree - full thickness burns involve epidermis and all of dermis (including dermal appendages), are painless, and require grafting.

NOTE: The extent and severity of burn injury may change over the first several days after injury; therefore be cautious in discussing prognosis with the victim's family.

ESTIMATION OF BODY SURFACE INVOLVED

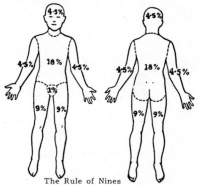

The Rule of Nines
(Not accurate for children <10 years of age.) The percentage of body surface involved must be modified according to age using the following chart.

Lund-Browder Chart

AGE - YEARS

| AREA | 0-1 | 1-4 | 4-9 | 10-15 | Adult | 2° | 3° | Total |
|------|-----|-----|-----|-------|-------|----|----|-------|
| Head | 19 | 17 | 13 | 10 | – | | | |
| Neck | 2 | 2 | 2 | 2 | 2 | | | |
| Trunk | 13 | 13 | 13 | 13 | 13 | | | |
| Buttock(R/L) | 2½ | 2½ | 2½ | 2½ | 2½ | | | |
| Genitalia | 1 | 1 | 1 | 1 | 1 | | | |
| Upper Arm (R/L) | 4 | 4 | 4 | 4 | 4 | | | |
| Lower Arm (R/L) | 3 | 3 | 3 | 3 | 3 | | | |
| Hand(R/L) | 2½ | 2½ | 2½ | 2½ | 2½ | | | |
| Thigh(R/L) | 5½ | 6½ | 8½ | 8½ | 9½ | | | |
| Leg(R/L) | 5 | 5 | 5 | 6 | 7 | | | |
| Foot(R/L) | 3½ | 3½ | 3½ | 3½ | 3½ | | | |
| | | | | | Total | | | |

III. Treatment

A. First-aid: Clean towels soaked in cold water may prevent progression of burn. Do not use grease, butter, etc.

B. Triage
   1) If burn is <10% (infants) or <15% (children) and involves no full thickness areas, the patient may be treated as an outpatient.
   2) Admission should be strongly considered for:
      a. burns larger than above
      b. electrical or chemical burns (full extent of burn may not be intially apparent)
      c. burns of critical areas such as face, hands, feet, or perineum
      d. if child abuse is suspected or home situation is not adequate to assure good care and follow-up
      e. child has another chronic illness
   3) Burns of >20-30% BSA, major burns to hand, face, joints, or perineum, and electrical burns require transfer to a Burn Center after initial stabilization.

C. Outpatient
   1) Cleanse with betadine and water (1:4) solution or synthetic detergent removing exudate, necrotic skin, etc.
   2) Apply sulfadiazine (Silvadene) in thin layer over burn then cover with bulky gauze dressing.
   3) Follow patient daily or every other day.

4) Home care - cleanse burn twice daily with mild soap followed with sulfadiazine and sterile dressing as above. Once epithelialization is underway, may be reduced to daily dressing change.

5) Tetanus toxoid 0.5 cc IM if needed.

D. Inpatient

Initial stabilization as detailed above.

1) Fluid resuscitation

The goal is to provide sufficient fluid for prevention of shock and renal failure secondary to excessive fluid losses and third spacing.

The two formulas listed below are only guidelines and adequacy of perfusion should be assessed using urine output (0.5-1.5 cc/kg/hr), BP, peripheral circulation, and sensorium. Frequent electrolytes and ABG's monitor acidosis.

a. Galveston Formula

(based on BSA since weight and surface area relationships are not constant in a growing child).

1st 24 hours - 5000 cc/m$^2$ of burned area (burn losses) plus 2000 cc/m$^2$ of total BSA (maintenance fluids) given over the first 24 hrs. with half of this amount being infused over the first 8 hrs. (Remember to include fluid already received enroute to referral center) Fluids in childrens > 1 year should be D5RL + 12.5 gm of 25% albumin per liter. For infants < 1 year, prepare a 1 liter solution of 930 ml of D5 1/3 NS, 20 mEq NaHCO$_3$ (1 mEq/ml) and 50 ml of 25% albumin.

2nd & subsequent days - 3750 cc/m$^2$ burned area/24 hrs. (burn losses) plus 1500 cc/m$^2$ of total BSA/24 hrs (maintenance fluids). Sodium requirements after the first 24 hrs. are lower and a solution of D5 1/3 NS with 20-30 meq/L of potassium phosphate is used. (Phosphate used because of frequent hypophosphatemia)

NOTE: Fluid requirements must be reevaluated as wounds heal. Wounds must be remapped weekly.

Beginning on day 2 homogenized milk or infant formula is begun hourly PO or NG and increased at 4 hr. intervals as tolerated while IV rate is decreased. Often by day 4-5 the pt. has IV only at keep open rate. Milk administration decreases the incidence of stress ulcers and helps to meet caloric demands. (Since the concentration of sodium in homogenized milk is only 25 meq/L most patients with burns >20% BSA require sodium

supplementation – 25 meq/L of milk consumed – given in 4-6 divided doses).
For burns >20% BSA, 100 gm albumin/m$^2$ burned/week in 3 divided doses are usually required to maintain serum albumin at 2-3 gm/100 ml.

b.  Parkland Formula
A guideline for replacement of deficits and ongoing losses; for infants maintenance fluids may need to be added to this:
4ml/kg/% burn of Ringer's Lactate (glucose may be added but beware stress hypergly-cemia) over the first 24 hours; 1/2 of total given over the first 8 hours calculated from the time of injury; the remaining half is given over the next 16 hours.
The second 24 hour fluid requirements average 50-75% of first day's requirement. Concentrations and rates best determined by monitoring weight, serum electrolytes, urine output, NG losses, etc.

Colloid may be added after 18-24 hrs. (1 gm/kg/day of albumin), to maintain serum albumin >2 gm/100 ml.

Withhold potassium generally for the first 48 hours because of large potassium release from damaged tissues. To most effectively manage electrolytes monitor urine electrolytes biweekly and replace urine losses accord-ingly.

2)  Wound Management/Infection Control
a.  Initial wound care is debridement, cleansing with mild betadine solution and application of silver sulfadiazine with dry dressing wrap. Escharotomies for vascular, respiratory or joint impairment may be needed.
b.  Daily care includes bed bath or hydro-therapy with 1:120 or 1:240 chlorox solution, application of silver sulfadiazine (may cause transient leukopenia) and dry wrap.
c.  Surveillance cultures of urine, wounds, respiratory tract. Use of prophylactic antibiotics is controversial but a short course of penicillin (3-5 days) may reduce the incidence of early streptococcal wound infections.
d.  "Burn fever" or post burn hypermetabolism represents a true resetting of central temp-

erature control mediated by interleukins released from burned tissues. Hyperpyrexia associated with <u>sepsis</u> is therefore more difficult to evaluate in the burned patient. Generally the child with T >103°F should be evaluated for sepsis.

e.  Early excision of burn wounds is now standard practice as soon as the child's medical condition is stable for surgery. Although no definite decrease in mortality has been shown, early excision and grafting has been shown to decrease morbidity, shorten hospital stays, and result in an increased level of long-term functioning for the burned child.

f.  Early splinting of upper and lower extremities and mobilization with range of motion exercises are critical to restoration of function after a major burn.

3) <u>Nutrition</u>

a.  Increase in metabolic rate can be as high as 100% in a major burn.

b.  Daily caloric requirements approximate: <2 yrs -- 80 cal/kg plus 30 cal/% burn, including 3-6 gm protein/kg/day; >2 yrs -- 60 cal/kg plus 30 cal/% burn, 2-8 gm protein/kg/day.

c.  Feeding may be met by enteral and/or parenteral hyperalimentation to promote healing, retard immune suppression, etc.

d.  Zinc deficiency is common - supplement feeds with poly-vi-sol with Fe, Zn acetate, and ascorbic acid. Monitor weekly Ca, Phos, total protein, albumin, transferrin, cholesterol, and triglycerides as a measure of sufficient nutrition. Daily weights and electrolytes are essential.

IV.  <u>Prevention</u>

The best treatment is prevention! Measures include child-proofing the home, smoke detectors, turning hot water tap temperature down to 49-54°C (requires 5 min immersion at 49° to cause full-thickness burn versus 5 seconds at 60°).

Ref: Carvajal HF, Parks DH. Burns in Children. Yearbook 1987, in press. Guzetta PC, Randolph J. Ped Review 1983; 4:271. Herndon DN. Pediatr Clin North Am 1985; 32:1311.

# N E U R O L O G Y

## I. Acute Shunt Malfunction

"Anything that goes wrong with a person with shunted
hydrocephalus is due to a shunt problem until proven
otherwise."
Freeman JM, D'Souza B. Pediatrics 1979; 64:111.

Consult neurosurgery if shunt obstruction or infection is
suspected. If unavailable, or patient is deteriorating, any
physician familiar with a shunt may tap it as follows:
  Procedure: Sterile preparation of site with betadine. Insert
  a 25 gauge needle into the pumping device to measure
  pressure and remove CSF. If blockage at the ventricular
  end is suspected and patient is deteriorating, insert an LP
  needle (up to 18g) through the burrhole which admits the
  shunt, aiming toward lateral ventricle. Measure pressure by
  manometry and send fluid for culture, cell count/differential,
  glucose and protein.

With suspicion of shunt malfunction or infection, admit patient
for revision and therapy. When delay in revision is
unavoidable, the patient may be medically managed with
hyperventilation and/or medication (see below) until surgery.

## II. Medical management of Hydrocephalus

Effective in any infant 2 weeks to 10 months with slowly
progressive hydrocephalus or an infant/child with a shunt and
signs of chronic malfunction without acute signs of
deterioration (rate of head circumference growth less than
three times the upper limit for age).

Acetazolamide - 25 mg/kg/day and increase by 25
mg/kg/day to a maximum 100 mg/kg/day divided tid, PO or
IV. (maximum of 2 gm/day)

Furosemide - 1 mg/kg/day divided tid, PO or IV

Polycitra - titrated to maintain bicarbonate > 18 mEq/L and
normal Na, K. Usual dose is 8-10 mEq/kg/day.

Side effects of therapy: mild lethargy; poor feeding;
occasional tachypnea; transient diarrhea; increased
susceptibility to dehydration (unable to concentrate urine)

Ref: Shinnar S, et al. J Pediatr 1985; 107:31-7.

## III. Seizures

A. A seizure is a sudden paroxysmal electrical discharge of
   neurons within the brain. Manifestations depend on age

and the state of brain maturation. <u>Epilepsy</u> is defined as two or more non-febrile seizures without known cause.

B.  Events that are not seizures:
Vasovagal syncope (breath holding spells), fainting, migraines, tics, behavioral disturbances.

C.  Febrile seizures - brief, generalized seizures, usually occurring between 3 months and 5 years of age, (at a stage of brain development when the cortex has a lower threshold for seizures than the adult), associated with fever but without evidence of intracranial infection or other definable cause.
Incidence:  3-4%

Work up:  Lumbar puncture is not routine but may be considered if: a) received medical care in the last 48 hours; b) focal seizure; c) suspicious PE; d) abnormal neurologic exam; e) already on antibiotics.  EEG is not predictive of febrile seizure recurrence or of later epilepsy.
Treatment:  Anticonvulsant prophylaxis is not recommended but may be considered if the febrile seizure is atypical, prolonged (> 15 min), focal or recurrent in 24 hours; if neurologic development is abnormal or if febrile seizures are recurrent.  Then: phenobarbital daily to maintain a serum level 15-25 mcg/ml.
Outcome:  30-40% with a first febrile seizure will have a second and 50% of this group will have a third.  Only 2% of children with febrile seizures will later have epilepsy compared with 0.5-1% of the general population.  There is no increased risk of mental retardation, cerebral palsy, or other neurologic sequelae.

D.  <u>Classification of Seizure Type</u>

|                                              |                             |
| -------------------------------------------- | --------------------------- |
| NEW                                          | OLD                         |
| Partial (focal hemisphere involvement)       |                             |
| Simple (consciousness not impaired)          | Focal motor/sensory         |
| Complex (consciousness impaired)             | Psychomotor/temporal lobe   |
| With secondary generalization                | Focal and/or grand mal      |
| Generalized (bi-hemispheric involvement)     |                             |
| Tonic/Clonic                                 | Grand mal                   |
| Tonic                                        | Grand mal                   |
| Clonic                                       | Grand mal                   |
| Absence                                      | Petit mal                   |
| Atonic                                       | Akinetic, drop attacks      |
| Myoclonic                                    | Minor motor                 |

E. <u>Commonly Used Drugs in the Treatment of Epilepsy</u>*

| Partial | Generalized | | |
|---|---|---|---|
| Focal motor or sensory; sensory; psychomotor; temporal lobe | Absence | Myoclonic; Atonic | Tonic-Clonic |
| Carbamazepine | Ethosuximide | Valproic acid | Carbamazepine |
| Phenobarbital | Valproic acid | Clonazepam | Phenobarbital |
| Phenytoin | Clonazepam | Phenobarbital | Phenytoin |
| Primidone | Acetazolamide | Ethosuximide | Primidone |
| Valproic acid | | Acetazolamide | Valproic acid |
| Clorazepate | | Ketogenic Diet | Mephobarbital |
| Mephobarbital | | ACTH/Cortico-steroids | |

*Drugs are listed in order of efficacy for each seizure type (see formulary for doses, therapeutic ranges). Monotherapy is the rule. When a single agent fails, add a second drug and taper the first when seizure control is obtained. Remember that the most frequent cause of treatment failure is lack of compliance.

<u>Ref</u>: Vining EPG, Freeman J. Pediatr Ann 1985; 14:741.

F. <u>Drug Interactions</u>: the following drug interactions occur with some frequency.
1) Phenytoin levels are increased by chloramphenicol, cimetidine, and isoniazid, and decreased by phenobarbital and valproate.
2) Phenobarbital levels predictably increase when valproate or chloramphenicol are added.
3) Carbemazapine levels are increased by erythromycin and decreased by phenytoin and other anticonvulsants.
For a more complete discussion see: Kutt H. Epilepsia 1984; 25:5118-31.

G. <u>Agents That May Cause Seizures</u>:

See Messing, et al. Neurology 1984; 34:1582-6.

## G. Status Epilepticus

General or partial seizure or series of seizures lasting more than 30 min. and during which consciousness is not regained. Guidelines for initial management:

| | | |
|---|---|---|
| I. | Stabilization 0 - 10 min. | Secure airway; obtain full vital signs; O2; intubate if necessary. Blood for ABG, CBC, electrolytes, BUN, calcium, magnesium, drug levels, toxicology screen, glucose and dextrostix (at bedside). Urine for toxicology screen. Consider NH3, lactate, Pb and LFT's. Start intravenous infusion with 5% dextrose in normal saline, (if indicated use 25% dextrose, 1 ml/kg). Institute volume restriction with signs of ICP. ICP management per acute brain insult protocol. Monitor vital signs and ECG closely. |
| II. | Control of seizures 10 - 25 min. | Diazepam, 0.2-0.5 mg/kg/dose IV (single dose maximum 5 mg for < 5 yrs, 10 mg > 5 yrs) no faster than 2 mg/min. May repeat every 10 min. to a maximum of 3 doses (or lorazepam 0.03-0.05 mg/kg/dose, up to a maximum of 4 mg Q6H). Be prepared to intubate patient. Phenytoin, start after 1st dose of diazepam; give 15-20 mg/kg in normal saline no faster than 50 mg/min.; if bradycardia or hypotension occur, slow infusion rate. |
| | 25 - 40 min. | If seizures persist, intubate and then continue phenytoin infusion until seizures stop or to a maximum dose of 25 mg/kg. |
| | 40 - 60 min. | If seizures continue, start infusion of phenobarbital, loading dose of 15-25 mg/kg no faster than 30 mg/min.; monitor vital signs closely. |
| | 60 - 90 min. | If seizures continue, start infusion of paraldehyde diluted in normal saline at a rate titrated to seizure control (see p. 183 for dose). |
| | 90 min. | If paraldehyde has not terminated seizures within 20 mins from the start of infusion, institute general anesthesia and neuromuscular blockade; EEG monitoring, and keep EEG near flat for at least 2 hours then begin slow withdrawal of anesthesia. |
| III. | Diagnostic | Should coincide with control of seizures and include; detailed history; physical exam; and consideration of treatable disease, i.e. meningitis, encephalitis, metabolic disorders, overdoses, mass lesions, and cerebral edema. |

Ref: Vining EPG, et al. Pediatr Ann 1985; 14:11; adapted from: Delgado-Escueta New Engl J Med 1982; 306:133.

## IV. The Ketogenic Diet

The ketogenic diet may be of value in the management of intractable tonic and/or clonic seizures and myoclonic seizures. Best results are obtained in children 2-5 years of age, although it has been used up to 20 years of age. This diet is reserved for patients whose seizures are uncontrolled by usual anticonvulsant drugs and for whom adequate parental supervision and patient cooperation can be assured. The anticonvulsant effect of the ketogenic diet is usually not maximal until after one or more weeks on a closely supervised diet. If seizure control has not been achieved within three months, this diet likely will not be effective. If seizure control is established, the diet can be effective for years.

### 1. Starting the Diet

A. An initial period of starvation and relative dehydration is necessary to establish adequate ketosis. This usually lasts 2-5 days. Initial lab tests include: electrolytes, BUN, Creat., Glucose, Dextrostick, (fasting), Cholesterol and Uric acid. Dextrosticks are followed BID or if symptomatic and electrolytes Q day over the starvation and diet initiation period. Weigh patient daily after voiding and check urine ketones BID. Vital signs Q4hr. Begin the diet after the urinary ketones have been 4+ for several days. (Serum bicarb level should now be 10-12 mEq/l.) Terminate the starvation period before 10% weight loss if the patient's bicarbonate is <10 mEq/l or if Kussmaul respirations are present.

B. Offer 1/3 of the calculated diet on the first day, then increase to 2/3, and finally to full diet on each successive day. Note: Treat symptomatic hypoglycemia and severe acidosis promptly.

C. If anticonvulsant drugs are being given, taper them one at a time when seizure control has been obtained. Phenobarbital should be gradually eliminated after 3 months. Note: Phenobarbital levels may rise without change in dosage with the ketogenic diet and thus should be monitored. Do not administer drugs which contain a carbohydrate vehicle. (Not even toothpaste, mouthwash, or cough syrups.)

### 2. Composition and Calculation of the 4:1 Diet

A. The diet consists of a ratio of 4 gm of fat (ketogenic), 1 gm of protein plus carbohydrate (antiketogenic). (Note: Rarely seizure control may require a 5 to 1 ratio)

B. Method of Calculation

1) 4 gm of fat plus 1 gm of protein and CHO (combined), is considered a "dietary unit"; or 36 cal + 4 cal = 40 calories/unit.

2) Daily caloric requirement: 75 cal/kg for 3yr
   68 cal/Kg for 6yr
   60 cal/Kg for 10yr

3) Determine number of "dietary units" required per day:

$$\frac{\text{Total Caloric Requirement}}{40 \text{ calories/dietary unit}}$$

4) Calculate gm of fat/day: number of "dietary units" x 4 gm fat/unit.

5) Calculate gm of protein/day: approximately 1gm/kg/day).

6) Obtain gm of CHO by subtracting total gms of protein from total number of dietary units since 1 unit = 1 gm protein + CHO.

7) Restrict fluids to 600-1200 cc/day, including liquids given as part of the meal, and apportion this throughout the day. Note: Fluid liberalization may be required in hot weather.

C. Example (for a 5 year old weighing 18 kg)

1) Daily requirement: 18 kg x 70 cal/kg = 1260 cal/day.

2) Number of "dietary units": 1260 cal ÷ 40 cal/unit = 31.5 units.

3) Number of gms of fat: 31.5 units x 4 gm fat/unit = 126 gm.

4) Number of gms of protein: 1.0 gm/kg x 18 kg = 18 gms.

5) Number of gms CHO: 31.5 gm - 18 gm (recall protein + CHO = 1 gm/unit) = 13.5 gm.

D. Supplementation

1) 1 gm bid of calcium carbonate.

2) Multivitamin with minerals and iron. (Again, avoid caloric containing preparations)

Note: Urine should be checked daily for ketones while on the diet and the time of maximal ketosis is in the afternoon. An abrupt decrease in ketosis may precipitate recurrence of seizures (one cookie can do it!). If ketonuria becomes negative or slight the child should be fed nothing except water or a calorie free beverage until urinary ketosis regains +4 positivity.

3. Method of Discontinuing Diet

After 2 years on the 4:1 ratio, reduce to a 3:1 (ketogenic: antiketogenic) ratio for 6 months, then to a 2:1 ratio for another 6 months, then resume a normal diet.

4.    Complications

      A.  Vomiting
      B.  Hypoglycemia
      C.  Severe acidosis
      D.  Urate nephropathy
      E.  Hyperlipidemia (although not thought to be
          atherogenic)
      F.  Decrease in hyperactivity
      G.  Elevation of Phenobarbital serum levels

(Note:  Valproic acid itself causes ketonuria thus there is
risk of decreased level of ketosis as valproate is
discontinued.)

Ref: Withrow CD in Glaser, et al, eds. Antiepileptic Drugs:
     Mechanism of Action.  New York: Raven Press, New York.
     1980:635-42; Barbosa E, et al. in Walser M, et al (eds.).
     Nutritional   management.   Philadelphia:   WB   Saunders,
     1984:272-92.
     The Department of Pharmacy at JHH Children's Center:
        personal communication R. Knudson, B.S. Pharmacist.

273

V. **Acute Brain Insult:** Coma and/or Severe Head Trauma (see Coma Scales on next page)

I. Stabilization

A) Immobilize cervical spine until cleared with AP and lateral neck films.

B) Airway control and ventilation - Ensure adequate and spontaneous respirations. Intubate patient with evidence of increased ICP, persistent seizures, inadequate respiratory effort, decreased gag, or a GCS of 8 or less.

C) Maintain adequate blood pressure - Gain IV access but avoid hypotonic fluids which may augment existing brain edema. ECG monitoring.

D) Brief history and physical exam.

E) Initial laboratory assessment - Lytes, BUN, Creat., Glucose, Ca, Dextrostick, Stat Na/K, spun HCT and CBC, ABG, (PT/PTT). For patients with coma, consider Mg, toxicology, LFT's, NH3, Pb, cultures.

F) Respond to initial labs - e.g. give glucose.

G) Suspect increased ICP with any brain insult: GCS of 8 or less; persistent seizures; abnormal vital signs (Cushing's Triad); dilated unresponsive pupils; decerebrate or decorticate posturing.

II. Management

Acutely - Place head in midline and at 20-30° to maximize venous drainage. Hyperventilate to a PCO2 of 20-25mm Hg. Give Mannitol IV 0.25 gm/kg and Lasix 1 mg/kg. Treat hypothermia, seizures, hypoglycemia, hyponatremia, acidosis.

III. Other Management

A) Respond to other pertinent lab results.

B) Thorough re-examination with attention to level of consciousness and other abnormal neurologic findings (e.g., signs of mass lesion effect).

C) If patient is stable, proceed to CT scan for evaluation of signs/symptoms of persistent focal neurologic deficit/mass effect or possible depressed skull fracture. Neurosurgery consult for ICP monitoring.

IV. Transfer to ICU setting for continued management.

Adapted in part from: James HE. Pediatr Ann 1986; 15:16-22; Dean M, Cohen S. JHH, personal communication.

## VI. Coma Scales

| Glasgow Coma Scale | | | Modified Coma Scale for Infants | | |
|---|---|---|---|---|---|
| Activity | Best Response | | Activity | Best Response | |
| Eye Opening | Spontaneous | 4 | Eye Opening | Spontaneous | 4 |
| | To speech | 3 | | To Speech | 3 |
| | To pain | 2 | | To pain | 2 |
| | None | 1 | | None | 1 |
| Verbal | Oriented | 5 | Verbal | Coos, babbles | 5 |
| | Confused | 4 | | Irritable | 4 |
| | Inappropriate words | 3 | | Cries to pain | 3 |
| | Nonspecific sounds | 2 | | Moans to pain | 2 |
| | None | 1 | | None | 1 |
| Motor | Follows commands | 6 | Motor | Normal spontaneous movements | 6 |
| | Localizes pain | 5 | | Withdraws to touch | 5 |
| | Withdraws to pain | 4 | | Withdraws to pain | 4 |
| | Abnormal flexion | 3 | | Abnormal flexion | 3 |
| | Extend | 2 | | Abnormal extension | 2 |
| | None | 1 | | None | 1 |

Ref: Jennett B, Teasdale G. Lancet 1977; 1:878; James HE. Pediatr Ann 1986; 15:16-22.

PERINATOLOGY

1. Fetal Assessment

A. Assessment of Fetal Maturity

1) Ultrasonography

Measurement of fetal parameters by ultrasound can be used to estimate gestational age. It is worthwhile to remember that ultrasound is no more than an estimate of fetal size, and that fetal size is at best an approximate indicator of gestational age. The accuracy of ultrasonographic estimates decreases with advancing gestation. Fetal crown-rump length in the first trimester is a good predictor of gestational age. In the second trimester, fetal biparietal diameter is used. During the third trimester, the rate of growth slows and isolated values of biparietal diameter are much less accurate. Second trimester measurements of fetal limb length, particularly femur length, correlate with gestational age. Standards for these measurements are available in the obstetric literature.

Ref: Campbell S, et al. Obset Gynecol 1985; 65: 613; Hohler C. Clin Obstet Gynecol 1984; 27:314.

2) Amniotic fluid phospholipids:

Measurement of amniotic fluid phospholipids provides information about lung surfactant characteristics and fetal lung maturity. The lecithin to sphingomyelin ratio (L/S ratio) is the most widely used index. An L/S ratio of 2.0 or greater indicates fetal lung maturity in most cases. However, an L/S ratio of less than 2 does not reliably exclude lung maturity.

Measurement of phosphatidyl glycerol provides further information about fetal lung development and improves the reliability of the L/S ratio. Its presence correlates well with functionally mature lungs.

Ref: Creasy G, Simon N. Am J Perinatol 1984; 1:302. Kulovitch M, Gluck L. Am J Obstet Gynecol 1979; 135: 64. Kulovitch M, et al. Am J Obstet Gynecol 1979; 135: 57.

B. Assessment of Fetal Well-Being Before Labor
   1) Fetal activity:
      The mother is asked to record each perceived fetal movement in a given period of time. Chronically low fetal activity, or a decrease or loss of fetal activity is a warning sign of possible fetal compromise or death.

      NOTE: Fetal activity should be used only as an adjunct to other determinations of fetal well-being. There is a marked variation between pregnant women; there is also significant influence by environmental factors.

   2) Maternal Serum Estriols:
      Abnormalities involving the fetus, placenta, or the mother can result in abnormally low estriol values. Serial estriol values reflect the integrity of the fetoplacental unit. Low estriol values, or serial falls in estriol values by 40% or more, may reflect fetal compromise. Monitoring estriols has become less popular but may have some use in postdate pregnancies or diabetic pregnancies.

   3) Non Stress Test (NST):
      The fetal heart rate is continuously monitored with the mother at rest. A normal or reactive non-stress test requires that there be at least two accelerations in fetal heart rate >15 beats/min above baseline, lasting 15 sec or more, occurring within a 10 min period. An abnormal or nonreactive pattern is one that does not meet these criteria. The NST is less specific for fetal distress than is the CST (see below), and becomes even less specific when assessing fetuses <32 weeks gestation.

   4) Contraction Stress Test:
      Baseline fetal heart and uterine activity are monitored. Adequate testing requires three uterine contractions, each lasting at least 40 sec, within a 10 minute period. Nipple stimulation or oxytocin administration may be needed to augment uterine activity. If late decelerations occur, the CST is positive and indicates possible decreased placental reserve. A negative CST, the absence of late decelerations, is a good prognostic finding. CST's have a false positive rate of 24 to 50 percent.

   5) Biophysical Profile
      Ultrasonography is used to assess fetal activity over a 30 min period, and to estimate amniotic fluid volume. The parameters examined are listed below and are scored 2 if normal or zero if abnormal. Low scores reflect fetal asphyxia.

a) Biophysical Profile Scoring: Technique

| Biophysical variable | Score = 2 | Score = 0 |
|---|---|---|
| 1. Fetal breathing movements | >1 episode of >30 s in 30 min | Absent or no episode of >30 s in 30 min |
| 2. Gross body movements | >3 discrete body/limb movements in 30 min (episodes of active continuous movement considered as single movement) | <2 episodes of body/limb movements in 30 min |
| 3. Fetal tone | >1 episode of active extension with return to flexion of fetal limb(s) or trunk. Opening and closing of hand considered normal tone | Either slow extension with return to partial flexion of limb in full extension or absent fetal movement |
| 4. Reactive fetal heart rate | >2 episodes of acceleration of >15 bpm and of >15 s associated with fetal movement in 10 min | <2 episodes of acceleration of fetal heart rate or acceleration of >15 bpm in in 20 min |
| 5. Qualitative amniotic fluid | >1 pocket of fluid measuring >1 cm in two perpendicular planes | Either no pockets or a pocket <1 cm in two perpendicular planes |

From: Manning F, et al. Eur J Obstet Gynecol Reprod Biol 1986; 21:331.

b) Biophysical Profile Scoring: Interpretation

| Score | Interpretation | Incidence of Low 5 min Apgar Scores (%) | Incidence of Fetal Distress in Labor (%) | Perinatal Mortality Rate (Per 1000 Live Births) |
|---|---|---|---|---|
| 10 | Normal infant, low risk for chronic asphyxia | 2 | 3 | 0 |
| 8 | Normal infant, low risk for chronic asphyxia | 9 | 9 | 40 |
| 6 | Suspected chronic asphyxia | 13 | 28 | 0 |
| 4 | Suspected chronic asphyxia | 27 | 27 | 91 |
| 2 | Strong suspicion of chronic asphyxia | 50 | 86 | 125 |
| 0 | Strong suspicion of chronic asphyxia | 80 | 100 | 600 |

Adapted from: Manning F, et al. Eur J Obstet Gynecol Reprod
Biol 1986; 2:331. Manning F, et al. Am J Obstet
Gynecol 1980; 136:787.

C.  Assessment of Fetal Well-Being During Labor
    1)  Fetal heart rate (FHR) monitoring:
        a)  Normal baseline FHR is 120-160 beats per min.
            Isolated accelerations >160 bpm suggest a good
            prognosis. Mild bradycardias (100-120 bpm)
            may be benign.
        b)  A normal tracing is characterized by both
            short term "beat to beat" variability (amplitude
            10-25 bpm), and slower oscillations in the
            heart rate (frequency 3-10 cycles per minute).
            Loss of variability suggests fetal distress.
            Drugs, fetal sleep, prematurity and other
            factors can also decrease variability.
        c)  Early decelerations represent head compression
            and are benign.
        d)  Variable decelerations represent cord
            compression and do not always indicate fetal
            distress. The following patterns suggest fetal
            distress: decelerations with duration >60 sec,
            decelerations to <70 bpm, associated loss of
            variability, associated tachycardia, slow return
            to baseline after deceleration, and "overshoot"
            patterns with gradual acceleration after
            deceleration.
        e)  Late decelerations are caused by uteroplacental
            insufficiency and indicate fetal distress.
        f)  A sinusoidal or undulating FHR pattern has
            been considered a sign of severe fetal compro-
            mise and is associated with a high rate of
            perinatal loss.
            Fetal heart rate patterns are illustrated on
            page 279.
    2)  Fetal scalp pH monitoring:
        Normal fetal pH is 7.25-7.35, approximately 0.1
        units lower than that of the mother. Normal fetal
        $PCO_2$ values are in the range of 40-45 mm Hg.
        Normal fetal $PO_2$ is 20-25 mm Hg. A fetal scalp pH
        of 7.20-7.25 may indicate fetal distress and is asso-
        ciated with an increased incidence of depression at
        delivery and lower 1 min Apgar scores. Fetal scalp
        pH <7.20 indicates significant fetal distress.

For references on fetal monitoring prior to and during
delivery, see Petre, R (ed): Clin Perinatol 1982: 9 (2).
Polin J, Frangipane W. Ped Clin North Amer 1986; 33:
621; Yeomans E, et al: Am J Obstet Gynecol 1985;
151:798.

# FETAL HEART RATE PATTERNS

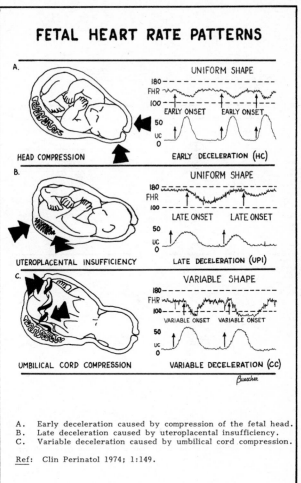

A. Early deceleration caused by compression of the fetal head.
B. Late deceleration caused by uteroplacental insufficiency.
C. Variable deceleration caused by umbilical cord compression.

<u>Ref</u>: Clin Perinatol 1974; 1:149.

2. <u>Assessment of the Neonate</u>

    A. <u>Apgar Scores:</u>
       The infant is rapidly assessed on five criteria at 1 and 5 min after delivery. In the compromised infant, continued assessment is important and Apgar scores at 10 and 20 min are valuable.

| APGAR SCORING | | | |
|---|---|---|---|
| SCORE | 0 | 1 | 2 |
| Heart Rate | Absent | <100 | >100 |
| Respiratory Effort | Absent | Slow Irregular | Good Crying |
| Muscle Tone | Limp | Some Flexion of Extremities | Active Motion |
| Reflex Irritability (nasal catheter) | No response | Grimace | Cough or sneeze |
| Color | Blue, pale | Extremities blue | Completely pink |

Adapted from Apgar V. <u>Anesth Analg</u> 1953; 32:260.

    B. <u>Assessment of Gestational Age in the Neonate</u>
       1) Examination of anterior lens vessels.

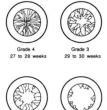

Grade 4
27 to 28 weeks

Grade 3
29 to 30 weeks

Grade 2
31 to 32 weeks

Grade 1
33 to 34 weeks

From: Hittner H, et al. J Pediatr 1977; 91:455.

2)    Assessment of gestational age by neurologic criteria

| NEUROLOGICAL SIGN | SCORE | | | | | |
|---|---|---|---|---|---|---|
| | 0 | 1 | 2 | 3 | 4 | 5 |
| POSTURE | | | | | | |
| SQUARE WINDOW | 90° | 60° | 45° | 30° | 0° | |
| ANKLE DORSIFLEXION | 90° | 75° | 45° | 20° | 0° | |
| ARM RECOIL | 180° | 90-180° | <90° | | | |
| LEG RECOIL | 180° | 90-180° | <90° | | | |
| POPLITEAL ANGLE | 180° | 160° | 130° | 110° | 90° | <90° |
| HEEL TO EAR | | | | | | |
| SCARF SIGN | | | | | | |
| HEAD LAG | | | | | | |
| VENTRAL SUSPENSION | | | | | | |

(Redrawn from Dubowitz.)   See legend, next page.

282

## TECHNIQUES OF ASSESSMENT OF
## NEUROLOGIC CRITERIA (Modified from Dubowitz)

POSTURE: Observe infant quiet, supine. Score 0: arms, legs extended; 1: beginning flexion of hips and knees, arms extended; 2: stronger flexion legs, arms extended; 3: arms slightly flexed, legs flexed and abducted; 4: full flexion arms, legs.

SQUARE WINDOW: Flex hand on forearm enough to obtain fullest possible flexion without wrist rotation. Measure angle between the hypothenar eminence and the ventral aspect of the forearm.

ANKLE DORSIFLEXION: Foot is dorsiflexed as much as possible onto anterior aspect of the leg. Measure the angle between the dorsum of the foot and the anterior aspect of the leg.

ARM RECOIL: With infant supine, flex forearms for 5 sec, then fully extend by pulling on hands, then release. Score 2: arms return briskly to full flexion; 1: response is sluggish or incomplete; 0: arms remain extended.

LEG RECOIL: With infant supine, flex hips and knees for 5 sec, then extend by pulling on feet, and release. Score 2: maximal response - full flexion of hips and knees; 1: partial flexion; 0: minimal flexion.

POPLITEAL ANGLE: Hold infant supine with pelvis flat, thigh held in the knee-chest position. Extend leg by gentle pressure and measure popliteal angle.

HEEL TO EAR MANEUVER: With baby supine, draw foot as near to the head without forcing it. Observe distance between foot and head, and degree of extension at the knee. Knee is free and may be down alongside abdomen.

SCARF SIGN: With baby supine, pull infant's hand around the neck around the opposite shoulder. See how far the elbow will go across. Score 0: Elbow reaches opposite axillary line; 1: past midaxillary line; 2: past midline; 3: elbow unable to reach midline.

HEAD LAG: With baby supine, grasp the hands and pull slowly towards the sitting position. Observe the position of head in relation to trunk. In small infant, head may initially be supported by one hand. Score 0: Complete lag; 1: partial control; 2: head in line with body; 3: head anterior to body.

VENTRAL SUSPENSION: Suspend infant in prone position. Note back extension, extremity flexion, and head and trunk alignment. Grade according to diagrams.

3) Assessment of gestational age by physical criteria

| External Sign | Score | | | | |
|---|---|---|---|---|---|
| | 0 | 1 | 2 | 3 | 4 |
| Edema | Obvious edema of hands and feet; pitting over tibia | No obvious edema of hands and feet; pitting over tibia | No edema | | |
| Skin texture | Very thin, gelatinous | Thin and smooth | Smooth; medium thickness. Rash or superficial peeling | Slight thickening. Superficial cracking and peeling especially of hands and feet | Thick and parchment-like; superficial or deep cracking |
| Skin color | Dark red | Uniformly pink | Pale pink; variable over body | Pale; only pink over ears, lips, palms, or soles | |
| Skin opacity (trunk) | Numerous veins, venules clearly seen, especially over abdomen | Veins and tributaries seen | A few large vessels clearly seen over abdomen | A few large vessels seen indistinctly over abdomen | No blood vessels seen |
| Lanugo (over back) | No lanugo | Abundant; long and thick over whole back | Hair thinning especially over lower back | Small amount of lanugo and bald area | At least 1/2 of back devoid of lanugo |
| Plantar creases | No skin creases | Faint red marks over anterior half of sole | Definite red marks over > anterior 1/2; indentations over < anterior 1/3 | Indentations over > anterior 1/3 | Definite deep indentations over > anterior 1/3 |

3) Assessment of gestational age by physical criteria (continued)

| External Sign | 0 | Score 1 | 2 | 3 | 4 |
|---|---|---|---|---|---|
| Nipple formation | Nipple barely visible; no areola | Nipple well defined; areola smooth and flat, diameter <0.75 cm | Areola stippled, edge not raised, diameter <0.75 cm | Areola stippled, edge raised, diameter >0.75 cm | |
| Breast size | No breast tissue palpable | Breast tissue on one or both sides, <0.5 cm diameter | Breast tissue both sides; one or both 0.5 - 1.0 cm | Breast tissue both sides; one or both >1 cm | |
| Ear form | Pinna flat, and shapeless; little or no incurving of edge | Incurving of part of edge of pinna | Partial incurving whole of upper pinna | Well-defined incurving whole of upper pinna | |
| Ear firmness | Pinna soft, easily folded, no recoil | Pinna soft, easily folded, slow recoil | Cartilage to edge of pinna, but soft in places, ready recoil | Pinna firm, cartilage to edge; instant recoil | |
| Genitals Male | Neither testis in scrotum | At least one testis high in scrotum | At least one testis right down | | |
| Female (with hips 1/2 abducted) | Labia majora widely separated, labia minora protruding | Labia majora almost cover labia minora | Labia majora completely cover labia minora | | |

4) Dubowitz score and estimation of gestational age
   The total Dubowitz score is the sum of the scores based on neurologic and physical criteria. Total score is plotted against gestational age below (redrawn from Dubowitz).

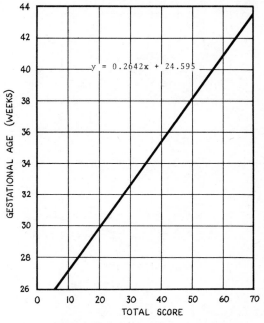

$$y = 0.2642x + 24.595$$

NOTE: Optimal timing for the Dubowitz exam is within the first 24 hours of life, preferably between 12 and 24 hours of age.

The original population on which Dubowitz scoring was based included only 2 infants with gestational age < 30 wks.

From: Dubowitz L, et al. J Pediatr 1970; 77:1.

C.  Blood Pressure Measurement in the Premature Infant

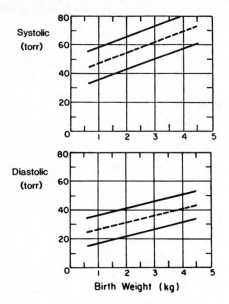

Predicted mean systolic and diastolic blood pressure (dashed lines) and 95% confidence limits for healthy newborns in the first 12 hours after birth.

From:  Versmold H, et al. Pediatrics 1981; 67:607.

D. Intrauterine Growth
Length and Weight

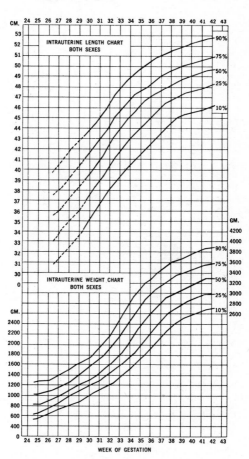

D.  Intrauterine Growth (continued)
    Head Circumference and Weight-Length Ratio

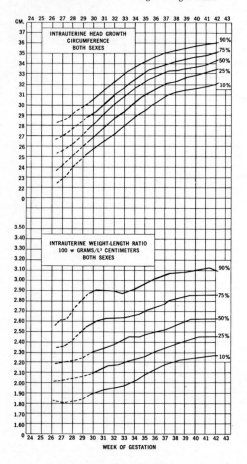

From:  Lubchenco L, et al.  Pediatrics 1966; 37:403.

E.  Premature Growth Chart

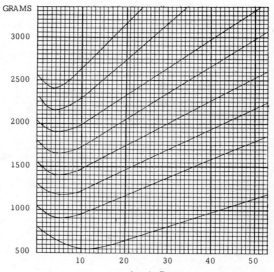

## F.  Head Circumference in the Premature Infant

HEAD CIRCUMFERENCE OF PREMATURE INFANTS
FROM BIRTH TO 16 WEEKS

| AGE | Head Circumferences (cm) | | |
|---|---|---|---|
| | Gestation 30-33 wks (healthy) | Gestation 34-37 wks (healthy) | Gestation various (sick) |
| 24 hrs | 27.0 ± 0.7 | 32.0 ± 0.7 | 30.9 ± 0.9 |
| 1 wk | 28.2 ± 0.7 | 32.7 ± 0.9 | 31.3 ± 1.0 |
| 2 wks | 29.5 ± 0.8 | 33.8 ± 0.8 | 31.7 ± 0.8 |
| 3 wks | 30.8 ± 0.8 | 35.0 ± 0.7 | 32.0 ± 0.8 |
| 4 wks | 32.0 ± 0.9 | 35.8 ± 0.8 | 32.4 ± 0.7 |
| 6 wks | 34.4 ± 0.7 | 37.1 ± 0.8 | 32.7 ± 0.8 |
| 8 wks | 35.8 ± 0.8 | 38.5 ± 1.0 | 33.3 ± 0.9 |
| 12 wks | 38.4 ± 1.1 | 40.3 ± 1.1 | 34.0 ± 0.9 |
| 16 wks | 40.2 ± 1.0 | 41.8 ± 0.9 | 34.5 ± 0.9 |

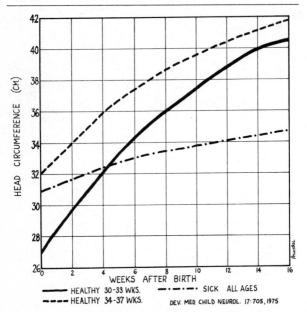

From Sher P, Brown S.  Dev Med Child Neurol 1975; 17:705.

3. Catheterization of the Umbilical Artery and Vein (Procedures for inserting umbilical catheters are found on pages 14-15).

   A. Catheter Placement by Graph Interpretation
      Umbilical artery catheters can be placed at either of two positions: low position, at the level of lumbar vertebrae 3 to 4; high position, at the level of thoracic vertebrae 6 to 9. The length of the catheter necessary to achieve either position is calculated from the graph below. Shoulder to umbilical length is measured as a perpendicular line dropped from the tip of the shoulder to a line extended from the umbilicus. A low line should be just above the bifurcation of the aorta. A high line should be above the diaphragm. Additional length must be added for the length of the umbilical stump.

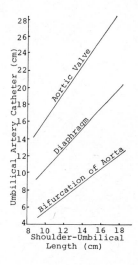

Adapted from: Dunn P. Arch Dis Child 1966; 41:69.

Placement of Umbilical Vein Catheter

An umbilical vein catheter should be placed in the inferior vena cava, above the level of the ductus venosus and the hepatic veins. The length of the catheter necessary to achieve this position is calculated from the graph below. Shoulder to umbilical length is measured as a perpendicular line dropped from the tip of the shoulder to a line extended from the umbilicus. The catheter tip should be placed between the levels of the diaphragm and the left atrium. Additional length must be added for the length of the umbilical stump.

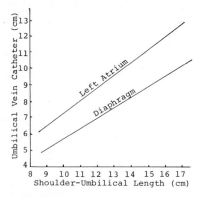

Adapted from: Dunn P. Arch Dis Child 1966; 41:69.

B.  Catheter Placement by Birthweight Regression Formulas

Umbilical Artery catheters may also be placed in the high position using the equation:

UA catheter length (cm) = [3 x Birthweight(kg)]+9 cm.

Similarly umbilical vein catheters may be placed above diaphragm and near or in the right atrium using the equation:

UV catheter length (cm) = [$\frac{1}{2}$ X UA length (cm)] + 1 cm.

Umbilical vessel catheterization by birthweight regression formulas may not be appropriate for SGA and LGA infants.

Ref: Shukla H, et al. Am J Dis Child 1986; 140:786.

## RESPIRATORY CARE AND PULMONARY FUNCTION

1.  Respiratory Rates of Normal Children*

| Age (yrs) | Boys | Girls | Age (yrs) | Boys | Girls |
|-----------|--------|--------|-----------|--------|--------|
| 0 - 1 | 31 ± 8 | 30 ± 6 | 9 - 10 | 19 ± 2 | 19 ± 2 |
| 1 - 2 | 26 ± 4 | 27 ± 4 | 10 - 11 | 19 ± 2 | 19 ± 2 |
| 2 - 3 | 25 ± 4 | 25 ± 3 | 11 - 12 | 19 ± 3 | 19 ± 3 |
| 3 - 4 | 24 ± 3 | 24 ± 3 | 12 - 13 | 19 ± 3 | 19 ± 2 |
| 4 - 5 | 23 ± 2 | 22 ± 2 | 13 - 14 | 19 ± 2 | 18 ± 2 |
| 5 - 6 | 22 ± 2 | 21 ± 2 | 14 - 15 | 18 ± 2 | 18 ± 3 |
| 6 - 7 | 21 ± 3 | 21 ± 3 | 15 - 16 | 17 ± 3 | 18 ± 3 |
| 7 - 8 | 20 ± 3 | 20 ± 2 | 16 - 17 | 17 ± 2 | 17 ± 3 |
| 8 - 9 | 20 ± 2 | 20 ± 2 | 17 - 18 | 16 ± 3 | 17 ± 3 |

* Mean ± 1 SD.

Ref: Iliff A, Lee V. Child Development 1952; 23:240.

2.  Pulmonary Function Tests (PFT's)

    A.  Usefulness of PFT's
        1)  To investigate pulmonary symptoms (such as cough, dyspnea, exercise tolerance).
        2)  To evaluate severity and follow progression of known pulmonary disorders (e.g. asthma, CF).
        3)  To follow and evaluate therapy of chronic pulmonary diseases.
        4)  For preoperative evaluation.

    B.  The Routine Pulmonary Function Tests
       (Interpretation of PFT's chart see page 299.)
        1)  Airway function measurements
           a)  Wright peak flow meter: to measure PFR - good standards, but relatively insensitive.
           b)  Forced expiratory spirometer (with and without bronchodilators): to measure forced expiratory volume in one second ($FEV_1$), max. mid-expiratory flow (MMEF).

c) Inspiratory-expiratory flow volume loops:

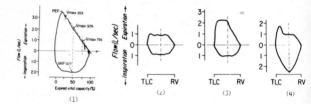

(1)  normal flow volume loop
(2)  fixed obstruction (e.g., postintubation tracheal stenosis) of the central airways (larynx, trachea, main stem bronchi)
(3)  variable obstruction of the extrathoracic central airways
(4)  variable obstructions of the intrathoracic central airways.

<u>Ref</u>: Ibid, p. 129.

2) Lung volume measurement
   a) static lung volume from spirometer:

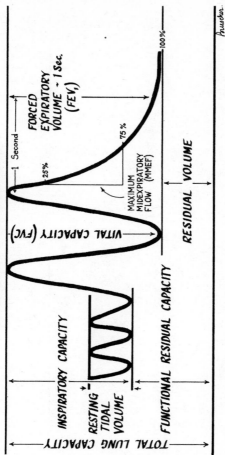

LUNG VOLUMES

b) Methods to measure lung volumes
   (1) Spirometer: cannot measure TLC and RV
   (2) Helium dilution
   (3) Nitrogen washout
   (4) Body plethysmography
   NOTE: (2), (3), and (4) are useful in calculating TLC and RV.

FORCED VITAL CAPACITY (FVC):
NORMAL VALUES

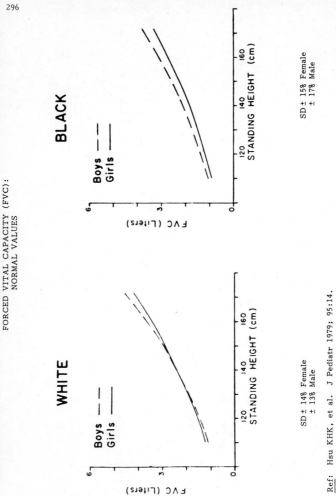

SD ± 14% Female
± 13% Male

SD ± 15% Female
± 17% Male

Ref: Hsu KHK, et al.  J Pediatr 1979; 95:14.

296

FORCED EXPIRATORY VOLUME IN ONE SECOND (FEV$_1$):
NORMAL VALUES

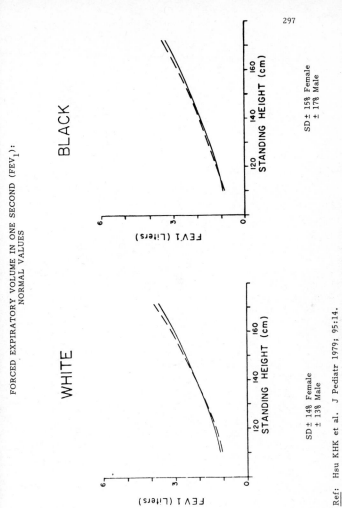

WHITE

SD $\pm$ 14% Female
$\pm$ 13% Male

BLACK

SD $\pm$ 15% Female
$\pm$ 17% Male

Ref: Hsu KHK et al. J Pediatr 1979; 95:14.

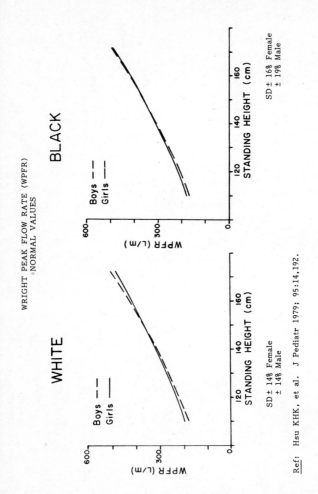

WRIGHT PEAK FLOW RATE (WPFR)
NORMAL VALUES

WHITE

BLACK

Boys - - -
Girls

WPFR (l/m)

STANDING HEIGHT (cm)

SD ± 14% Female
± 14% Male

SD ± 16% Female
± 19% Male

Ref: Hsu KHK, et al. J Pediatr 1979; 95:14,192.

# INTERPRETATION OF PULMONARY FUNCTION TESTS

| | OBSTRUCTIVE; e.g. asthma, cystic fibrosis | RESTRICTIVE; e.g. pleural disease, muscle weakness |
|---|---|---|
| **Spirometry** | | |
| Forced vital capacity (FVC)* | normal or reduced | reduced |
| Forced expired volume in one second (FEV$_1$)* | reduced | reduced |
| FEV$_1$/FVC (%)** | reduced | normal **** |
| Maximal midexpiratory flow rate (MMFR)* | reduced | |
| Wright peak flow rate (WPFR) | normal or reduced | |
| **Lung volumes** | | |
| Total lung capacity (TLC)* | normal or increased | reduced |
| Residual volume (RV)* | normal or increased | normal or increased |
| RV/TLC (%)*** | normal or increased | |
| FRC* | normal or increased | normal |

*Normal range: predicted ± 20%
**Predicted normal: >85%
***Predicted normal: 20 ± 10%
****Cannot diagnose restriction when there is obstruction by spirometry alone. In this case, lung volumes should be calculated by other methods (such as He dilution or N$_2$ washout). Lung volumes for blacks are lower than for whites (see charts on pages 296-298) when referenced to standing height.

3) Pulmonary gas exchange measurements
   a) Arterial blood gas

| NORMAL CONDITIONS | | pH | $PCO_2$ | $HCO_3^-$ (mEq/L) | $CO_2$ |
|---|---|---|---|---|---|
| Child | | 7.35-7.45 | 35-45 | 24-26 | 25-28 |
| Term Infant | – birth | 7.26-7.29 | 54.5 | | |
| | – 1 hr | 7.30 | 38.8 | | 20.6 |
| | – 3 hr | 7.34 | 38.3 | | 21.9 |
| | – 1 to 3 d | 7.38-7.41 | 34-35 | | 21.4 |
| Premature >1250 g – 1 to 3 d | | 7.38-7.39 | 38-39 | | |
| <1250 g – 1 to 3 d | | 7.35-7.36 | 37-44 | | |

| ABNORMAL CONDITIONS | |
|---|---|
| Metabolic Acidosis: | $PCO_2$ falls by 1-1.5 x the ↓ in $HCO_3$ |
| Metabolic Alkalosis: | $PCO_2$ rises by 0.25-1 x the ↑ in $HCO_3$ |
| Acute Resp. Acidosis: | $HCO_3$ rises 1mEq/L for each 10 mm Hg ↑ in $PCO_2$ |
| Chronic Resp. Acidosis: | $HCO_3$ rises 4mEq/L for each 10mm Hg ↑ in $PCO_2$ |
| Acute Resp. Alkalosis: | $HCO_3$ falls 1-3mEq/L for each 10mm Hg ↓ in $PCO_2$ |
| Chronic Resp. Alkalosis: | $HCO_3$ falls 2-5mEq/L for each 10mm Hg ↓ in $PCO$, but usually not to <14 mEq/L |

Adapted from: Schrier RW, Renal and Electrolyte Disorders, 3rd ed. Boston:Little, Brown, 1986:146.

b) Pulse oximetry
   Noninvasive method for monitoring beat-to-beat arterial oxygen saturation.

   Note: Refer to the oxyhemoglobin dissociation curve to convert arterial oxygen saturation to arterial oxygen tension ($PaO_2$).

Ref: Fanconi S, et al. J Pediatr 1985;107:362-6.

c) Diffusing capacity measurement using carbon monoxide (CO): (single breath method or steady state)

   $D_{LCO}$ in ml/min/mm Hg = amount of carbon monoxide uptake by the lungs over a known amount of pressure.
   $D_{LCO}$ is normal in asthma and bronchitis.

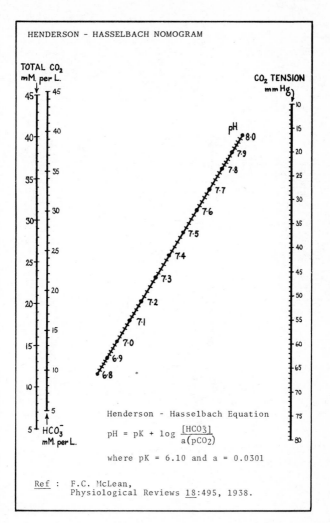

HENDERSON - HASSELBACH NOMOGRAM

TOTAL CO₂
mM. per L.

CO₂ TENSION
mm Hg.

pH

8.0
7.9
7.8
7.7
7.6
7.5
7.4
7.3
7.2
7.1
7.0
6.9
6.8

HCO₃⁻
mM. per L.

Henderson - Hasselbach Equation

$$pH = pK + \log \frac{[HCO_3]}{a(pCO_2)}$$

where pK = 6.10 and a = 0.0301

Ref : F.C. McLean,
Physiological Reviews 18:495, 1938.

$D_{LCO}$ is decreased in restrictive lung diseases with thickened alveolar capillary membrane, emphysema, anemia, lung resection, carbon monoxide intoxication, pulmonary microembolization.

$D_{LCO}$ is increased in early left ventricular failure, polycythemia.

3. Oxygen Delivery Devices
   A. Low-Flow Oxygen Systems: do not provide sufficient gas to supply the entire inspired atmosphere. (e.g. nasal cannula or catheter, oxygen mask, and mask with reservoir bag).

      1) Nasal cannula or catheter – delivers approximately 24-44% $FIO_2$ with commonly used oxygen flow rates in infants of 1/8-2 liters per minute (LPM) and older children to adults of 1-6 LPM.

      2) Oxygen mask – delivers approximately 40-60% $FIO_2$ with commonly used oxygen flow rates of 5-8 LPM.

      3) Mask with reservoir bag – delivers approximately 60-99+% $FIO_2$ with commonly used oxygen flow rates of 6-10 LPM.

   Note: 1) In a low-flow system, the larger the tidal volume, the lower the $FIO_2$; or, the smaller the tidal volume, the higher the $FIO_2$. The oxygen flow and device used must be titrated to the patient's need using either arterial blood gas or pulse oximeter measurements.

      2) Nasal cannula or catheter flows above 6 LPM are uncomfortable and do little to increase inspired oxygen concentrations.

      3) An oxygen mask should never be run at less than 5 LPM to prevent accumulation of exhaled air in the mask reservoir.

   B. High-Flow Oxygen Systems: provide sufficient flow rate and reservoir capacity to supply the entire inspired atmosphere (e.g. venturi mask and nebulizer systems including hood, aerosol mask, face tent, T-piece and trach mask).

Note: 1) High-flow systems can provide consistent concentrations of oxygen from 24-100%, which are independent of patient ventilatory pattern.
2) The temperature and humidity of the gas in a high-flow system may be controlled since the entire inspired atmosphere is provided.

Ref: Shapiro BA, et al. Clinical Application of Respiratory Care. Chicago: Year Book Medical Publishers, 1975: 130-6. Fan LL, et al J Pediatr 1983; 103:923-5.

4.  Reference Data

A.  Minute Ventilation ($\dot{V}_E$) = respiratory rate x tidal volume (TV)

$$\dot{V}_E \times P_A CO_2 = \text{constant}; \qquad TV = 10\text{-}15 \text{ ml/kg}$$

B.  Alveolar Gas Equation:

$$P_A O_2 = P_I O_2 - \frac{P_A CO_2}{R} \qquad P_I O_2 = F_I O_2 \times (P_B - 47 \text{ mm Hg})$$

Note: $P_I O_2$ = 150 mm Hg at sea level in room air

R = respiratory exchange quotient = 0.8 in most cases
(↑ with glucose intake, ↓ with fat)

PB = 760 mmHg

Ref: Kendig EL, Chernick V. Disorders of the Respiratory Tract in Children. Philadlephia: WB Saunders, 1983:27.

C.  Oxyhemoglobin Dissociation Curves

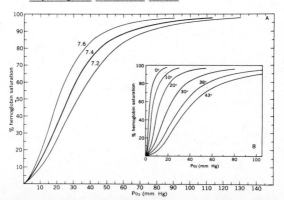

Note:   1)  Increased hemoglobin affinity for oxygen (shift to the left) is the result of alkalemia, hypothermia, hypocarbia, decreased 2,3-diphosphoglycerate, increased concentration of fetal hemoglobin, and anemia.

2)  Decreased hemoglobin affinity for oxygen (shift to the right) is the result of acidemia, hyperthermia, hypercarbia, and increased 2,3-diphosphoglycerate.

Ref:  From Lambersten CJ  Transport of Oxygen, Carbon Dioxide, and Inert Gases by the Blood.  In:  Mountcastle VB (ed).  Medical Physiology, 14th Edition St. Louis:  C V Mosby, 1980:1725.

D.   SHUNT AT DIFFERENT INSPIRED OXYGEN MIXTURES

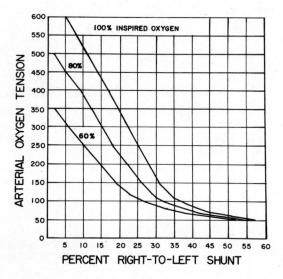

Calculations are based on an assumed hemoglobin of 16 gm%, an arteriovenous difference of 4 volumes per cent, a respiratory quotient of 0.8 and an arterial $PCO_2$ of 40 mmHg.

Ref:  Avery ME, et al.  The Lung and Its Disorders in the Newborn Infant, 4th Edition.  Philadelphia:  W B Saunders 1981:69.

# INFECTIOUS DISEASES

<u>NOTE:</u>

For more detailed and updated information on immunizations and isolation protocols, please refer to the current
issues of Morbidity and Mortality World Report or the
current edition of the "Red Book" - the Report of the
Committee on Infectious Diseases (RCID) of the American
Academy of Pediatrics.

### RECOMMENDED SCHEDULE FOR ACTIVE
### IMMUNIZATION OF INFANTS AND CHILDREN
### 1986

| AGE | PREPARATION |
|---|---|
| 2 months | DTP/TOPV |
| 4 months | DTP/TOPV |
| 6 months | DTP/(TOPV Optional) |
| 12 months | Tuberculin (TB) Test* |
| 15 months | Measles/Mumps/Rubella (MMR)** |
| 18 months | DTP/TOPV** |
| 24 months | Haemophilus Influenzae b (HIB)*** |
| 4-6 years | DTP/TOPV |
| 14-16 years | Td (and every 10 years thereafter) |

### RECOMMENDED SCHEDULE FOR PRIMARY
### IMMUNIZATION FOR CHILDREN NOT IMMUNIZED
### IN EARLY INFANCY

| Under 7 Years of Age | |
|---|---|
| First Visit | DTP/TOPV/TB Test/MMR if > 15mo. |
| Interval After First Visit | |
| 1 month | HIB if 24-60 months |
| 2 months | DTP/TOPV |
| 4 months | DTP/(TOPV Optional) |
| 10-16 months or preschool | DTP/TOPV |
| 14-16 years | Td (repeat every 10 years) |

*Intradermal PPD (Mantoux) preferred. Tuberculin test may be
given at 15 months (with MMR). Frequency of repeated tests
depends on risk of exposure. Testing once every one to two
years is generally recommended.
**18 month DTP/TOPV can be given simultaneously with MMR at
15 months.
***Can be given at 18-23 months for children at high risk. Can
be given with DTP or pneumovax. Pneumovax is administered at
24 months in high risk groups.

7 Years of Age and Over

| First Visit | Td/TOPV/TB Test/MMR |
|---|---|
| Interval After First Visit | |
| 2 months | Td/TOPV |
| 8-14 months | Td/TOPV |
| 14-16 years | Td-repeat every 10 yrs |

Interruption of immunizations does not require restarting of the series. The only restriction is that live virus vaccines (TOPV and MMR) be spaced at least 1 month apart. This timing requirement may be waived in certain unusual circumstances.

1. Active Immunization

   A. General Information
      1) Live virus vaccines prepared in chick embryo cell culture (mumps, measles, yellow fever) are virtually devoid of allergic substances, but a few egg-sensitive children have been reported to have developed anaphylaxis after measles vaccine. (See RCID, 1986: 18-20).
      2) Care should be exercised in the administration of live virus vaccines in children with immunodeficiency or immunosuppressed states. Leukemics in remission who have not had chemotherapy for at least three months may receive live virus vaccines for infections to which they have not previously been immunized. Live virus vaccines are contraindicted for children with congenital immune deficiency.
      3) Immunization of premature infants may be based on chronological age. However, if the child remains hospitalized, TOPV should not be initiated to prevent cross-infection in the nursery. [Do not use reduced dose.]
      4) Live virus vaccines should not be given to individuals who have received gamma globulin within the previous three months because of possible interference with the desired immune response.
      5) Administration of all live virus vaccines is contraindicated in pregnant women.
      6) Defer immunizations in the presence of a febrile illness.

   B. Diphtheria/Tetanus/Pertussis (DTP)
      Adsorbed triple vaccine: usual dose is 0.5 ml. Injections should be given approximately eight weeks apart.
      1) Precautions:
         a) Common side effects of pertussis vaccination include: redness, swelling or pain at site, and fever, and are not contraindications to further immunizations.

        b)    There are few specific guidelines for immunizations in children with a history of febrile convulsion or other neurologic disorders. The value of immunization must be weighed against the possibility of adverse reactions. Prophylactic antipyretics and anticonvulsants may be considered for children deemed to be at high risk for convulsions.

        c)    Children with evolving neurologic disorders or severe reactions to DTP (fever > 40.5°C, screaming, somnolence, shock, convulsions) should not receive further pertussis immunizations.

    2)    Special Situations:

        a)    If a child under age 6 years has had proven pertussis, use DT only. (Parapertussis has no cross-immunity).

        b)    Over the age of 7 years use Td antigen.

        c)    In the face of a pertussis outbreak, give 0.25 ml pertussis vaccine, adsorbed, as a booster dose.

    3)    Guide to Tetanus Prophylaxis in Wound Management: (see page 315 also)

| Previous Tetanus Immunization (Doses) | Clean, Minor Wounds | | Tetanus-Prone Wounds | |
|---|---|---|---|---|
| | Toxoid (Td) | Tetanus Immune Globulin (TIG) | Toxoid (Td) | Tetanus Immune Globulin (TIG) |
| Uncertain or Less than 3 | Yes | No | Yes | Yes |
| 3 or more* | No** | No | No*** | No |

  *If only 3 doses, give 4th dose of toxoid.
  **Unless more than 10 years since last dose
***Unless more than 5 years since last dose

    C.    Haemophilus Influenzae b Polysaccharide Vaccine (HIB)

        1)    Immunize all children at 24 months of age, including those with previous H.flu disease.

        2)    Immunize all children 24-60 months unless child had invasive H.flu disease after age 24 months.

        3)    Uncertain protection 18-23 months, may need booster at 24 months (at least 2 months after first dose).

        4)    Not recommended for children less than 18 months.

        5)    Recommended for children with functional or anatomic asplenia, nephrotic syndrome, and cytoreduction/Hodgkins.

D.  Recommendations are now under discussion for the use of hepatitis B vaccine. However, children at substantial risk of hepatitis B infection should be considered for vaccination on a case by case basis.

Those at risk include:
1)  Clients of institutions for the mentally retarded
2)  Hemodialysis patients
3)  Homosexually active males
4)  Illicit injectable drug abusers
5)  Recipients of blood products with a high risk of hepatitis B transmission (Factor VIII, cryoprecipitate, prothrombin complex concentrate)
6)  Household and sexual contact of HBV carriers
7)  Infants of mothers who are hepatitis B chronic carriers
8)  Medical and dental personnel.

Dosage recommendations
Under 10 years of age: 3 doses of 0.5 ml IM (10 mcg) at 0, 1, and 6 months. Over 10 years of age: 1.0 ml (20 mcg) doses IM at 0, 1, and 6 months. HBIG and hepatitis vaccine should be given simultaneously to infants when transplacental transmission is likely. (See page 314 for HBIG.) Immunosuppressed patients (e.g. renal dialysis) should get twice the dose.

Typical profile of serological markers in adult patients with acute type-B hepatitis. Many HBV infections in children are asymptomatic, and children have a higher incidence of chronic carriage.

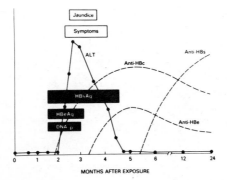

MONTHS AFTER EXPOSURE

Ref: Schafer DF, et al. Viewpoints on Digestive Diseases 1982; 14:5, with permission.

| **HBsAg** | **anti-HBc** | **anti-HAV** | **Interpretation** |
|:---:|:---:|:---:|---|
| | | | **Test Result** |
| − | − | + | Recent acute hepatitis A infection |
| + | + | − | Acute hepatitis B infection |
| + | − | − | Early acute or chronic hepatitis B |
| − | + | − | Confirms acute or recent hepatitis B |
| − | − | − | Possible non-A, non-B hepatitis, other virus, or toxin |
| + | + | + | Acute hepatitis B superimposed on recent hepatitis A |

Ref: Perspectives on Viral Hepatitis. North Chicago Abbott Laboratories, 1983, with permission.

E. Influenza
   Multivalent A and B vaccine is available, but the antigenic makeup of the vaccine varies from year to year, as do recommendations for its use.

   Indications
1) Not routinely recommended for normal children.

2) Target high-risk children should be immunized if 6 months or older including chronic pulmonary disease (moderate-severe asthma, bronchopulmonary dysplasia); hemodynamically significant cardiac disease, sickle cell disease, and children receiving immunosuppressive therapy.

3) Other high-risk children should be considered, including chronic renal and metabolic diseases, diabetes, and those receiving chronic aspirin therapy.

4) Influenza vaccine should be administered in the fall. It may be administered simultaneously (separate site) with MMR, HIB, pneumovax, and TOPV, but should not be given within 7 days of DTP. If child with chicken or egg allergy has hypersensitivity to skin test, do not use vaccine. Administer split virus in children <12 years.

F.  Measles
    Give live, attenuated measles virus vaccine 0.5 ml SQ
    into deltoid area.
    Contraindications
    1)  Febrile illness
    2)  Pregnancy
    3)  Leukemia or other malignancy
    4)  Defects of cell-mediated immunity
    5)  Immunosuppression
    6)  Untreated active tuberculosis
    7)  Administration of plasma or immune globulin in
        previous 8 weeks

G.  Mumps
    Live attenuated virus is recommended for children 15
    months and above and for adolescents and adults who
    have not had clinical disease. Do not give within 3
    months of blood/immune globulin transfusion.

    Contraindications
    1)  Agammaglobulinemia
    2)  Malignancy, antimetabolite, or steroid therapy,
        immunodeficiency or immunosuppressed states
    3)  Pregnancy
    4)  Hypersensitivity on skin test in cases of
        chicken/egg allergy.

H.  Pneumococcal Polysaccharide Vaccine (0.5 ml SQ): Indi-
    cated in children >2 years old with sickle cell anemia,
    splenectomy, chronic nephrotic syndrome, chronic liver
    disease, malignancy, or primary immunodeficiency.

    Contraindications:
    1)  Pregnant women (effect on fetus unkown)
    2)  Children <2 years old (inconsistent antibody
        responses).
    3)  Revaccination with new 23-valent vaccine in patients
        who received old 14-valent vaccine not recommended
        due to risk of adverse reactions.

I.  Poliomyelitis
    The live vaccine is provided as a trivalent vaccine and
    administered orally. Storage and dose instructions vary
    with manufacturer. Oral polio vaccine virus is excreted
    by the vaccinee, so that it should not be used by
    household contacts of immunodeficient or immunosup-
    pressed individuals. Injectable polio vaccine should be
    used instead.

    1)  Contraindications for live polio vaccine
        a)  Immunodeficiency disease or immunosuppressive
            therapy
        b)  Malignancy

2) Injectable polio vaccine (Salk) may be given to immunodeficient or immunosuppressed patients; response will be limited by underlying condition. Administer at 2, 4, and 6 months.

J. Rabies
The decision to treat for rabies must be based on whether the attack was provoked, the type of animal and its availability for observation, the immunization status of the animal, and the presence of rabies in the state or community.
   1) Persons not previously immunized: Inject Human Rabies Immune Globin (HRIG) 20 IU/kg, one-half infiltrated at the bite site, if possible, and the remainder IM. Administer Human Diploid Cell Vaccine (HDCV) 1.0 ml IM on days 0, 3, 7, 14, and 28. Give HRIG as soon as possible after exposure, but no later than day 8 of the HDCV schedule. When HRIG is not available use equine serum RIG in a dose of 40 IU/kg after a SC test dose.
   2) Persons previously immunized: Give HDCV 1.0 ml IM on days 0 and 3. HRIG should not be given.

Postexposure Antirabies Treatment Guide

| Species of Animal | Condition of Animal at Time of Attack | Treatment of Exposed Human |
|---|---|---|
| Wild* | Regard as rabid | HRIG + HDCV |
| Domestic: (Dog, Cat)** | Healthy | None |
| | Unknown (escaped) or rabid or suspected rabid | HRIG + HDCV Call Public Health Official |

*Skunk, fox, coyote, raccoon, bat, other carnivores

**Other: (Livestock, rodents, rabbits) - consider individually

K. Rubella
Live rubella vaccine is currently recommended by the American Academy of Pediatrics. It should be given at 15 months of age , and should be given in a single subcutaneous dose of 0.5 ml. Antibody levels appear to have declined minimally over the 10 years the vaccine has been in use, but the duration of immunity is as yet uncertain.

Contraindications
1) Pregnancy
2) Immunosuppression, immunodeficiency or generalized malignancy
3) Ig or blood transfusion in past 3 months.

L. Tuberculosis
    1) Guide to treating

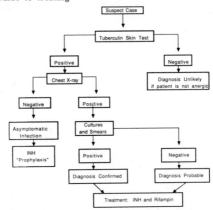

2) When the population of tubercle bacilli is large
   (e.g. miliary, extensive cavitary lesions, meningitis, or renal disease) or the patient is from an
   area where drug-resistant tuberculosis is prevalent,
   streptomycin should be included, but for no longer
   than 3 months.

3) Newborn infants of mothers with tuberculosis:
      See RCID, 1986: 387-8.

| Mother's Status | Infant | Other |
|---|---|---|
| I. + PPD, no evidence of infection | No therapy | PPD to infant at 4-6 wks, 3-4 mo, 12 mo. Investigate household contacts. |
| II. Newly diagnosed Tb, minimal disease or Rx >2 wks and non-contagious. | INH until ⊟ PPD demonstrated at 6 mo. and no active cases in household. *BCG vaccine if compliance cannot be assured. | -Report to Public Health Department<br>-Refer mother for therapy<br>-Follow-up PPD and chest x-ray on infant at 4-6 wks, 3-4 mo, and 6 mo.<br>-Evaluate household contacts and clear home before discharge |

| Mother's Status | Infant | Other |
|---|---|---|
| III. Contagious Tb infection | INH as above<br><br><br><br>BCG as above | –Same as Category II above.<br>–Isolate mother from infant until mother is not contagious. |
| IV. Hematogenous spread of Tb | INH + rifampin<br>-Stop at 6 mo if ⊞ PPD, ⊟ CXR<br>-Stop at 12 mo if ⊞ PPD, ⊞ CXR | –Congenital Tuberculosis possible<br>–CXR and PPD at birth<br>–investigate household |

*BCG (0.1 ml) is given SQ as superficially as possible over the right deltoid, or by the multiple puncture technique. If infant is non-reactive to PPD at 8 weeks, repeat BCG until reactive. Do not give BCG during INH administration, BCG organisms are inhibited by INH.

      4)    Active disease should be considered in a person who received BCG if a PPD yields >10 mm induration or there is clinical evidence of TB. Infections with atypical mycobacteria may also give PPD reactions of 5-10 mm induration.

  M.    Other
        Cholera, yellow fever, plague, Rocky Mountain Spotted Fever and typhus vaccines are used only in foreign travel to affected countries and/or in other high risk situation.

2.   Passive Immunization

  A.    Hepatitis A
        Give 0.02 ml/kg of Immune Serum Globulin (ISG) to:
        1)   Anyone inoculated with a needle or who has had open lesions directly in contact with material (blood, serum, saliva or other body fluids) from a patient known to have hepatitis A.
        2)   Persons sharing common living quarters such as family members, roommates, sex partners, or individuals who dine regularly or use common plates or glasses with a patient with known hepatitis A.
        3)   Schoolmates in any class where more than one case of hepatitis A has been established.
        4)   Infants of mothers with HAA⊖ hepatitis.
        5)   Daycare - all employees and children when one case established.

NOTE: For prolonged continuous exposure, give 0.06 ml/kg of ISG and repeat in 4-5 months. If no clinical evidence of disease has occurred in 10-12 months of intensive exposure, subclinical infection has probably occurred.

B.  Hepatitis B
    Hepatitis B Immune Globulin (HBIG) is the treatment of choice. IG has had detectable anti-HBs after 1972 and may be used with variable effectiveness for passive immunization to hepatitis B when HBIG is not available.
    1)  Give 0.06 ml/kg HBIG (max 5ml) to person with percutaneous exposure (within 24 hours) or with sexual contact (within 14 days). HB Vaccine recommended for persons with perinatal percutaneous exposure, and for homosexually active males or sexual contacts of hepatitis B carriers. If unable to administer vaccine, repeat the dose of HBIG 1 month later.
    2)  Infants born to mothers with known third trimester hepatitis B or who are HBsAg positive at delivery should receive HBIG 0.5 ml IM, and HB vaccine (see page 308).

    Ref: MMWR, 1984; 33:285.

C.  Immunodeficiency Disorders
    1)  Intramuscular Immune Serum Globulin: 0.6-1.0 ml/kg IM every 2-4 weeks. A double dose is given at the onset of therapy. Indicated only for humoral immunodeficiency syndromes involving IgG. Dose and interval adjusted for each individual based on clinical response and IgG level.
    2)  Intravenous immunoglobulin (IVIG): 300-500 mg/kg IV every 3-5 weeks for immunodeficiency diseases. The dose is modified as needed depending on the child's IgG levels and clinical course. (Ref: Lederman H, personal communication, 1987).
        IVIG may be effective in Kawasaki Disease and idiopathic thrombocytopenic purpura in doses of 400 mg/kg/day for 4-5 days. It may be effective in preventing secondary bacterial infections in AIDS.

    Ref: Newburger JW et al. New Eng J Med 1986; 315:341; Calvelli TA, et al. Pediatr Inf Dis 1986; 5:S207; Imbach, et al. Lancet 1985; 2:464.

D.  Measles
    "Preventive" dose of Immune Globulin is 0.25 ml/kg IM for otherwise normal unvaccinated infants and children within 6 days of exposure. Especially indicated in contacts less than 1 year old. Give measles vaccine 3 months after Ig administration.

For unvaccinated children with malignancies, immuno-deficiency, or those on immunosuppressive therapy give 0.5 ml/kg (15 ml max.) IM.

E.  Rabies
(see page 311 under Active Immunizations)

F.  Rubella
The use of Immune Serum Globulin, 0.55 ml/kg, may be considered for pregnant women exposed during the first trimester only if termination of pregnancy is not an option, as this Ig is of questionable benefit.

G.  Tetanus
(See page 305 for recommendations for use of vaccine and globulin.)  Use a TIG dose of 250 to 500 units IM for susceptible wounds and 3,000 to 6,000 units IM (with some placed into the wound) for the clinical illness.  If TIG is not available, use equine antitoxin after testing for hypersensitivity.  Dosage is 3,000 to 5,000 units for those with susceptible wounds and 50,000 to 100,000 units (20,000 given IV, the rest IM) for clinical illness.

H.  Varicella-Zoster
Zoster Immune Globulin (ZIG) is effective if given to immunocompromised patients within 96 hours of exposure but is optimal if given within 48 hours.  It is available from the American Red Cross and is indicated in the following exposed populations:

1)  Immunocompromised children (and non-immune adults).
2)  Normal adolescents and adults if non-immune.
3)  Newborn of mother with onset of chicken pox within 5 days before or 2 days after delivery.
4)  Premature infant >28 weeks gestation with non-immune mother.
5)  Premature infant <28 weeks gestation regardless of maternal history.
6)  Pregnant women.  Note - protection for fetus is unknown.

3.  Prophylaxis - Haemophilus Influenzae and Meningococcus

H. Flu disease:  Rifampin should be given to all household contacts (including adults) in households with at least one contact less than 48 months of age who has not received HIB vaccine (or if the HIB vaccine was given at less than 24 months of age or within the preceding 3 weeks).  Initiate prophylaxis as soon as possible.  The management of daycare and nursery school contacts should be individualized.

Meningococcal disease:
Those who have had contact with the patient's oral secretions, as well as all household, day care, and nursery school contacts, should receive sulfisoxazole or Rifampin prophylaxis within 24 hours.

Prophylaxis is not routinely recommended for medical personnel unless they have had contact with the patient's oral secretions. See Formulary for rifampin doses.

ISOLATION TECHNIQUES FOR VARIOUS ILLNESSES

| | Respiratory | Enteric | Wound and Skin | Strict | Blood & Body Fluids |
|---|---|---|---|---|---|
| Disease | Rubella[1] Hemophilus influenza Meningitis[2] Meningococcemia Mumps Pertussis Tuberculosis | Cholera Diarrhea Enteropathic or enterotoxigenic E. coli Hepatitis A Salmonella Shigella Staph enterocolitis Typhoid Fever Yersinia | Extensive wound Gas gangrene Localized zoster Melioidosis Plague Staph skin or wound Strep skin or wound | Cong. Rubella[3] Disseminated Zoster/ Varicella Extensive burn staph or strep Herpes simplex neonatorum Rabies Staph pneumonia | AIDS, Hepatitis B, Syphilis, Malaria, Leptospirosis |
| Handwashing | Upon entering and leaving room | Upon entering and leaving room | Upon entering and leaving room | Upon entering and leaving room | Upon entering and leaving room |
| Single Room | Yes, door closed | Desirable, esp. with incontinent children | Desirable | Yes, door closed | Desirable, esp. if extensive bleeding |
| Gown | No | Yes | Yes with contact | Yes | Yes, with contact |
| Mask | Yes | No | Staph or Strep | Yes | No |
| Gloves | No | Yes with contact | Yes with contact | Yes | Yes with contact |
| Excretions | No | Yes | No | Yes | Yes |
| Secretions | Yes | Hepatitis, AIDS | Yes | Yes | Yes |

[1] Pregnant women should avoid contact.
[2] Until 24 hours after effective treatment is begun.
[3] Requires gown, no gloves.

PART IV

REFERENCE DATA

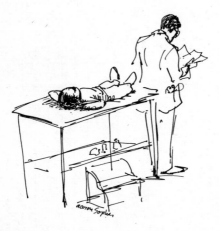

GIRLS
BIRTH TO 36 MONTHS
LENGTH AND WEIGHT

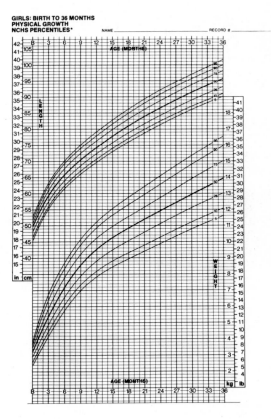

**GIRLS: BIRTH TO 36 MONTHS**
**PHYSICAL GROWTH**
**NCHS PERCENTILES\***       NAME _____       RECORD # _____

Adapted from National Center for Health Statistics data.  Copyright Ross Laboratories, 1976.

320

GIRLS
2 TO 18 YEARS
STATURE AND WEIGHT

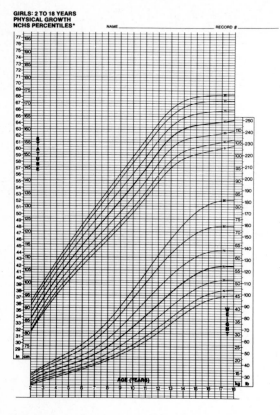

Adapted from National Center for Health Statistics data. Copyright Ross Laboratories, 1976.

# BOYS
## BIRTH TO 36 MONTHS
## LENGTH AND WEIGHT

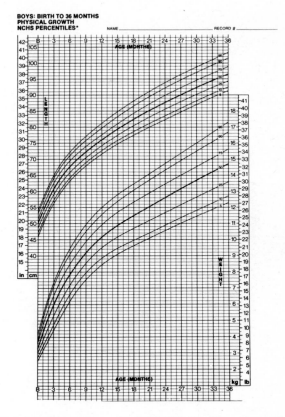

Adapted from National Center for Health Statistics data. Copyright Ross Laboratories, 1976.

322

BOYS
2 TO 18 YEARS
STATURE AND WEIGHT

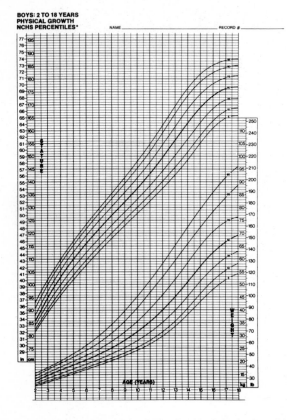

# HEAD CIRCUMFERENCE - GIRLS

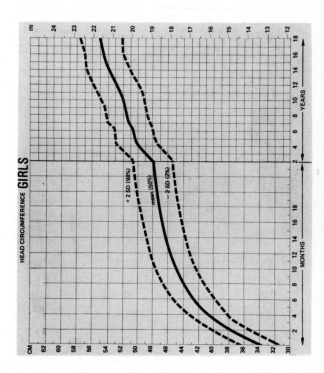

Ref: Nellhaus G, Pediatrics, 1968; 41:106.

## HEAD CIRCUMFERENCE - BOYS

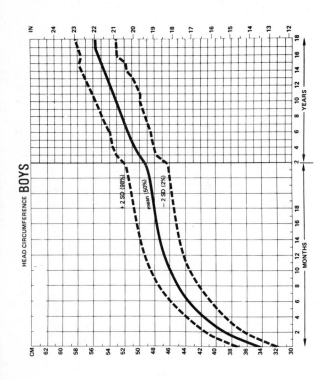

Ref: Nellhaus G, Pediatrics, 1968; 41:106.

## INCREMENTAL GROWTH CHARTS*
### (GROWTH VELOCITY)

# INSTRUCTIONS

1. Measure the child at the beginning and the end of a 6-month interval, if possible.

2. Subtract the initial measurement from the follow-up measurement to obtain the increment.

3. If the interval between measurements is not exactly 6 months (182 days), divide the increment by the interval in days and multiply by 182 to obtain the adjusted 6-month increment. The Table of Consecutively Numbered Days can be used to determine the interval between the measurements. If measurements are made in different years, add 365 to the day of the year for the follow-up measurement. Extrapolating increments from intervals of 3 months or less is not recommended.

4. Locate the intersection of the increment and the child's age at the *end* of the interval to determine the 6-month incremental percentile.

**Interpretation:** The accompanying charts permit definition of growth rate (growth velocity) relative to current reference data. Further investigation is indicated for children growing at rates markedly different from the 50th incremental percentile or for children whose incremental percentile changes rapidly.

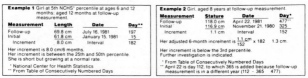

**Example 1** Girl at 5th NCHS* percentile at ages 6 and 12 months; aged 12 months at follow-up measurement.

| Measurement | Length | Date | Day** |
|---|---|---|---|
| Follow-up | 69.8 cm | July 16, 1981 | 197 |
| Initial | 61.8 cm | January 15, 1981 | 15 |
| Increment | 8.0 cm | Interval | 182 |

Her increment is 8.0 cm/6 months.
Her increment is between the 25th and 50th percentile.
She is short but growing at a normal rate.

* National Center for Health Statistics
** From Table of Consecutively Numbered Days

**Example 2** Girl, aged 8 years at follow-up measurement.

| Measurement | Stature | Date | Day* |
|---|---|---|---|
| Follow-up | 118.0 cm | April 22, 1981 | 477** |
| Initial | 116.9 cm | November 21, 1980 | 325 |
| Increment | 1.1 cm | Interval | 152 |

Her adjusted 6-month increment is $\frac{1.1 cm}{152} \times 182$   1.3 cm

Her increment is below the 3rd percentile.
Further investigation is indicated.

* From Table of Consecutively Numbered Days
** April 22 is day 112, to which 365 is added because follow-up measurement is in a different year (112 · 365   477).

### Table of Consecutively Numbered Days

| Day | JAN | FEB | MAR | APR | MAY | JUN | JUL | AUG | SEP | OCT | NOV | DEC | Day |
|---|---|---|---|---|---|---|---|---|---|---|---|---|---|
| 1 | 1 | 32 | 60 | 91 | 121 | 152 | 182 | 213 | 244 | 274 | 305 | 335 | 1 |
| 2 | 2 | 33 | 61 | 92 | 122 | 153 | 183 | 214 | 245 | 275 | 306 | 336 | 2 |
| 3 | 3 | 34 | 62 | 93 | 123 | 154 | 184 | 215 | 246 | 276 | 307 | 337 | 3 |
| 4 | 4 | 35 | 63 | 94 | 124 | 155 | 185 | 216 | 247 | 277 | 308 | 338 | 4 |
| 5 | 5 | 36 | 64 | 95 | 125 | 156 | 186 | 217 | 248 | 278 | 309 | 339 | 5 |
| 6 | 6 | 37 | 65 | 96 | 126 | 157 | 187 | 218 | 249 | 279 | 310 | 340 | 6 |
| 7 | 7 | 38 | 66 | 97 | 127 | 158 | 188 | 219 | 250 | 280 | 311 | 341 | 7 |
| 8 | 8 | 39 | 67 | 98 | 128 | 159 | 189 | 220 | 251 | 281 | 312 | 342 | 8 |
| 9 | 9 | 40 | 68 | 99 | 129 | 160 | 190 | 221 | 252 | 282 | 313 | 343 | 9 |
| 10 | 10 | 41 | 69 | 100 | 130 | 161 | 191 | 222 | 253 | 283 | 314 | 344 | 10 |
| 11 | 11 | 42 | 70 | 101 | 131 | 162 | 192 | 223 | 254 | 284 | 315 | 345 | 11 |
| 12 | 12 | 43 | 71 | 102 | 132 | 163 | 193 | 224 | 255 | 285 | 316 | 346 | 12 |
| 13 | 13 | 44 | 72 | 103 | 133 | 164 | 194 | 225 | 256 | 286 | 317 | 347 | 13 |
| 14 | 14 | 45 | 73 | 104 | 134 | 165 | 195 | 226 | 257 | 287 | 318 | 348 | 14 |
| 15 | 15 | 46 | 74 | 105 | 135 | 166 | 196 | 227 | 258 | 288 | 319 | 349 | 15 |
| 16 | 16 | 47 | 75 | 106 | 136 | 167 | 197 | 228 | 259 | 289 | 320 | 350 | 16 |
| 17 | 17 | 48 | 76 | 107 | 137 | 168 | 198 | 229 | 260 | 290 | 321 | 351 | 17 |
| 18 | 18 | 49 | 77 | 108 | 138 | 169 | 199 | 230 | 261 | 291 | 322 | 352 | 18 |
| 19 | 19 | 50 | 78 | 109 | 139 | 170 | 200 | 231 | 262 | 292 | 323 | 353 | 19 |
| 20 | 20 | 51 | 79 | 110 | 140 | 171 | 201 | 232 | 263 | 293 | 324 | 354 | 20 |
| 21 | 21 | 52 | 80 | 111 | 141 | 172 | 202 | 233 | 264 | 294 | 325 | 355 | 21 |
| 22 | 22 | 53 | 81 | 112 | 142 | 173 | 203 | 234 | 265 | 295 | 326 | 356 | 22 |
| 23 | 23 | 54 | 82 | 113 | 143 | 174 | 204 | 235 | 266 | 296 | 327 | 357 | 23 |
| 24 | 24 | 55 | 83 | 114 | 144 | 175 | 205 | 236 | 267 | 297 | 328 | 358 | 24 |
| 25 | 25 | 56 | 84 | 115 | 145 | 176 | 206 | 237 | 268 | 298 | 329 | 359 | 25 |
| 26 | 26 | 57 | 85 | 116 | 146 | 177 | 207 | 238 | 269 | 299 | 330 | 360 | 26 |
| 27 | 27 | 58 | 86 | 117 | 147 | 178 | 208 | 239 | 270 | 300 | 331 | 361 | 27 |
| 28 | 28 | 59 | 87 | 118 | 148 | 179 | 209 | 240 | 271 | 301 | 332 | 362 | 28 |
| 29 | 29 | — | 88 | 119 | 149 | 180 | 210 | 241 | 272 | 302 | 333 | 363 | 29 |
| 30 | 30 | — | 89 | 120 | 150 | 181 | 211 | 242 | 273 | 303 | 334 | 364 | 30 |
| 31 | 31 | — | 90 | — | 151 | — | 212 | 243 | — | 304 | — | 365 | 31 |
| Day | JAN | FEB | MAR | APR | MAY | JUN | JUL | AUG | SEP | OCT | NOV | DEC | . . |

*Courtesy of Ross Laboratories, Columbus, OH, 43216, 1981.

## INCREMENTAL GROWTH CHARTS
### GIRLS: 0-36 MONTHS

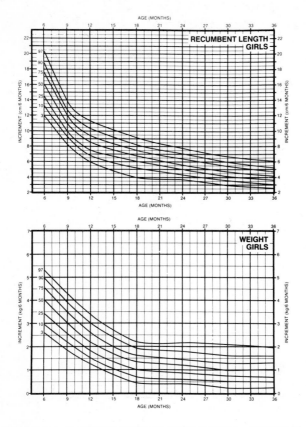

Adapted from the National Center for Health Statistics. Courtesy of Ross Laboratories, Columbus, OH, 43216, 1981.

# INCREMENTAL GROWTH CHARTS
## GIRLS: 2-18 YEARS

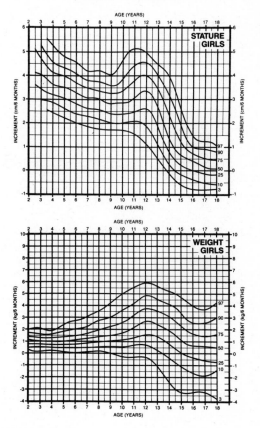

Adapted from the National Center for Health Statistics. Courtesy of Ross Laboratories, Columbus, OH, 43216, 1981.

## INCREMENTAL GROWTH CHARTS
### BOYS: 0-36 MONTHS

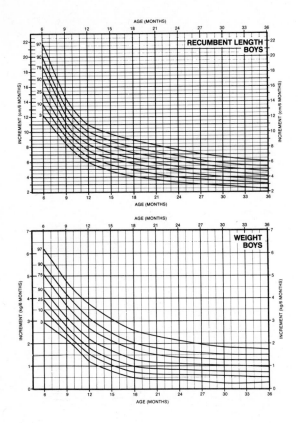

Adapted from the National Center for Health Statistics.  Courtesy of
Ross Laboratories, Columbus, OH, 43216, 1981.

# INCREMENTAL GROWTH CHARTS
## BOYS: 2-18 YEARS

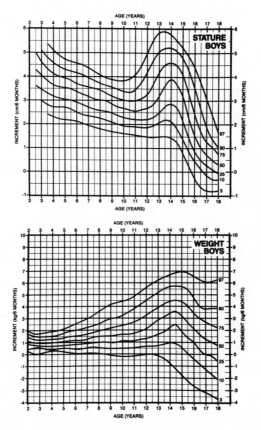

Adapted from the National Center for Health Statistics. Courtesy of
Ross Laboratories, Columbus, OH, 43216, 1981.

330

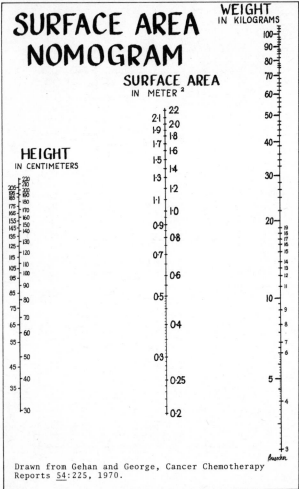

# SURFACE AREA NOMOGRAM

**WEIGHT**
IN KILOGRAMS

**SURFACE AREA**
IN METER²

**HEIGHT**
IN CENTIMETERS

Drawn from Gehan and George, Cancer Chemotherapy
Reports 54:225, 1970.

BONE AGE

Age-at-Appearance Percentiles for Epiphyses and Round Bones

| | Boys Percentiles | | | Girls Percentiles | | |
|---|---|---|---|---|---|---|
| | 5th | 50th | 95th | 5th | 50th | 95th |
| **Wrist** | | | | | | |
| Capitate | birth | 3m | 7m | birth | 2m | 7m |
| Hamate | 2w | 4m | 10m | birth | 2m | 7m |
| Distal radius | 6w | 1y1m | 2y4m | 5m | 10m | 1y8m |
| Triquetral | 6m | 2y5m | 5y6m | 3m | 1y8m | 3y9m |
| Lunate | 1y6m | 4y1m | 6y9m | 1y1m | 2y7m | 5y8m |
| Scaphoid | 3y7m | 5y8m | 7y10m | 2y4m | 4y1m | 6y |
| Trapezium | 3y6m | 5y10m | 9y | 1y11m | 4y1m | 6y4m |
| Trapezoid | 3y1m | 6y3m | 8y6m | 2y5m | 4y2m | 6y |
| Distal Ulna | 5y3m | 7y1m | 9y1m | 3y3m | 5y4m | 7y8m |
| **Elbow** | | | | | | |
| Capitulum | 3w | 4m | 1y1m | 3w | 3m | 9m |
| Radial head | 3y | 5y3m | 8y | 2y3m | 3y10m | 6y3m |
| Medial epicondyle | 4y3m | 6y3m | 8y5m | 2y1m | 3y5m | 5y1m |
| Olecranon of ulna | 7y9m | 9y8m | 11y11m | 5y7m | 8y | 9y11m |
| Lateral epicondyle | 9y3m | 11y3m | 13y8m | 7y2m | 9y3m | 11y3m |
| **Shoulder** | | | | | | |
| Head of humerus | 37w* | | 16w | 37w* | | 16w |
| Coronoid | birth | 2w | 4w | birth | 2w | 5m |
| Tubercle of humerus | 3m | 10m | 2y4m | 2m | 6m | 1y2m |
| Acromion of scapula | 12y2m | 13y9m | 15y6m | 10y4m | 11y11m | 15y6m |
| Acromion of clavicle | 12y | 14y | 15y11m | 10y10m | 12y9m | 15y4m |

*Prenatal age

BONE AGE (continued)

Age-at-Appearance Percentiles for Epiphyses and Round Bones

| | Boys Percentiles | | | Girls Percentiles | | |
|---|---|---|---|---|---|---|
| | 5th | 50th | 95th | 5th | 50th | 95th |
| **Hip** | | | | | | |
| Head of femur | 3w | 4m | 8m | 2w | 4m | 7m |
| Greater trochanter | 1y11m | 3y | 4y4m | 1y | 1y10m | 3y |
| Os Acetabulum | 11y11m | 13y6m | 15y4m | 9y7m | 11y6m | 13y5m |
| Iliac crest | 12y | 14y | 15y11m | 10y10m | 12y9m | 15y4m |
| Ischial tuberosity | 13y7m | 15y3m | 17y1m | 11y9m | 13y11m | 16y |
| **Knee** | | | | | | |
| Distal femur | 31w* | | 40w* | 31w* | | 39w* |
| Proximal tibia | 34w* | | 5w | 34w* | | 2w |
| Proximal fibula | 1y10m | 3y6m | 5y3m | 1y4m | 2y7m | 3y11m |
| Patella | 2y7m | 4y | 6y | 1y6m | 2y6m | 4y |
| Tibial tubercle | 9y11m | 11y10m | 13y5m | 7y11m | 10y3m | 11y10m |
| **Foot** | | | | | | |
| Calcaneus | 22w* | | 25w* | 22w* | | 25w* |
| Talus | 25w* | | 31w* | 25w* | | 31w* |
| Cuboid | 37w* | | 16w | 37w* | | 8w |
| Third cuneiform | 3w | 6m | 1y7m | birth | 3m | 1y3m |
| Os calcis, apophysis | 5y2m | 7y7m | 9y7m | 3y6m | 5y4m | 7y4m |

*Prenatal age

Modified from Garn, SM, Rohman, CG and Silverman, FN: Med Radiogr Photogr 43:45, 1967.

## DENTAL DEVELOPMENT

| | DECIDUOUS TEETH | | | | PERMANENT TEETH | |
| | Eruption | | Shedding | | Eruption | |
| | Maxillary | Mandibular | Maxillary | Mandibular | Maxillary | Mandibular |
|---|---|---|---|---|---|---|
| Central Incisors | 6-8 mo | 5-7 mo | 7-8 yr | 6-7 yr | 7-8 yr | 6-7 yr |
| Lateral Incisors | 8-11 mo | 7-10 mo | 8-9 yr | 7-8 yr | 8-9 yr | 7-8 yr |
| Cuspids | 16-20 mo | 16-20 mo | 11-12 yr | 9-11 yr | 11-12 yr | 9-11 yr |
| 1st Premolar | – | – | – | – | 10-11 yr | 10-12 yr |
| 2nd Premolar | – | – | – | – | 10-12 yr | 11-13 yr |
| 1st Molars | 10-16 mo | 10-16 mo | 10-11 yr | 10-12 yr | 6-7 yr | 6-7 yr |
| 2nd Molars | 20-30 mo | 20-30 mo | 10-12 yr | 11-13 yr | 12-13 yr | 12-13 yr |
| 3rd Molars | – | – | – | – | 17-22 yr | 17-22 yr |

NOTE: Sexes are combined although girls tend to be slightly advanced over boys. Averages are approximate values derived from various studies.

Ref: Vaughn, VC, et al (eds): Nelson's Textbook of Pediatrics. Philadelphia: W.B. Saunders, 1979, p. 32.

334

BLOOD PRESSURES, AGES 0-12 MONTHS

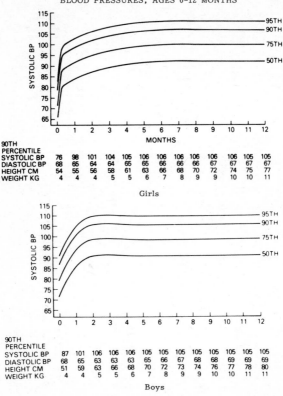

| 90TH PERCENTILE | | | | | | | | | | | | | |
|---|---|---|---|---|---|---|---|---|---|---|---|---|
| SYSTOLIC BP | 76 | 98 | 101 | 104 | 105 | 106 | 106 | 106 | 106 | 106 | 106 | 105 | 105 |
| DIASTOLIC BP | 68 | 65 | 64 | 64 | 65 | 65 | 66 | 66 | 66 | 67 | 67 | 67 | 67 |
| HEIGHT CM | 54 | 55 | 56 | 58 | 61 | 63 | 66 | 68 | 70 | 72 | 74 | 75 | 77 |
| WEIGHT KG | 4 | 4 | 4 | 5 | 5 | 6 | 7 | 8 | 9 | 9 | 10 | 10 | 11 |

Girls

| 90TH PERCENTILE | | | | | | | | | | | | | |
|---|---|---|---|---|---|---|---|---|---|---|---|---|
| SYSTOLIC BP | 87 | 101 | 106 | 106 | 106 | 105 | 105 | 105 | 105 | 105 | 105 | 105 | 105 |
| DIASTOLIC BP | 68 | 65 | 63 | 63 | 65 | 66 | 67 | 68 | 68 | 69 | 69 | 69 | 69 |
| HEIGHT CM | 51 | 59 | 63 | 66 | 68 | 70 | 72 | 73 | 74 | 76 | 77 | 78 | 80 |
| WEIGHT KG | 4 | 4 | 5 | 5 | 6 | 7 | 8 | 9 | 9 | 10 | 10 | 11 | 11 |

Boys

Ref: Horan MJ. Pediatrics 1987; 79:1-25. With permission.

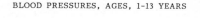

## BLOOD PRESSURES, AGES, 1-13 YEARS

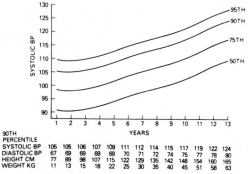

**90TH PERCENTILE**

| | 1 | 2 | 3 | 4 | 5 | 6 | 7 | 8 | 9 | 10 | 11 | 12 | 13 |
|---|---|---|---|---|---|---|---|---|---|---|---|---|---|
| SYSTOLIC BP | 105 | 105 | 106 | 107 | 109 | 111 | 112 | 114 | 115 | 117 | 119 | 122 | 124 |
| DIASTOLIC BP | 67 | 69 | 69 | 69 | 69 | 70 | 71 | 72 | 74 | 75 | 77 | 78 | 80 |
| HEIGHT CM | 77 | 89 | 98 | 107 | 115 | 122 | 129 | 135 | 142 | 148 | 154 | 160 | 165 |
| WEIGHT KG | 11 | 13 | 15 | 18 | 22 | 25 | 30 | 35 | 40 | 45 | 51 | 58 | 63 |

Girls

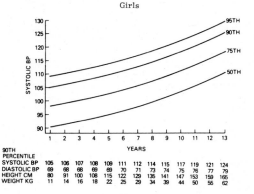

**90TH PERCENTILE**

| | 1 | 2 | 3 | 4 | 5 | 6 | 7 | 8 | 9 | 10 | 11 | 12 | 13 |
|---|---|---|---|---|---|---|---|---|---|---|---|---|---|
| SYSTOLIC BP | 105 | 106 | 107 | 108 | 109 | 111 | 112 | 114 | 115 | 117 | 119 | 121 | 124 |
| DIASTOLIC BP | 69 | 68 | 68 | 69 | 69 | 70 | 71 | 73 | 74 | 75 | 76 | 77 | 79 |
| HEIGHT CM | 80 | 91 | 100 | 108 | 115 | 122 | 129 | 135 | 141 | 147 | 153 | 159 | 165 |
| WEIGHT KG | 11 | 14 | 16 | 18 | 22 | 25 | 29 | 34 | 39 | 44 | 50 | 55 | 62 |

Boys

Ref: Horan MJ. Pediatrics 1987; 79:1-25. With permission.

BLOOD PRESSURES, AGES, 13-18 YEARS

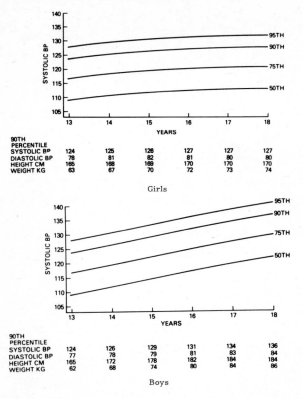

| 90TH PERCENTILE | | | | | | |
|---|---|---|---|---|---|---|
| SYSTOLIC BP | 124 | 125 | 126 | 127 | 127 | 127 |
| DIASTOLIC BP | 78 | 81 | 82 | 81 | 80 | 80 |
| HEIGHT CM | 165 | 168 | 169 | 170 | 170 | 170 |
| WEIGHT KG | 63 | 67 | 70 | 72 | 73 | 74 |

Girls

| 90TH PERCENTILE | | | | | | |
|---|---|---|---|---|---|---|
| SYSTOLIC BP | 124 | 126 | 129 | 131 | 134 | 136 |
| DIASTOLIC BP | 77 | 78 | 79 | 81 | 83 | 84 |
| HEIGHT CM | 165 | 172 | 178 | 182 | 184 | 184 |
| WEIGHT KG | 62 | 68 | 74 | 80 | 84 | 86 |

Boys

Ref: Horan MJ. Pediatrics 1987; 79:1-25. With permission.

# RECOMMENDED DAILY DIETARY ALLOWANCES

| | Age | Wt | Ht | Energy | Prot. | Fat-Soluble Vitamins | | | Water-Soluble Vitamins | | | | Minerals | | |
|---|---|---|---|---|---|---|---|---|---|---|---|---|---|---|---|
| | | | | | | Vit. A | Vit. D | Vit. E | Vit. C | Nia-cin | Ribo-flavin | Thia-min | Ca | P | Fe |
| | (yrs) | (kg) | (cm) | (kcal) | (g/kg) | (µg RE)[1] | (µg)[2] | (mg αTE)[3] | (mg) | (mg) | (mg) | (mg) | (mg) | (mg) | (mg) |
| In-fants | 0–½ | 6 | 60 | kg × 115 | 2.2 | 420 | 10 | 3 | 35 | 6 | 0.4 | 0.3 | 360 | 240 | 10 |
| | ½–1 | 9 | 71 | kg × 105 | 2.0 | 400 | 10 | 4 | 35 | 8 | 0.6 | 0.5 | 540 | 360 | 15 |
| Chil-dren | 1–3 | 13 | 90 | kg × 100 | 1.8 | 400 | 10 | 5 | 45 | 9 | 0.8 | 0.7 | 800 | 800 | 15 |
| | 4–6 | 20 | 112 | kg × 85 | 1.5 | 500 | 10 | 6 | 45 | 11 | 1.0 | 0.9 | 800 | 800 | 10 |
| | 7–10 | 28 | 132 | kg × 86 | 1.2 | 700 | 10 | 7 | 45 | 16 | 1.4 | 1.2 | 800 | 800 | 10 |
| Boys | 11–14 | 45 | 157 | kg × 60 | 1.0 | 1000 | 10 | 8 | 50 | 18 | 1.6 | 1.4 | 1200 | 1200 | 18 |
| | 15–18 | 66 | 176 | kg × 42 | 0.85 | 1000 | 10 | 10 | 60 | 18 | 1.7 | 1.4 | 1200 | 1200 | 18 |
| Girls | 11–14 | 46 | 157 | kg × 48 | 1.0 | 800 | 10 | 8 | 50 | 15 | 1.3 | 1.1 | 1200 | 1200 | 18 |
| | 15–18 | 55 | 163 | kg × 38 | 0.85 | 800 | 10 | 8 | 60 | 14 | 1.3 | 1.1 | 1200 | 1200 | 18 |
| Pregnant | | | | +300[4] | +30g/day | +200 | +5 | +2 | +20 | +2 | +0.3 | +0.4 | +400 | +400 | * |
| Lactating | | | | +500 | +20g/day | +400 | +5 | +3 | +40 | +5 | +0.5 | +0.5 | +400 | +400 | * |

[1] Retinol equivalents (1 retinol equivalent = 1 µg retinol or 6 µg β carotene)

[2] As cholecalciferol (10 µg cholecalciferol = 400 IU vitamin D)

[3] αTocopherol equivalents (1 αTE = 1 mg d-α-tocopherol)

[4] + in addition to normal recommended dietary allowances

Reproduced from "Recommended Dietary Allowances," 9th Edition, 1980 with permission of the National Academy of Sciences, Washington, DC.

*30–60 mg supplemental iron per day for lactating or pregnant females.

## COMPOSITION OF INFANT FORMULAS

| Formula | Calories per oz. | per ml. | Percentage wt/vol (grams/100 ml) Protein *() | Fat *() | CHO *() | mEq/L Na | K | mg/L Ca | P | Ca/P ratio | mg/L Fe | Approx. Solute Load Renal (mOsm/L) | Cl‡ |
|---|---|---|---|---|---|---|---|---|---|---|---|---|---|
| Cow's milk | 20 | .67 | 3.30(21) | 3.30(49) | 4.70(30) | 21 | 39 | 1190 | 930 | 1.30/1 | 0.5 | 220 | 260 |
| Enfamil 20** | 20 | .67 | 1.50(9) | 3.80(50) | 6.98(41) | 8 | 18 | 465 | 317 | 1.47/1 | 1.1 | 100 | 270 |
| Enfamil premature | 20 | .67 | 2.00(12) | 3.40(44) | 7.40(44) | 11 | 19 | 793 | 402 | 2.00/1 | 1.7 | 180 | 220 |
| Evaporated milk with karo syrup see page 340. | 23 | .67 | 3.04(18) | 3.38(45) | 6.12(37) | 22 | 35 | 1165 | 909 | 1.28/1 | 0.9 | | |
| Human milk | 21 | .70 | 1.00(6) | 4.40(55) | 6.90(39) | 7 | 13 | 320 | 140 | 2.3/1 | 0.3 | 75 | 273 |
| Isomil | 20 | .67 | 1.80(11) | 3.69(49) | 6.80(40) | 14 | 24 | 700 | 500 | 1.40/1 | 12 | 122 | 230 |
| Isomil SF | 20 | .67 | 2.00(12) | 3.60(48) | 6.80(40) | 14 | 20 | 700 | 500 | 1.40/1 | 12 | 131 | 140 |
| Lofenalac | 20 | .67 | 2.20(13) | 2.60(35) | 8.80(52) | 14 | 18 | 634 | 475 | 1.33/1 | 13 | 134 | 310 |
| MJ 3232A (mixed as 81g diet powder plus 59g added carbohydrate per quart) | 20 | .67 | 1.90(11) | 2.80(36) | 9.10(54) | 12 | 19 | 634 | 423 | 1.50/1 | 13 | 124 | – |
| MJ 80056 (per 100g of diet powder) | 490 | | 0.00(0) | 22.5(41) | 71.8(59) | 3 | 9 | 540 | 300 | 1.80/1 | 11 | – | 182 |

*() Percentage calories supplied by · · ·

** also comes with Fe (12 mg/L)

‡ vapor pressure method as determined by manufacturers method: Ernst JA, et al. Pediatrics 1983; 72:350.

Ref: values listed were provided by manufacturers except when indicated otherwise.

## COMPOSITION OF INFANT FORMULAS (continued)

| Formula | Calories per oz. | per ml. | Percentage wt/vol (grams/100 ml) Protein *() | Fat *() | CHO *() | mEq/L Na | K | mg/L Ca | P | Ca/P ratio | mg/L Fe | Approx. Solute Renal Load (mOsm/L) Renal | GI‡ |
|---|---|---|---|---|---|---|---|---|---|---|---|---|---|
| Nursoy | 20 | .67 | 2.10(12) | 3.60(48) | 6.90(40) | 9 | 19 | 630 | 440 | 1.40/1 | 12 | 122 | 266 |
| Nutramigen | 20 | .67 | 1.90(11) | 2.64(35) | 9.09(54) | 14 | 19 | 634 | 423 | 1.50/1 | 13 | 130 | 430 |
| Portagen | 20 | .67 | 2.30(14) | 3.17(41) | 7.82(45) | 14 | 22 | 635 | 475 | 1.33/1 | 13 | 150 | 200 |
| Pregestimil | 20 | .67 | 1.90(11) | 2.75(35) | 9.10(54) | 14 | 19 | 634 | 423 | 1.50/1 | 13 | 120 | 310 |
| Prosobee | 20 | .67 | 2.00(12) | 3.60(48) | 6.80(40) | 11 | 21 | 634 | 500 | 1.26/1 | 13 | 130 | 180 |
| RCF | *** | | 2.00(20) | 3.60(80) | 0 (0) | 14 | 20 | 700 | 500 | 1.4/1 | 1.5 | 131*** | 60 |
| Similac 20** | 20 | .67 | 1.50(9) | 3.63(48) | 7.23(43) | 10 | 21 | 510 | 390 | 1.30/1 | 1.5 | 105 | 260 |
| Similac 24 LBW | 24 | .80 | 2.20(11) | 4.49(42) | 8.49(42) | 16 | 31 | 730 | 560 | 1.30/1 | 3.0 | 161 | 260 |
| Similac PM 60/40 | 20 | .67 | 1.58(9) | 3.76(50) | 6.88(41) | 7 | 15 | 400 | 200 | 2.00/1 | 1.5 | 96 | 240 |
| Similac special care | 20 | .67 | 1.83(11) | 3.67(47) | 7.17(42) | 13 | 24 | 1200 | 600 | 2.00/1 | 2.5 | 128 | 230 |
| Similac whey plus iron | 20 | .67 | 1.50(9) | 3.63(48) | 7.23(43) | 10 | 19 | 400 | 300 | 1.33/1 | 12 | 101 | 270 |
| SMA 20 | 20 | .67 | 1.50(9) | 3.60(48) | 7.20(43) | 6.5 | 14.3 | 440 | 330 | 1.33/1 | 12.7 | 126 | 271 |
| SMA Preemie | 24 | .80 | 2.00(10) | 4.40(48) | 8.60(42) | 14 | 19 | 750 | 400 | 1.88/1 | 3 | 175 | 300 |

*() Percentage calories supplied by . . .
** also comes with Fe (12 mg/L)
*** varies with amount carbohydrate added
‡ vapor pressure method as determined by manufacturers method: Ernst JA, et al. Pediatrics 1983; 72:350.
Ref: values listed were provided by manufacturers except when indicated otherwise.

INGREDIENTS OF INFANT FORMULAS

| Product | Protein | Fat | Carbohydrate | Comments |
|---|---|---|---|---|
| Cow's milk | 80% casein, 20% whey | Butterfat | Lactose | |
| Enfamil | 40% casein; 60% whey | 45% soy, 55% coconut oils | Lactose | |
| Enfamil premature | 40% casein; 60% whey | 40% MCT oil, soy and coconut oil | Corn syrup solids, lactose | Premature infants |
| Evaporated milk based | 80% casein; 20% whey | Butterfat | Lactose | Add 17 oz. water and 15 cc Karo syrup to a 13 oz. can. Supplement with multivitamins and iron. |
| Human milk | 40% casein, 60% whey | Human milk fat | Lactose | |
| Isomil | Soy protein | Coconut and soy oils | *Corn syrup solids and sucrose | For cow's milk protein and/or lactose intolerance |
| Isomil SF | Soy protein | Coconut and soy oils | Corn syrup solids | For cow's milk protein, lactose, and/or sucrose intolerance |
| Lofenalac | Processed casein hydrolysate to remove most of the phenylalanine | Corn oil | Corn syrup solids and modified tapioca starch | For phenylketonuria (PKU) - low in phenylalanine |
| (MJ)80056 | none | Corn oil | Corn syrup solids and modified tapioca starch | Protein free formula for amino acid disorders. |
| (MJ)3232A | casein hydrolysate | MCT oil | Tapioca starch, mono- and disaccharide free | Management of disaccharidase deficiencies. |

*Corn syrup solids = dextrose, maltose, other glucose polymers

INGREDIENTS OF INFANT FORMULAS (continued)

| Product | Protein | Fat | Carbohydrate | Comments |
|---------|---------|-----|--------------|----------|
| Nursoy | Soy protein | Coconut, saf-flower and soy-bean oils | Sucrose | For cow's milk protein and/or lactose intolerance |
| Nutramigen | Casein hydrolysate | Corn oil | Corn syrup solids, modified corn starch | Use for sensitivity to intact milk protein, or for lactose intolerance |
| Portagen | Sodium caseinate | 88% MCT oil, 12% corn oil | Corn syrup solids, sucrose | Use in fat malabsorption states, lactose intolerance (liver disease) |
| Pregestimil | Casein hydro-lysate with added L-cystine, L-tyrosine, L-tryptophan | 60% corn oil, 40% MCT oil | corn syrup solids, modified tapioca starch | Suitable for many malabsorption syndromes |
| Prosobee | Soy protein isolate and methionine | soy oil, coconut oil | 100% corn syrup solids (glucose polymers) | Use for lactose and cow's milk protein intolerance; sucrose intolerance; galactosemia |
| RCF (Ross Carbohydrate Free) | Soy protein isolate | coconut and soy oils | None | Contains no carbohydrates |
| Similac | Non-fat cow's milk | Coconut and soy oils | Lactose | |

INGREDIENTS OF INFANT FORMULAS (continued)

| Product | Protein | Fat | Carbohydrate | Comments |
|---|---|---|---|---|
| Similac 24 LBW | Non-fat cow's milk | MCT oil, coconut and soy oils | lactose and corn syrup solids | Dilute initial feedings. For premature infants with fluid intolerance. |
| Similac PM 60/40 | Casein and whey (60/40 ratio whey/casein) | Coconut and soy oils | Lactose | (Ca:P = 2:1) For those predisposed to hypocalcemia; low salt content |
| Similac special care | 60% whey 40% casein | MCT oil, soy oil, coconut oil | 50% lactose 50% corn syrup solids | Premature infants Ca:P=2:1 |
| Similac whey plus iron | 60% whey 40% casein | Coconut and soy oils | Lactose | |
| SMA | non-fat cow's milk, demineralized whey | Coconut and safflower and soybean oil | Lactose | Low salt content |
| SMA preemie | 60% whey 40% casein | MCT oil, coconut and soy oils | Lactose and glucose polymers | Premature infants |

TUBE FEEDING FORMULAS - SUPPLEMENTAL FEEDINGS

| PRODUCT | CHO SOURCE | PROTEIN SOURCE | FAT SOURCE | CHO gm/L | PRO-TEIN gm/L | FAT gm/L | mOsm/kg | Na/K+ mEq/L | RESIDUE | VITAMIN§ CONTENT | FEATURE | CAL/ML |
|---|---|---|---|---|---|---|---|---|---|---|---|---|
| CRITI-CARE HN | Malto-dextrin corn starch | enzymatic-ally hydro-lyzed casein with added L-methionine L-tyrosine, L-tryptophan | saf-flower oil | 222 | 38 | 3 | 650 | 27/34 | Low | 1890 cc | Lactose free, elemental | 1.06 |
| ENSURE | Corn syrup, sucrose | Na and Ca caseinates, soy protein | Corn oil | 145 | 37 | 37 | 450 | 37/40 | Low | 1925 cc | Supplemental feeding, lactose free; requires digestion | 1.06 |
| ENSURE PLUS | Corn syrup, sucrose | Na and Ca caseinates, soy protein | Corn oil | 200 | 55 | 53 | 600* | 50/59 | Low | 1420 cc | Same as ENSURE | 1.5 |
| ENRICH | Hydro-lyzed corn starch, sucrose, soy, polysac-charides | Na and Ca caseinates, soy protein | Corn oil | 160 | 40 | 37 | 480 | 37/40 | Low | 1390 cc | High dietary fiber, lactose free | 1.1 |
| ISOCAL | Malto-dextrins | Na - Ca caseinates, soy protein | Soy oil, MCT oil | 133 | 34 | 44 | 300 | 23/34 | Low | 1890 cc | Requires digestion, low Na, lactose free | 1.06 |

*⁂ Unflavored formulas. Flavored formulas add mOsm.
§ Volume needed to meet or exceed RDA for Vitamin and Mineral needs of children 4-18 years.

TUBE FEEDING FORMULAS - SUPPLEMENTAL FEEDINGS (continued)

| PRODUCT | CHO SOURCE | PROTEIN SOURCE | FAT SOURCE | CHO gm/L | PRO-TEIN gm/L | FAT gm/L | mOsm/kg | Na/K+ mEq/L | RES-IDUE | VITAMINS CONTENT | FEATURE | CAL/ML |
|---|---|---|---|---|---|---|---|---|---|---|---|---|
| MAGNA-CAL | Malto-dextrin sucrose | Na - Ca caseinates | Soy oil | 250 | 70 | 80 | 590 | 44/32 | Low | 1000 cc | Lactose free, high calorie, requires digestion and absorption | 2 |
| OSMO-LITE | Hydro-lyzed corn starch | Ca - Na caseinate, soy protein | MCT, corn & soy oils | 143 | 37 | 38 | 300 | 24/26 | Low | 1925 cc | Lactose free, low Na, requires digestion | 1.06 |
| PRECISION LR | Malto-dextrin sucrose | Egg albumin | Soy oil, MCT oil | 247 | 26 | 2 | 510* | 30/22 | Low | 1730 cc | Lactose free, absorbed upper gut | 1.1 |
| PRECISION HN | Malto-dextrin, sucrose | Egg albumin | Soy oil | 218 | 44 | 1 | 525* | 42/23 | Low | 2730 cc | Lactose free, high protein, absorbed upper gut | 1.1 |
| PULMO-CARE | Hydro-lyzed corn starch and sucrose | Na-Ca caseinate | Corn oil | 104 | 62 | 90 | 490 | 56/48 | Low | 1000 cc | Lactose free, high fat and low carbohydrate to reduce $CO_2$ production | 1.5 |
| SUS-TACAL | Sucrose, corn syrup | Na and Ca caseinates, soy protein | Par-tially hydro-genated soy oil | 140 | 61 | 23 | 620* | 41/54 | Low | 1080 cc | High protein, requires digestion, lactose free | 1 |

*Unflavored formulas. Flavored formulas add mOsm.

§ Volume needed to meet or exceed RDA for Vitamin and Mineral needs of children 4-18 years.

TUBE FEEDING FORMULAS - SUPPLEMENTAL FEEDINGS (continued)

| PRODUCT | CHO SOURCE | PROTEIN SOURCE | FAT SOURCE | CHO gm/L | PROTEIN gm/L | FAT gm/L | mOsm/kg | Na/K+ mEq/L | RESIDUE | VITAMIN CONTENT | FEATURE | CAL/ML |
|---|---|---|---|---|---|---|---|---|---|---|---|---|
| SUSTACAL HC | Sucrose, corn syrup | Ca and Na caseinate | soy oil | 190 | 61 | 58 | 650 | 36/38 | Low | 1180 cc | Same as sustacal | 1.5 |
| TRAVASORB MCT | corn syrup | lactalbumin K caseinate | MCT, sunflower oil | 123 | 49 | 33 | 250 | 15/45 | Low | 2000 cc | Low osmolality | 1.0 |
| TRAVASORB RENAL | Glucose, oligosaccharides, sucrose | Crystalline L-amino acids | Sunflower oils, MCT oil | 271 | 23 | 18 | 590 | 0/0 | Low | Inadequate | Electrolyte + lactose free, essential amino acids | 1.4 |
| VIVONEX | Glucose, oligosaccharides | L-amino acids | Safflower oil | 226 | 21 | 1 | 550* | 20/30 | Low | 1800 cc | Lactose free, no pancreatic stimulus, absorbed upper gut | 1 |
| VIVONEX T.E.N. | Glucose, oligosaccharides | L-amino acids | Safflower oil | 206 | 38 | 3 | 630* | 20/20 | Low | 2100 cc | Lactose free, absorbed upper gut, high protein | 1 |
| VITAL HN | Hydrolyzed corn starch, sucrose | Whey, soy and meat protein hydrolysate, free essential amino acids | Safflower oil and MCT oil | 185 | 42 | 11 | 460 | 20/34 | Low | 1500 cc | Absorbed in upper gut, low Na, lactose free, 45% MCT | 1 |

Unflavored formulas. Flavored formulas add mOsm.
*§ Volume needed to meet or exceed RDA for Vitamin and Mineral needs of children 4-18 years.

# NUTRITION SUPPLEMENTS

Protein:
1. Casec; calcium caseinate in powder form.
   100g of powder provides 88g protein and 370 calories.
2. Promod; whey protein concentrate in powder form.
   100 g of powder provides 75g protein and 425 calories.
3. Propac; whey protein concentrate in powder form.
   100 g of powder provides 75g protein and 395 calories.

Carbohydrate:
1. Moducal; corn starch hydrolysate in powder form.
   100 g of powder provides 95g carbohydrate and 380 calories.
2. Polycose; corn starch hydrolysate in powder and liquid form.
   100g of powder provides 94g carbohydrate and 380 calories. 100cc liquid provides 50g carbohydrate and 200 calories.

Fat:
1. MCT oil; fractionated coconut oil with 90% of the triglycerides as $C_8$ and $C_{10}$ saturated fatty acids.
   Provides 8.3 cal/gram or 7.7 cal/cc.
   (15cc = 14g = 115 cal)
2. Microlipid; a 50% fat emulsion with safflower oil.
   1000 cc provides 500g of fat and 4500 calories.

## GUIDE TO THE INTRODUCTION OF SUPPLEMENTAL FEEDINGS IN INFANCY

1.  Introduce supplemental foods at about 4-6 months of age.

2.  Use single ingredient (not mixed) foods.

3.  Introduce foods one at a time at intervals of 3-7 days.

4.  Add water to the diet when solids are introduced (higher renal solute load with solids).

5.  Begin juices when the infant can drink from a cup.


## GUIDE TO MINERAL AND VITAMIN SUPPLEMENTATION

| Age | Vitamins | | | | Minerals | |
| --- | --- | --- | --- | --- | --- | --- |
| | multi | D | E | Folate | Fe | Fluoride* |
| 0-6 mo | | | | | | |
| (breast fed) | | + | | | | ± |
| (formula fed) | | | | | | ± |
| Preterm | | | | | | |
| (breast fed) | + | + | ± | ± | + | ± |
| (formula fed) | + | + | ± | ± | + | ± |
| >6 mo | | + | | | ±** | ± |
| Children | | | | | | ± |

*Depends on local drinking water supply. For doses see
  Formulary.
**Cereal and formulas are possible sources.

Ref: AAP. Pediatric Nutrition Handbook, 2nd ed, 1985.

# PARENTERAL NUTRITION GUIDELINES

Parenteral alimentation is indicated when a patient is unable to feed or is unable to meet established caloric requirements by the enteral route.

A. Specific Requirements
   1. Protein

   |  | neonate | infant | child | adult |
   |---|---|---|---|---|
   | (g/kg/day) | 2.0-2.5 | 1.5-2.5 | 1.0-2.0 | 0.8-1.0 |

   NOTE: For neonates, begin with 0.5 g/kg/day and increase by 0.5-1 g/kg/day. For infants, children, and adults, begin with 1 g/kg/day and increase by 0.5-1 g/kg/day to maximum of 3 g/kg/day. The percent of total calories supplied by protein should be 8-15%.

   2. Fat
   Begin with 0.5 g/kg/day and advance by 0.5-1 g/kg/day to maximum of 4 g/kg/day (40% of total calories). Due to risk of hypersensitivity reactions give a test dose of 1.0 ml/kg of 10% lipid emulsions over 1 hour for infants less than 5 kg, or 0.1 ml/minute over 10-15 minutes for patients weighing more than 5 kg.

   3. Carbohydrate
   Begin with 7-8 mg/kg/min and advance to 12-14 mg/kg/min. Up to 12.5% dextrose can be infused peripherally and 25% dextrose centrally.

   4. Electrolytes and minerals
   Refer to Fluids section, pp. 231-33.

B. Monitoring (a suggested protocol follows):
   1. Baseline CBC with differential, electrolyte panel, chemistry panel (LFT'S, protein, albumin, cholesterol & triglycerides), and magnesium.

   2. Daily weight, fluid and caloric intake, and output.

   3. Twice weekly CBC, electrolytes, BUN, creatinine, calcium, and phosphorous.

   4. Weekly chemistry panel and head circumference

   5. Biweekly anthropometrics, magnesium, and transferrin.

Ref: The Johns Hopkins Hospital Clinical Nutrition Manual, July 1986.

# BLOOD CHEMISTRIES

These values are compiled from the published literature and from the Johns Hopkins Hospital Department of Laboratory Medicine. Normal values vary with the analytic method used. If any doubt exists, consult your laboratory for its analytical method and normal range of values. The values between the parentheses are normal values according to the International System (SI) of measurement.

Ref: Meites S, ed. Pediatric Clinical Chemistry, 2nd Edition. The American Association for Clinical Chemistry, 1981; Tietz NW. Textbook of Clinical Chemistry, 1981; Lundberg GD, et al. JAMA 1986; 255:2329-39; Scully RE, et al. New Eng J Med 1986; 314:39-49.

Acid phosphatase:
| | | |
|---|---|---|
| Newborn | 7.4-19.4 U/ml | (7.4-19.4 U/ml) |
| 2-13 yrs | 6.4-15.2 U/ml | (6.4-15.2 U/ml) |
| Adult | M: 0.5-11.0 U/ml | (0.5-11.0 U/ml) |
| | F: 0.2-9.5 U/ml | (0.2-9.5 U/ml) |

Alanine Aminotransferase (ALT):
| | | |
|---|---|---|
| Infants | <54 U/L | (<54 U/L) |
| Children/Adults | 1-30 U/L | (1-30 U/L) |

Aldolase:
| | | |
|---|---|---|
| Adult | <8 U/L | (<8 U/L) |
| Children | <16 U/L | (<16 U/L) |
| Newborn | <32 U/L | (<32 U/L) |

Alkaline phosphatase:
| | | |
|---|---|---|
| Infant | 150-400 U/L | (150-400 U/L) |
| 2-10 yrs | 100-300 U/L | (100-300 U/L) |
| 11-18 yrs male | 50-375 U/L | (50-375 U/L) |
| female | 30-300 U/L | (30-300 U/L) |
| Adult | 30-100 U/L | (30-100 U/L) |

Alpha 1-Antitrypsin: 2.1-5.0 gm/L

Alpha Fetoprotein: <10 mg/dl  (<0.1 gm/L)

Ammonia Nitrogen (Venous Sample): (Heparinized specimen in ice water and analyzed within 30 min)
| | | |
|---|---|---|
| all ages | 13-48 µg/dl | (9-34 µmol/L) |

Amylase:
| | | |
|---|---|---|
| Newborn: | 5-65 U/L | (5-65 U/L) |
| >1 yr: | 25-125 U/L | (25-125 U/L) |

Arsenic: <30 µg/dl  (<0.4 mmol/L)

Aspartate Aminotransferase (AST):

| | | |
|---|---|---|
| Newborn/Infant | 25-75 U/L | (25-75 U/L) |
| Child/Adult | 0-40 U/L | (0-40 U/L) |

Bicarbonate:

| | | |
|---|---|---|
| Premature | 18-26 mEq/L | (18-26 mmol/L) |
| Infant | 20-26 mEq/L | (20-26 mmol/L) |
| 1-2 yrs | 20-25 mEq/L | (20-25 mmol/L) |
| >2 yrs | 22-26 mEq/L | (22-26 mmol/L) |

Bilirubin (total):

| | | |
|---|---|---|
| Cord | <1.8 mg/dl | (<30.6 μmol/L) |
| 24 hrs | | |
|   Preterm | ≤6 mg/dl | (<103 μmol/L) |
|   Term | ≤6 mg/dl | (≤103 μmol/L) |
| 48 hrs | | |
|   Preterm | <8 mg/dl | (<137 μmol/L) |
|   Term | ≤7 mg/dl | (≤120 μmol/L) |
| 3-5 days | | |
|   Preterm | <12 mg/dl | (<205 μmol/L) |
|   Term | ≤12 mg/dl | (≤205 μmol/L) |
| 1 mo-Adult | ≤1.5 mg/dl | (≤26 μmol/L) |
| Conjugated: | ≤0.5 mg/dl | (≤9 μmol/L) |

Calcium (Total):

| | | |
|---|---|---|
| Premature <1 week | 6-10 mg/dl | (1.5-2.5 mmol/L) |
| Full term <1 week | 7.0-12.0 mg/dl | (1.75-3 mmol/L) |
| Child | 8-10.5 mg/dl | (2-2.6 mmol/L) |
| Adult | 8.5-10.5 mg/dl | (2.1-2.6 mmol/L) |

Calcium (Ionized):    4.4-5.4 mg/dl         (0.1-1.35 mmol/L)

Carbon Dioxide ($CO_2$ content):

| | | |
|---|---|---|
| Cord blood | 15-20 mmol/L | (15-20 mmol/L) |
| Child | 18-27 mmol/L | (18-27 mmol/L) |
| Adult | 24-35 mmol/L | (24-35 mmol/L) |

Carbon Monoxide (carboxyhemoglobin):

| | |
|---|---|
| Nonsmoker | <2% of total Hemoglobin |
| Smoker | <10% of total Hemoglobin |
| Lethal | >60% of total Hemoglobin |

Carotenoids (Carotenes):

| | | |
|---|---|---|
| Infant | 20-70 μg/dl | (0.37-1.30 μmol/L) |
| Child | 40-130 μg/dl | (0.74-2.42 μmol/L) |
| Adult | 60-200 μg/dl | (1.12-3.72 μmol/L) |

Ceruloplasmin:       23-58 mg/dl         (1.32-3.83 μmol/L)

Chloride:            94-106 mEq/L        (94-106 mmol/L)

Cholesterol:         (See Lipids)

Copper:

| | | |
|---|---|---|
| 0-6 mos | <70 µg/dl | (<11 µmol/L) |
| 6 mos-5 yrs | 27-153 µg/dl | (4.2-24.1 µmol/L) |
| 5-17 yrs | 94-234 µg/dl | (14.2-36.8 µmol/L) |
| Adult | 70-155 µg/dl | (11-24.4 µmol/L) |

Creatine Kinase (Creatine Phosphokinase):

| Age | Upper 95th percentile values, U/L | |
|---|---|---|
| | M | F |
| 1 d | 600 | 500 |
| 2-10 d | 440 | 440 |
| <1 yr | 170 | 170 |
| 1-7 yr | 109 | 100 |
| 7-9 yr | 103 | 85 |
| 9-11 yr | 109 | 88 |
| 11-13 yr | 108 | 85 |
| 13-15 yr | 129 | 85 |
| 15-17 yr | 247 | 74 |
| 17-19 yr | 190 | 68 |

Creatinine (Serum):

| Age, yr | Upper limits, mg/dl (µmol/L) | |
|---|---|---|
| | M | F |
| 1 | 0.6 (53) | 0.5 (44) |
| 2-3 | 0.7 (62) | 0.6 (53) |
| 4-7 | 0.8 (71) | 0.7 (62) |
| 8-10 | 0.9 (80) | 0.8 (71) |
| 11-12 | 1.0 (88) | 0.9 (80) |
| 13-17 | 1.2 (106) | 1.1 (97) |
| 18-20 | 1.3 (115) | 1.1 (97) |
| Adult | 1.2 (106) | 1.4 (124) |

Ferritin:

| | | |
|---|---|---|
| Children | 7-144 ng/ml | (7-144 µg/L) |
| Adult | F: 10-110 ng/ml | (10-110 µg/L) |
| | M: 30-265 ng/ml | (30-265 µg/L) |

Fibrin Degradation Products:
Titer:            1:50=positive

Fibrinogen:       200-400 mg/dl        (2-4 g/L)

Folic Acid (Folate):    1.9-14 ng/L       (4.3-23.6 nmol/L)

Galactose:

| | | |
|---|---|---|
| Newborn | 0-20 mg/dl | 0-1.11 mmol/L |
| Thereafter | <5 mg/dl | <0.28 mmol/L |

Gammaglutamyl Transferase (GGT):

| | | |
|---|---|---|
| Cord | 19-270 U/L | (19-270 U/L) |
| Premature | 56-233 U/L | (56-233 U/L) |
| 0-3 wks | 0-130 U/L | (0-130 U/L) |
| 3 wks-3 mos | 4-120 U/L | (4-120 U/L) |
| >3 mos | M: 5-65 U/L | (5-65 U/L) |
| | F: 5-35 U/L | (5-35 U/L) |
| 1-15 yrs | 0-23 U/L | (0-23 U/L) |
| 16 yrs-Adult | 0-35 U/L | (0-35 U/L) |

Gastrin:      <300 pg/ml      (<300 ng/L)

Glucose (Serum):

| | | |
|---|---|---|
| Premature | 20-65 mg/dl | (1.1-3.6 mmol/L) |
| Full term | 20-110 mg/dl | (1.1-6.4 mmol/L) |
| 1 wk-16 yrs | 60-105 mg/dl | (3.3-5.8 mmol/L) |
| >16 yrs | 70-115 mg/dl | (3.9-6.4 nmol/L) |

Haptoglobin:
     400-1800 mg/L      0.4-1.8 g/L
(Note: detectable in only 10-20% of newborns)

Iron:

| | Iron | | Iron Binding Capacity | | %Saturation |
|---|---|---|---|---|---|
| | (µg/dl) | (µmol/L) | (µg/dl) | (µmol/L) | (µg/dl) |
| Newborn | 110-270 | (19.7-48.3) | 59-175 | (10.6-31.3) | 65% |
| 4-10 mos | 30-70 | (5.4-12.5) | 250-400 | (45-72) | 25% |
| 3-10 yrs | 53-119 | (9.5-27.0) | 250-400 | (45-72) | 30% |
| Adult | 72-186 | (12.9-33.3) | 250-400 | (45-72) | 35% |

Ketones:

| | |
|---|---|
| Qualitative: | negative |
| Quantitative: | up to 3 mg% |

Lactate:

| | | |
|---|---|---|
| Capillary blood | | |
| (Newborn) | <30 mg/dl | (<3.0 mmol/L) |
| (Child) | 5-20 mg/dl | (0.56-2.25 mmol/L) |
| Venous | 5-18 mg/dl | (0.5-2.0 mmol/L) |
| Arterial | 3-7 mg/dl | (0.3-0.8 mmol/L) |

Lactate Dehydrogenase (37°C):

| | | |
|---|---|---|
| Newborn | 160-1500 U/L | (160-1500 U/L) |
| Infant | 150-360 U/L | (150-360 U/L) |
| Child | 150-300 U/L | (150-300 U/L) |
| Adult | 100-250 U/L | (100-250 U/L) |

Lactate Dehydrogenase Isoenzymes (% total):

| | |
|---|---|
| $LD_1$ Heart | 24-34% |
| $LD_2$ Heart, Erythrocytes | 35-45% |
| $LD_3$ Muscle | 15-25% |
| $LD_4$ Liver, trace muscle | 4-10% |
| $LD_5$ Liver, muscle | 1-9% |

Lead   See page 252.

Lipase                        20-180 U/L                (20-180 U/L)

Lipids

<table>
<tr><th></th><th colspan="2">Normal Upper Limits<br>Total Serum<br>Cholesterol mg/dl (mmol/L)</th><th colspan="2">Serum<br>Triglycerides mg/dl (g/L)</th></tr>
<tr><th>Age</th><th>Males</th><th>Females*</th><th>Males</th><th>Females*</th></tr>
<tr><td>0-4 yrs</td><td>203 (5.28)</td><td>200 (5.2)</td><td>99 (0.99)</td><td>112 (1.12)</td></tr>
<tr><td>5-9</td><td>203 (5.28)</td><td>205 (5.33)</td><td>101 (1.01)</td><td>105 (1.05)</td></tr>
<tr><td>10-14</td><td>202 (5.25)</td><td>201 (5.22)</td><td>125 (1.25)</td><td>131 (1.31)</td></tr>
<tr><td>15-19</td><td>197 (5.12)</td><td>200 (5.2)</td><td>148 (1.48)</td><td>124 (1.24)</td></tr>
<tr><td>20-24</td><td>218 (5.67)</td><td>216 (5.62)</td><td>201 (2.01)</td><td>131 (1.31)</td></tr>
<tr><td>25-29</td><td>244 (6.34)</td><td>222 (5.77)</td><td>249 (2.49)</td><td>144 (1.44)</td></tr>
<tr><td>30-34</td><td>254 (6.60)</td><td>230 (5.98)</td><td>266 (2.66)</td><td>150 (1.50)</td></tr>
<tr><td>35-39</td><td>270 (7.02)</td><td>242 (6.24)</td><td>321 (3.21)</td><td>176 (1.76)</td></tr>
<tr><td>40-44</td><td>268 (6.97)</td><td>252 (6.55)</td><td>320 (3.20)</td><td>191 (1.91)</td></tr>
<tr><td>45-49</td><td>276 (7.18)</td><td>265 (6.89)</td><td>327 (3.27)</td><td>214 (2.14)</td></tr>
</table>

*Use of oral contraceptives significantly raises both total serum cholesterol and serum triglyceride levels.

<table>
<tr><th></th><th colspan="6">Normal Upper Limits mg/dl* (mmol/L)</th></tr>
<tr><th>Age</th><th colspan="2">HDL - Cholesterol</th><th colspan="2">LDL</th><th colspan="2">VLDL</th></tr>
<tr><th></th><th>males</th><th>females</th><th>males</th><th>females</th><th>males</th><th>females</th></tr>
<tr><td>0- 4</td><td>-</td><td>-</td><td>-</td><td>-</td><td>-</td><td>-</td></tr>
<tr><td>5- 9</td><td>74(1.91)</td><td>73(1.89)</td><td>129(3.34)</td><td>140(3.62)</td><td>18(0.47)</td><td>24(0.62)</td></tr>
<tr><td>10-14</td><td>74(1.91)</td><td>70(1.81)</td><td>132(3.41)</td><td>136(3.52)</td><td>22(0.57)</td><td>23(0.59)</td></tr>
<tr><td>15-19</td><td>63(1.63)</td><td>73(1.89)</td><td>130(3.36)</td><td>135(3.49)</td><td>26(0.67)</td><td>24(0.62)</td></tr>
<tr><td>20-24</td><td>63(1.63)</td><td>-</td><td>147(3.80)</td><td>- -</td><td>28(0.72)</td><td>- -</td></tr>
<tr><td>25-29</td><td>63(1.63)</td><td>81(2.09)</td><td>165(4.27)</td><td>151(3.90)</td><td>36(0.93)</td><td>24(0.65)</td></tr>
<tr><td>30-34</td><td>63(1.63)</td><td>75(1.94)</td><td>185(4.78)</td><td>150(3.88)</td><td>48(1.24)</td><td>25(0.65)</td></tr>
<tr><td>35-39</td><td>62(1.60)</td><td>82(2.12)</td><td>189(4.89)</td><td>172(4.45)</td><td>56(1.49)</td><td>35(0.91)</td></tr>
<tr><td>40-44</td><td>67(1.73)</td><td>87(2.25)</td><td>186(4.81)</td><td>174(4.50)</td><td>56(1.49)</td><td>29(0.75)</td></tr>
<tr><td>45-49</td><td>64(1.66)</td><td>86(2.22)</td><td>202(5.22)</td><td>187(4.84)</td><td>51 1.32)</td><td>38(0.98)</td></tr>
</table>

Magnesium:              1.5-2.0 mEq/L            (0.75-1 mmol/L)

Manganese (Blood):
  Newborn              2.4-9.6 µg/dl            (2.44-1.75 µmol/L)
  2-18 yrs             0.8-2.1 µg/dl            (0.15-0.38 µmol/L)

Methemoglobin:       <0.3 g/dl or <3% of total Hb    (<46.5 µmol/L)

5' Nucleotidase:        2.2-15.0 U/L      (2.2-15.0 U/L)

Osmolality:             285-295 mOsm/kg    (270-285 mOsm/L plasma)

Phenylalanine:
<u>Newborn</u>                       <4 mg/dl                   (<0.24 mmol/L)
  Child                        <3 mg/dl                   (<0.18 mmol/L)

Phosphorus:
  <u>Newborn</u>                4.2-9.0 mg/dl         (1.36-2.91 mmol/L)
  1 yr                      3.8-6.2 mg/dl         (1.23-2.0 mmol/L)
  2-5 yrs               3.5-6.8 mg/dl         (1.13-2.2 mmol/L)
  Adult                    3.0-4.5 mg/dl         (0.97-1.45 mmol/L)

<u>Porcelain</u>:                10-25 mg/dl          (no SI conversion factor)

Potassium:
  <u><10 days of age</u>      3.5-6.0 mEq/L         (3.5-6.0 mmol/L)
  >10 days of age       3.5-5.0 mEq/L         (3.5-5.0 mmol/L)

Prolactin:

| Age | ng/ml | μg/L |
|---|---|---|
| Newborn | <200 | (<200) |
| Adult | <20 | (<20) |

<u>Proteins</u> Average (Range) in grams/dl:

| Age | Total | Albumin | Globulin | Gamma Globulin |
|---|---|---|---|---|
| Premature | 5.5 | 3.7 | 1.8 | 0.7 |
| | (4.0-7.0) | (2.5-4.5) | (1.2-2.0) | (0.5-0.9) |
| FT Newborn | 6.4 | 3.4 | 3.1 | 0.8 |
| | (5.0-7.1) | (2.5-5.0) | (1.2-4.0) | (0.7-0.9) |
| 1-3 mos | 6.6 | 3.8 | 2.5 | 0.3 |
| | (4.7-7.4) | (3.0-4.2) | (1.0-3.3) | (0.1-0.5) |
| 3-12 mos | 6.8 | 3.9 | 2.6 | 0.6 |
| | (5.0-7.5) | (2.7-5.0) | (2.0-3.8) | (0.4-1.2) |
| 1-15 yrs | 7.4 | 4.0 | 3.1 | 0.9 |
| | (6.5-8.6) | (3.2-5.0) | (2.0-4.0) | (0.6-1.2) |

<u>Pyruvate</u>:                                  (50-140 mmol/L)

Sodium:
  <u>Premature</u>              130-140 mEq/L       (130-140 mmol/L)
  Older                    135-145 mEq/L       (135-145 mmol/L)

<u>Transaminase</u> (SGOT):  See AST (Aspartate Aminotransferase)

<u>Transaminase</u> (SGPT):  See ALT (Alanine Aminotransferase)

<u>Triglycerides</u>:  See Lipids

<u>Urea</u> <u>Nitrogen</u>:        5-25 mg/dl            (1.8-9.0 mmol/L)

Uric Acid:

| Age, yr | mg/dl | (mmol/L) |
|---|---|---|
| 0-2 | 2.0-7.0 | (0.12-0.42) |
| 2-12 | 2.0-6.5 | (0.12-0.39) |
| 12-14 | 2.0-7.0 | (0.12-0.42) |
| 14-adult, M | 3.0-8.0 | (0.18-0.48) |
| F | 2.0-7.0 | (0.12-0.42) |

Vitamin A (Retinol):

| | | |
|---|---|---|
| 0-1 yr | 20-90 µg/dl | (0.7-3.14 µmol/L) |
| 1-5 yrs | 30-100 µg/dl | (1.05-3.50 µmol/L) |
| 5-16 yrs | 60-100 µg/dl | (2.09-3.50 µmol/L) |
| Adult | 20-80 µg/dl | (0.70-2.79 µmol/L) |

Vitamin B1 (Thiamine):

| | | |
|---|---|---|
| | 5.3-7.9 µg/dl | (0.16-0.23 µmol/L) |

Vitamin B2 (Riboflavin):

| | | |
|---|---|---|
| | 3.7-13.7 µg/dl | (98-363 mmol/L) |

Vitamin B12 (Cobalamin):

| | | |
|---|---|---|
| | 130-785 pg/ml | (96-579 pmol/L) |

Vitamin C (Ascorbic Acid):

| | | |
|---|---|---|
| | 0.2-2.0 mg/dl | (11.4-113.6 µmol/L) |

Vitamin D (1,25 Dihydroxy):

| | | |
|---|---|---|
| Newborn | 21 ± 2 pg/ml | (50 ± 4.8 nmol/L) |
| Child | 43 ± 3 pg/ml | (103 ± 7.2 nmol/L) |
| Adult | 29 ± 2 pg/ml | (69.6 ± 4.8 nmol/L) |

Vitamin E:

| | | |
|---|---|---|
| | 5-20 µg/dl | (8.4-23 µmol/L) |

Zinc:

| | | |
|---|---|---|
| | 55-150 µg/dl | (8.4-23 µmol/L) |

## NORMAL SEROLOGIC REFERENCE VALUES

| | | |
|---|---|---|
| Antinuclear antibody | | <1:160 |
| | | |
| Anti-Streptolysin O Titer | | |
| Preschool | | <1:85 |
| School ages and adults | | <1:170 |
| Older adults | | <1:85 |

NOTE: Significant if rising titer can be demonstrated at weekly intervals.

| | | |
|---|---|---|
| Anti-Hyaluronidase | | <1:256 |
| Anti-Nuclear Antibody | | <1:40 |
| | | |
| C-Reactive Protein | | Negative |
| | | |
| $C_1$ esterase inhibitor | | 17.4-24 mg/dl |
| | | |
| $C_3$ | 1-6 mos | 53-175 mg/dl |
| | 7-12 mos | 75-180 mg/dl |
| | 1-5 yr | 77-166 mg/dl |
| | 6-10 yr | 88-199 mg/dl |
| | adult | 83-177 mg/dl |
| | | |
| $C_4$ | 1-6 mos | 7-42 mg/dl |
| | 7-12 mos | 9.5-39 mg/dl |
| | 1-5 yr | 9-40 mg/dl |
| | 6-10 yr | 12-40 mg/dl |
| | adult | 15-45 mg/dl |
| | | |
| $C_{H50}$ | | 75-160 u/ml |
| | | |
| Rheumatoid factor | | <20 negative |
| | | 20-40 suggestive |
| | | $\geq$80 positive |
| | | |
| Rheumaton titer | | |
| (modified Waaler-Rose slide test) | | negative |
| | | $\geq$10 may be significant |
| | | |
| Total B cells | | 5-20% of lymphocytes |
| Total T cells | | 50-80% of lymphocytes |
| T helper cells | | 34-56% of lymphocytes |
| T suppressor cells | | 18-32% of lymphocytes |
| helper/suppressor ratio | | 1.1-2.5 |

## LEVELS OF IMMUNOGLOBULINS

| | IgG (mg/dl) | IgM (mg/dl) | IgA (mg/dl) | IgE (u/ml) |
|---|---|---|---|---|
| **Serum*** | | | | |
| Newborn | 640 – 1600 | 6 – 24 | 0 – 5 | 0 – 10 |
| 1-3 mo | 300 – 1000 | 15 – 150 | 3 – 66 | – |
| 3-6 mo | 140 – 1000 | 15 – 110 | 4 – 90 | – |
| 6-12 mo | 400 – 1150 | 43 – 225 | 45 – 225 | – |
| 1-2 yr | 350 – 1200 | 36 – 240 | 35 – 240 | – |
| 2-6 yr | 500 – 1300 | 50 – 199 | 40 – 190 | 0 – 200 |
| 6-12 yr | 700 – 1650 | 50 – 260 | 40 – 270 | – |
| 12-16 yr | 700 – 1550 | 45 – 240 | 50 – 232 | 0 – 400 |
| Adult | 650 – 1500 | 40 – 345 | 70 – 390 | – |
| **Secretions** | | | | |
| Colostrum | 10 | 61 | 1234 | – |
| Stimulated parotid saliva | 0.036 | 0.043 | 3.9 | – |
| Unstimulated whole saliva | 4.86 | 0.55 | 30.4 | – |
| Jejunal fluid | 34 | 70 | – | – |
| Seminal fluid | 510 | 90 | 116 | – |
| **Cerebrospinal fluid** | | | | |
| Normal | 3 ± 1 | 0 | 0.4±0.5 | – |
| Purulent infection | 9 | 4 | 4 | – |
| Viral infection | 4 | 0.5 | 1 | – |

*Values represent mean ± 2 standard deviations.
Adapted from Meites S, ed. Pediatric Clinical Chemistry, 2nd ed., 1981; Tietz NW. Textbook of Clinical Chemistry, 1981; Fosarelli P, et al. Clin Pediatr 1985; 24:84-8.

## CEREBROSPINAL FLUID

| Cell Count | | %PMNs |
|---|---|---|
| Preterm mean | 9.0 (0-25.4 WBC/mm$^3$) | 57% |
| Term mean | 8.2 (0-22.4 WBC/mm$^3$) | 61% |
| >1 mo | 0-7 | 0 |

| Glucose | | |
|---|---|---|
| Preterm | 24-63 mg/dl | (mean 50) |
| Term | 34-119 mg/dl | (mean 52) |
| Child | 40-80 mg/dl | |

| CSF Glucose/Blood Glucose (%) | |
|---|---|
| Preterm | 55-105 |
| Term | 44-128 |
| Child | 50% |

Lactic Acid Dehydrogenase:   Mean 20 U/ml (range 5-30 U/ml)

Myelin Basic Protein:   <4 ng/ml

Pressure:   Initial L.P.   (mm H$_2$0)
  Newborn                 80-110 (<110)
  Infant/Child            <200 (lateral recumbent position)
  Respiratory movements   5-10

| Protein | | |
|---|---|---|
| Preterm | (mean 115) | 65-150 mg/dl |
| Term | (mean 90) | 20-170 mg/dl |
| Children | Ventricular | 5-15 mg/dl |
| | Cisternal | 5-25 mg/dl |
| | Lumbar | 5-40 mg/dl |

Ref:   Sarff LD et al. J Pediatr 1976; 88:473.

## NORMAL VALUES - HEMATOLOGY

| Age | Hgb (gm%) mean (-2SD) | Hct (%) mean (-2SD) | MCV (fl) mean (-2SD) | MCHC (gm/%RBC) mean (-2SD) | Retic (%) | WBC/mm³ x 100 mean (-2SD) | Plts (10³/mm³) mean (±2SD) |
|---|---|---|---|---|---|---|---|
| 26-30 wk gestation[1] | 13.4 (11) | 41.5 (34.9) | 118.2 (106.7) | 37.9 (30.6) | – | 4.4 (2.7) | 254 (180-327) |
| 28 wks | 14.5 | 45 | 120 | 31 | (5-10) | – | 275 |
| 32 wks | 15.0 | 47 | 118 | 32 | (3-10) | – | 290 |
| Term[2] | | | | | | | |
| (cord) | 16.5 (13.5) | 51 (42) | 108 (98) | 33 (30) | (3-7) | 18.1 (9-30)[3] | 290 |
| 1-3 days | 18.5 (14.5) | 56 (45) | 108 (95) | 33 (29) | (1.8-4.6) | 18.9 (9.4-34) | 192 |
| 2 wk | 16.6 (13.4) | 53 (41) | 105 (88) | 31.4 (28.1) | (0.1-1.7) | 11.4 (5-20) | 252 |
| 1 month | 13.9 (10.7) | 44 (33) | 101 (91) | 31.8 (28.1) | | 10.8 (5-19.5) | |
| 2 months | 11.2 (9.4) | 35 (28) | 95 (84) | 31.8 (28.3) | (0.7-2.3) | | |
| 6 months | 12.6 (11.1) | 36 (31) | 76 (68) | 35 (32.7) | | 11.9 (6-17.5) | |
| 6m-2yrs | 12 (10.5) | 36 (33) | 78 (70) | 33 (30) | | 10.6 (6-17) | (150-350) |
| 2-6 yrs | 12.5 (11.5) | 37 (34) | 81 (75) | 34 (31) | (0.5-1.0) | 8.5 (5-15.5) | " |
| 6-12 yrs | 13.5 (11.5) | 40 (35) | 86 (77) | 34 (31) | (0.5-1.0) | 8.1 (4.5-13.5) | " |
| 12-18 yrs | | | | | | | |
| male | 14.5 (13) | 43 (36) | 88 (78) | 34 (31) | (0.5-1.0) | 7.8 (4.5-13/5) | " |
| female | 14 (12) | 41 (37) | 90 (78) | 34 (31) | (0.5-1.0) | 7.8 (4.5-13.5) | " |
| Adult | | | | | | | |
| male | 15.5 (13.5) | 47 (41) | 90 (80) | 34 (31) | (0.8-2.5) | 7.4 (4.5-11) | " |
| female | 14 (12) | 41 (36) | 90 (80) | 34 (31) | (0.8-4.1) | 7.4 (4.5-11) | " |

[1]Values are from fetal samplings. [2]Under 1 month, capillary Hgb exceeds venous: 1 hr-3.6 gm difference; 5 days-2.2 gm difference; 3 wks-1.1 gm difference. [3]Mean (95% confidence limits).

Ref: Adapted from: Forestier F, et al. Pediatr Res 1986; 20:342-6; Oski FA, Naiman JL. Hematological Problems in the Newborn Infant. WB Saunders, 1982; Nathan D, Oski FA. Hematology of Infancy and Childhood. WB Saunders, 1981; Metoth Y, et al. Acta Paed Scand 1971; 60:317; Wintrobe. Clinical Hematology. Lea & Febiger, 1981.

NORMAL RANGES FOR HEMOGLOBIN AND MCV

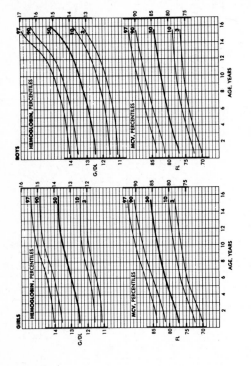

Ref: Dallman PR, and Siimes MA: J Pediatr 1979; 94:26.

## CONVERSION FORMULAS

Weight

| Grams | Pounds |
|-------|--------|
| 454   | 1.0    |
| 1000  | 2.2    |

To change pounds to grams, multiply by 454.

To change kilograms to pounds, multiply by 2.2.

Length

To convert inches to cms, multiply by 2.54.

Temperature

To convert degrees Celsius to degrees Fahrenheit: (9/5 x temperature) + 32

To convert degrees Fahrenheit to degrees Celsius (temperature - 32) x 5/9

## TEMPERATURE EQUIVALENTS

| Centigrade | Fahrenheit | Centigrade | Fahrenheit |
|------------|------------|------------|------------|
| 34.0 | 93.2  | 38.6 | 101.4 |
| 34.2 | 93.6  | 38.8 | 101.8 |
| 34.4 | 93.9  | 39.0 | 102.2 |
| 34.6 | 94.3  | 39.2 | 102.5 |
| 34.8 | 94.6  | 39.4 | 102.9 |
| 35.0 | 95.0  | 39.6 | 103.2 |
| 35.2 | 95.4  | 39.8 | 103.6 |
| 35.4 | 95.7  | 40.0 | 104.0 |
| 35.6 | 96.1  | 40.2 | 104.3 |
| 35.8 | 96.4  | 40.4 | 104.7 |
| 36.0 | 96.8  | 40.6 | 105.1 |
| 36.2 | 97.1  | 40.8 | 105.4 |
| 36.4 | 97.5  | 41.0 | 105.8 |
| 36.6 | 97.8  | 41.2 | 106.1 |
| 36.8 | 98.2  | 41.4 | 106.5 |
| 37.0 | 98.6  | 41.6 | 106.8 |
| 37.2 | 98.9  | 41.8 | 107.2 |
| 37.4 | 99.3  | 42.0 | 107.6 |
| 37.6 | 99.6  | 42.2 | 108.0 |
| 37.8 | 100.0 | 42.4 | 108.3 |
| 38.0 | 100.4 | 42.6 | 108.7 |
| 38.2 | 100.7 | 42.8 | 109.0 |
| 38.4 | 101.1 | 43.0 | 109.4 |

CONVERSION OF POUNDS AND OUNCES TO GRAMS

| Ounces | 1 lb. | 2 lb. | 3 lb. | 4 lb. | 5 lb. | 6 lb. | 7 lb. | 8 lb. |
|---|---|---|---|---|---|---|---|---|
| | | | | GRAMS | | | | |
| 0 | 454 | 907 | 1,361 | 1,814 | 2,268 | 2,722 | 3,175 | 3,629 |
| 1 | 482 | 936 | 1,389 | 1,843 | 2,296 | 2,750 | 3,204 | 3,657 |
| 2 | 510 | 964 | 1,418 | 1,871 | 2,325 | 2,778 | 3,232 | 3,686 |
| 3 | 539 | 992 | 1,446 | 1,899 | 2,353 | 2,807 | 3,260 | 3,714 |
| 4 | 567 | 1,021 | 1,474 | 1,928 | 2,381 | 2,835 | 3,289 | 3,742 |
| 5 | 595 | 1,049 | 1,503 | 1,956 | 2,410 | 2,863 | 3,317 | 3,771 |
| 6 | 624 | 1,077 | 1,531 | 1,985 | 2,438 | 2,892 | 3,345 | 3,799 |
| 7 | 652 | 1,106 | 1,559 | 2,013 | 2,466 | 2,920 | 3,374 | 3,827 |
| 8 | 680 | 1,134 | 1,588 | 2,041 | 2,495 | 2,948 | 3,402 | 3,856 |
| 9 | 709 | 1,162 | 1,616 | 2,070 | 2,523 | 2,977 | 3,430 | 3,884 |
| 10 | 737 | 1,191 | 1,644 | 2,098 | 2,552 | 3,005 | 3,459 | 3,912 |
| 11 | 765 | 1,219 | 1,673 | 2,126 | 2,580 | 3,033 | 3,487 | 3,941 |
| 12 | 794 | 1,247 | 1,701 | 2,155 | 2,608 | 3,062 | 3,515 | 3,969 |
| 13 | 822 | 1,276 | 1,729 | 2,183 | 2,637 | 3,090 | 3,544 | 3,997 |
| 14 | 851 | 1,304 | 1,758 | 2,211 | 2,665 | 3,119 | 3,572 | 4,026 |
| 15 | 879 | 1,332 | 1,786 | 2,240 | 2,693 | 3,147 | 3,600 | 4,054 |

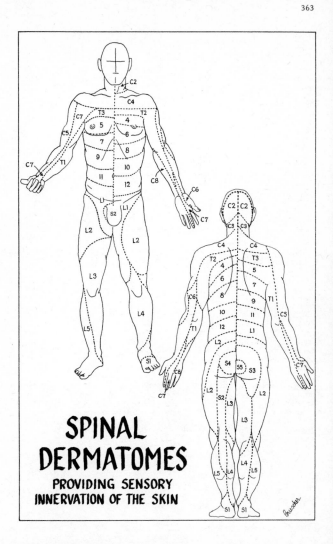

# SPINAL DERMATOMES
## PROVIDING SENSORY INNERVATION OF THE SKIN

# INDEX